ASSESSING AND TREATING SUICIDAL THINKING AND BEHAVIORS IN CHILDREN AND ADOLESCENTS

Assessing and Treating Suicidal Thinking and Behaviors in Children and Adolescents is a guide to working with children and young people who present with either obvious or hidden suicidal thoughts, preoccupations, or plans.

Chapters explore a range of treatment approaches and focus on how to support parents, caregivers, families, and schools. Expressive therapies are highlighted, but the chapters also cover evidence-based models such as cognitive-behavioral therapy (CBT), dialectical behavior therapy (DBT), and prescriptive play therapy.

Expressive therapists, school-based counselors, and other clinicians who work with at-risk children and adolescents from diverse communities and backgrounds will come away from this book with the tools they need to integrate an individual child's capabilities, sources of distress, and internal and external resources in order to build a developmentally sensitive treatment plan.

Leslie W. Baker is the CEO and owner of Therapy2Thrive® Ruby Hill Marriage and Family Counseling Center, an outpatient clinic in California.

Mary Ruth Cross is the CEO and owner of Treehouse Family Counseling Services, an outpatient clinic focused on play therapy treatment with children and families.

ASSESSING AND TREATING SUICIDAL THINKING AND BEHAVIORS IN CHILDREN AND ADOLESCENTS

A Play Therapy Guide for Mental Health Professionals in Clinical and School-Based Settings

Edited by Leslie W. Baker and Mary Ruth Cross

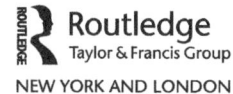

Routledge
Taylor & Francis Group

NEW YORK AND LONDON

Designed cover image: master1305 © Getty Images

First published 2025
by Routledge
605 Third Avenue, New York, NY 10158

and by Routledge
4 Park Square, Milton Park, Abingdon, Oxon, OX14 4RN

Routledge is an imprint of the Taylor & Francis Group, an informa business

ISBN: 978-1-032-41084-5 (hbk)
ISBN: 978-1-032-41082-1 (pbk)
ISBN: 978-1-003-35856-5 (ebk)

DOI: 10.4324/9781003358565

Typeset in Baskerville
by Apex CoVantage, LLC

We dedicate this book to the children, adolescents, and the "littles" in us all who may experience what it is to struggle with thoughts and behaviors of suicide, creating a connection to survive. We dedicate this to all those whose support is a beacon of hope for suicidal youth, including parents, caregivers, and families. This dedication is to our brave clients whose gifts of courage and stories of resiliency allow our many allies in mental health and education to grow and shed light on darkness.

I, Leslie W. Baker, dedicate this book to my co-editor and co-author, Mary Ruth Cross. Thank you for your positivity, friendship, and fortitude through this project. This book is a testament to our resilience! I also wish to dedicate the book to my family, especially my mom; as an English Teacher, she inspired me! Further dedication goes to my extended family, Vicki Penny, Leslie Johnson, Camille Troup, Georgina Higgins, Cathy Wagner, Patty Graham, and my faith for being present with me during a dark time many years ago. I am deeply grateful for this life experience, which has allowed me a window into this topic. Thank you to my children, Paul and Tori, for their patience and love as they witnessed that mental health prevails. Last but never least, I dedicate this book to my husband, Tom English, who has healed my soul, lifted my heart, and held my hand through this life journey. I am forever grateful to you, my love.

And I, Mary Ruth Cross, dedicate this book to my dear friend, co-editor, co-author, and travel buddy Leslie W. Baker, whose wisdom, innovation, and grace made this book a reality. We are stronger than we know. I also wish to thank my daughter Susie, who is a constant reminder that life is worth every minute, and my husband James for his honest and loving support from start to finish.

~ Leslie W. Baker and Mary Ruth Cross

CONTENTS

Foreword   *xii*

Acknowledgments   *xv*

About the Editors   *xvi*

About the Contributors   *xviii*

Preface: Perspectives on Suicide   *xxii*

PART 1   UNDERSTANDING YOUTH SUICIDE   1

1   INTRODUCTION: SUICIDE ASSESSMENT, TREATMENT,
    AND PREVENTION FOR YOUTH   3

    Mary Ruth Cross and Leslie W. Baker

2   LAW AND ETHICS, RESEARCH, MEDIA, AND LOOKING
    FORWARD TOWARD ZERO SUICIDE   11

    Leslie W. Baker and Mary Ruth Cross

3   INTEGRATING PSYCHIATRY INTO TREATMENT OF SUICIDAL
    YOUTH: INFORMATION FOR CLINICIANS   32

    Daniel Jon Kostalnick

4   COUNTERTRANSFERENCE IN THE TREATMENT OF YOUTH
    SUICIDE AND INTERVENTIONS FOR PROVIDING INNER AND
    EXTERNAL SUPPORT   39

    Leslie W. Baker and Mary Ruth Cross

PART 2   ASSESSMENT, THEORY, AND TREATMENT OF
         YOUTH SUICIDE   57

5   ASSESSMENT OF SUICIDE FOR YOUTH   59

    Mary Ruth Cross and Leslie W. Baker

6   PLAY THERAPY THEORIES: APPLICATIONS TO SUICIDE
    IN YOUTH   78

    Mary Ruth Cross and Leslie W. Baker

7   TREATMENT OF SUICIDAL THINKING AND BEHAVIORS IN
    CHILDREN AND ADOLESCENTS USING PLAY THERAPY   99
    Leslie W. Baker, Mary Ruth Cross, and Kim Vander Dussen

8   IMPACTS OF DIVERSITY IN SUICIDE ASSESSMENT,
    TREATMENT, AND PREVENTION FOR CHILDREN AND
    ADOLESCENTS   129

    8.1 OVERVIEW   130
         Rebekah Byrd and Yumiko Ogawa

    8.2 BLACK AMERICAN CHILDREN AND ADOLESCENTS   133
         Althea T. Simpson

    8.3 HISPANIC/LATINE CHILDREN AND ADOLESCENTS   138
         Matthew Nicholas Schramm and Jose Luis Tapia-Fuselier, Jr.

    8.4 NATIVE AMERICAN AND ALASKAN NATIVE CHILDREN
         AND ADOLESCENTS   143
         Ruben Colon

    8.5 ASIAN AMERICANS AND PACIFIC ISLANDER CHILDREN
         AND ADOLESCENTS   148
         Yung-Wei Dennis Lin

    8.6 UNDERSTANDING SUICIDALITY IN LGBTQ YOUTH
         THROUGH THE LENS OF QUEER-PRYSM   154
         Leslie W. Baker

    8.7 AUTISTIC AND NEURODIVERGENT CHILDREN AND
         ADOLESCENTS   159
         Robert Jason Grant

    8.8 SUMMARY   166
         Rebekah Byrd and Yumiko Ogawa

9   THE ROLE OF SCHOOLS IN SUICIDE: RESPONSE,
    RESOURCING, AND PREVENTION FOR CHILDREN   175
    Nichole Vernon

**10 TECHNOLOGY'S EMERGING ROLE FROM ASSESSMENT TO
     PREVENTION IN CHILDREN AND ADOLESCENTS**   **188**

Jessica Stone

Epilogue   *203*

Appendix   *204*

Index   *210*

FOREWORD

I know for sure there is a need to get professionals better trained, more empathic, and more competent when it comes to suicidal thoughts and behaviors in children and teens. I know this because I was a teen in crisis, complete with dramatic flares, who desperately needed empathy, nurturing, and guidance. And I recognize that I spun a web around me, thick and impenetrable, that kept others at arm's length. The thing I wished and hoped for the most was the very thing I fought to keep away.

At this stage of my life, it's not important to think about the why's of it all. What seems more relevant is to explain the isolated despair, the behavioral communication, and, most importantly, the professional opportunities that were missed by others. I truly believe I could have gotten the help I needed, which might have spared me and my family a lot of pain. But the professionals I met along the way were woefully unprepared to help me. YES, I attended family and individual therapy, and in the context of those settings, I managed to dig in my heels and wait for someone to come find me. But other clients in my family were more cooperative, talkative, and eager to answer questions. And the attention towards me was fleeting; I was not worth the effort it took to get me to provide monosyllabic answers. In retrospect, I believe I had one good friend, and that's the only person I wanted to speak with about anything important. However, she also modeled a lot of the provocative behavior that I assumed, so she was the least likely person to help me find my way out of the maze where I spent my time in those days.

I can think of many stressors: my parent's divorce, my relocation to the US, the loss of my grandmother, my identity issues, low self-esteem, acculturation challenges, and my tendency to bury my head in books with topics that required more maturity than I possessed at the time. The result was that no specific place seemed safe. The school offered little comfort, and kids teased me because I had a "funny name" and my English was imperfect. After school, my brother tormented me, although he remembers it as benign, whereas I think of it as emotional and physical abuse. When my mother came home, she was exhausted and had to prepare a meal and get ready for her next workday. She was painfully non-existent to me through no fault of her own. She was a single mom trying to provide for three kids in a new country. Whatever sweetness and lightness my mother had ever possessed was firmly underground due to all the burdens of her life.

I hope that gives a flavor of who I was back then: isolated, uncertain, grieving, and lacking a sense of who I was. By the time I was 17, my relationship with my mother was overtly conflictual, and I experienced her as someone who was constantly disappointed in me. It seemed nothing I did was right. I had also discovered that my oldest brother was gay, and I felt consumed with questions, worry, and confusion that had nowhere to go. I was about to finish high school, I was in love with someone distant and unavailable, and I could not envision any kind of future for myself. To add to this picture, my good friend had recently introduced me to drinking and parties, and I found immediate relief in being high. Being inebriated was one of the nicest experiences I had ever had, providing these amazing euphoric feelings. When I was high, I didn't care about anything or anyone, especially myself, and I was constantly putting myself in harm's way.

I was enjoying a bottle of Tanqueray alone in my room when the pain of being me felt overwhelming, and when I tried to envision my future, nothing appeared. I grabbed a razor blade and got into a bubble bath with my clothes on. I slit one wrist and watched the water get red. I closed my eyes, and when I pulled my arm out of the water, I could feel pain. I called out to my roommate, and she did not respond. I felt confused, tired, and sleepy. As I started closing my eyes, my roommate opened the front door, entered the bathroom, and freaked out. She called 911 and helped me out of the tub. She wrapped up my wrist and helped me get into dry clothes. When they put me on the gurney, I passed out, waking up in the ER, under the big lights, with lots of people hovering around me. I felt nauseous but never did throw up. My head was spinning without mercy.

They stitched up my wrist, and suddenly, I was alone in a small room with people coming in and out for one thing or another. I remember someone asking for my mother's name and phone number, which I provided without thinking. Suddenly, my mother and oldest brother were outside; I could hear them talking to a doctor. I could hear my mother crying, and through a small opening, I could see my brother hugging her.

The doctor came in to see me. I could feel his disdain immediately. He said, "Well, looks like you couldn't even get this right!" I didn't understand what he meant; it took a while. But his next words are etched in my brain until this very moment: "Next time you want to do yourself in, cut *up* on your arm, not across." I started to cry, and he stood up. "You have just put your mother through a lot of pain for nothing! You need to get your shit together and grow up!" I had no words to say back to him before my mother came in. I think he told me that someone would take out my stitches next week.

Maybe this was some kind of "tough love" approach. My experience of it was that I didn't matter to anyone, that this doctor was encouraging me to try again and get it right, and that I had caused immeasurable pain to my family. To say I felt low was an understatement. My mother was indeed in pain and told me she didn't understand, blamed this, that, and the other thing, and told me she wanted me to return home with her (which, of course, I did not).

This experience likely contributed to my becoming a mental health professional. Over the years, I have been very attuned to any child or teen who talks about wanting to disappear, be invisible, and shrink into nothingness. I have been acutely interested in children and youth's behavioral communication, much more than the words they use. I have practiced compassion and empathy, always focusing on the youth in front of me and making sure they feel seen and heard. And most importantly, I have tried to identify and implement effective ways of being with kids who have the desire to die and leave this earth. And believe me, children can feel this desire deeply because their pain is felt deeply, too, and they can't visualize options. It goes without saying that I maintain a systemic lens with a deep comprehension that if children are feeling this much pain, their parents need to know how to respond in ways that can send positive messages of love and comfort.

I am so excited to see this topic gain more and more attention, especially in this cultural climate of great stress and uncertainty. It is definitive that youth suicide appears to be much more common as children's stressors are so much more acute. This book provides a solid foundation for clinicians and educators to become better informed about spotting children who might need help, conducting adequate clinical assessments, and addressing their suicidal thoughts and behaviors. This topic is explored from many angles, including racial and cultural differences, age and gender differences, and makes a comprehensive effort to find ways to establish rapport with children who are often guarded and distrustful.

I can tell you with certainty that all suicide gestures and attempts are a call for help, an invitation for connection. We cannot afford to be angry or dismissive of children. We need to be incredibly cautious to see the danger and the opportunities that become available to us if we are in privileged positions to assist. I never hurt myself again, but I thought about it a lot. There were moments of distress in which I played the ER doctor's words in my head. In my 30s, I tried to track down my medical records so that I could locate that doctor and give him feedback, but my efforts failed. Here I am in my 70s, finally calling him out for his gross "treatment." In the moment of closure, the circle closed. I am grateful to have the chance to provide this context as you read Cross and Baker's useful and thorough book about connecting and helping children who long to die.

I would be remiss not to mention that someone did "save my life" after this event: a Jesuit priest named Lou Savary. Lou always seemed to listen to me without judgment; he came to my apartment every week for months just to see how I was. Even when I was drinking, I knew I could call him, and he wouldn't hang up. With him by my side, I became clear-headed, made decisions that were in my best interests, and started reaching out more to my family. I have had a chance to tell Lou directly that he pulled me up from the depths of despair and provided real help, and I only hope he gets it. His willingness to reach out and make himself present made all the difference. He was the perfect antithesis to my ER doctor, and this story would not be complete without adding this last important paragraph.

by Eliana Gil

ACKNOWLEDGMENTS

Suicide touches so many so profoundly. Those we have lost, those who almost died and instead survived, those who cope with suicidal thoughts and behaviors daily, those we stand alongside to support, guide, and protect and care for oneself in moments, sometimes dark moments, only to prevail because of someone's concern or care in lifting and supporting us through the darkness to the light. Our hearts are touched deeply by the children and adolescents who find their way back to living.

Writing about suicide in children and adolescents is no easy task. We completed this book with the support and guidance of our families, friends, the play therapy community, and those who contributed to expanding our knowledge and understanding of suicide and how to empower play therapists, school-based counselors, families, caretakers, and mental health allies. We especially would like to thank our publisher and the staff at Routledge Publishing for their guidance and support.

We would also like to thank all of the contributing authors who worked tirelessly to support children and adolescents through the challenges of assisting in assessing and treating mental health concerns. Each of these authors has provided insight into the specific populations they work with to help all of us address suicide from a culturally and developmentally sensitive perspective.

We thank James Cross for his editing and feedback expertise, Tom English for his technological prowess in digital and organizational support, and Angelina Anderson and Mary Labarre for their research support. These talented and caring people helped inform and assisted in completing this book. We would also like to thank Eliana Gil for guiding and supporting us throughout this project. Her own story is a beacon of hope for us all.

Lastly, our deepest thanks go to all children, adolescents, adults, and families who have trusted us with their stories and emotional pain. We have listened and hope this book will bring healing and light to those in the darkness of despair through the healing power of play.

Leslie and Mary Ruth

ABOUT THE EDITORS

Leslie W. Baker, LMFT, NCC, RPT-S™

Leslie W. Baker is a Licensed Marriage and Family Therapist, National Board-Certified Counselor, Gottmann Certified Therapist, and a Registered Play Therapist – Supervisor™.

She is the CEO and Owner of Therapy2Thrive® Ruby Hill Marriage and Family Counseling Center. Leslie has over 30 years of practical experience as a clinician and supervisor. She has presented workshops on the topic of suicide for 11 years. Her background includes more than 13 years as Adjunct Faculty at the University of Phoenix in the College of Social Sciences, Master of Counseling program, and nine years as the Lead Area Chair for the Master's in Counseling Program. For an additional ten years, she has been an Adjunct Faculty and Associate Professor for John F. Kennedy University in Campbell, CA, and an Adjunct Professor for Antioch University in Santa Barbara, CA. Leslie is an active member of the California Association for Marriage and Family Therapy (CAMFT), East Bay Association for Marriage and Family Therapists (EBCAMFT), Association for Play Therapy (APT), and the California Association for Play Therapy (CALAPT).

Leslie served on the Committee for Technology as a clinical member of the San Francisco Chapter of the CALAPT. Recently, Leslie has presented to local, national, and international groups focusing on using play therapy and integrating expressive play-based therapies for trauma treatment, treatment of suicide, and incorporating technology into treating youth. A Certified Suicide Bereavement-trained Clinician since 2017, Leslie has worked with suicide loss survivors, treating those who cope with suicidal thoughts and behaviors. Leslie is the author of a children's book for children coping with a grown-up mental illness and co-author of a children's book to assist youth in coping with no good, very bad things. She is also a contributing author to two book chapters on advancing technology use in play therapy.

Mary Ruth Cross, LMFT, NCC, RPT-S™

Mary Ruth Cross is a licensed Marriage and Family Therapist, a National Board-Certified Counselor, and a Registered Play Therapist – Supervisor™.

She is the CEO and Owner of Treehouse Family Counseling Services in San Ramon, CA, where she and her staff work together using play therapy to address clinical issues for the entire family. She has over 30 years of clinical experience working with abused and traumatized children and adolescents in outpatient settings. She has advanced training in Critical Incident Stress Debriefing, EMDR, grief and loss, death and dying, and suicide assessment and treatment. Mary Ruth also owns the Academy for Play Therapy Training™, where she provides clinical training in play therapy. She also supports the play therapy community through Cross Play Therapy Consulting, where her tailor-made program supports clinicians working towards full credentialing as play therapists through the Association for Play Therapy.

She has been a counselor educator for John F. Kennedy University and the University of Phoenix, bringing awareness and training in play therapy to graduate students.

She is the former President of the California Association for Play Therapy (CALAPT) and the San Francisco Bay Area Chapter of CALAPT. As a graduate of the Leadership Academy through the Association for Play Therapy, Mary Ruth serves on the Credentialing Committee and previously served on the Conference Committee. She is an active advocate for play therapy. She is a sought-after lecturer and has presented workshops to local, national, and international audiences. She is co-authoring a children's book called *Snug and Rug and the 'No Good Very Bad Thing': A Story of coping, calming and courage for children.*

ABOUT THE CONTRIBUTORS

Rebekah Byrd, Ph.D., LPC, LCMHC, NCC, RPT-S™, ACS

Dr. Byrd (she/her) is an Associate Professor of Counseling and Director of the Institute for Play Therapy and Expressive Arts Education and Research at Sacred Heart University. Dr. Byrd has been a counselor educator for over 13 years and has over 20 years of experience working in the mental health field in varying capacities and settings. Her research specialization falls primarily in issues pertaining to children/adolescent counseling, play therapy, LGBTGEQQIA+ advocacy, school counseling, social justice/multicultural concerns, self-injury, and women's wellness. She recently co-authored a textbook on counseling children and adolescents. She serves on many national and statewide committees and was recently awarded the Counselor Educator Advocacy Award from the Association for Child and Adolescent Counseling (ACAC).

Ruben Colon, LCSW

Ruben Xochicuauhtli Colon, LCSW, is a graduate of San Jose State University, where he earned both his BSW and MSW. Ruben worked in a public multidisciplinary behavioral health clinic setting, moving from there to being the Diversity and Inclusion Specialist for the San Andreas Regional Center, where he successfully obtained grant funding from the state to start the agency's "Engaging Native American Families Initiative." He has been dedicating himself to full-time private practice, seeing clients at his office near his hometown of Santa Clara (Land of the Muwekma Ohlone) and in the Central Valley of California. He has been involved in indigenous healing circles in the San Francisco Bay Area for the past 30 years and is a founding member of Calpulli Tonalehqueh Cultural Diffusion Group based in San Jose, CA. For individuals who identify as indigenous to the Americas, he can also integrate Native Wellness Concepts into his sessions through the use of the medicine wheel, the red road to sobriety, and historical trauma frameworks.

Robert Jason Grant, Ph.D., RPT-S™

Dr. Grant is the creator of AutPlay® Therapy. He is a therapist, supervisor, and consultant and utilizes several years of advanced training and his own lived neurodivergent experience to provide affirming services to children and their families. He is an international trainer, keynote presenter, and multi-published author of several articles and books. He is currently serving as past chair on the board of directors for the Association for Play Therapy.

Daniel Jon Kostalnick, M.D., F.A.P.A.

Dr. Kostalnick is a Board-Certified Physician by the American Board of Psychiatry and Neurology and the National Board of Physicians and Surgeons with extensive training and expertise in psychopharmacology and psychotherapy – incorporating the biological and psychological aspects of psychiatric health and wellness. Additionally, Dr. Kostalnick is a Fellow of the American Psychiatric Association and a Fellow of the International College of

Neuropsychopharmacology (CINP) Scotland, United Kingdom. He lives in California with his family and enjoys writing poetry and exploring the intersection of science, spirituality, and the arts.

Yung-Wei Dennis Lin, Ph.D., NCC

Dr. Lin Yung Wei is an Associate Professor in the Department of Counselor Education at the University of Iowa. Dr. Lin has served on multiple editorial boards for professional journals, including the *Journal of Counseling and Development* (JCD), the *Journal of Child and Adolescent Counseling* (JCAC), the *International Journal of Play Therapy*, and the *Journal of Counseling Outcome Research and Evaluation* (CORE), and is currently the associate editor of JCD, the flagship journal of the counseling profession. In addition to editorial work, Dr. Lin also served as the Chair of the Research Committee in the Association for Play Therapy (APT), a member of the Research Taskforce in the Association for Assessment and Research in Counseling (AARC) and is an Executive Committee member in the New Jersey Association for Play Therapy (NJAPT).

Dr. Lin is also a certified master trainer of Applied Suicide Intervention Skills Training (ASIST; Trainer ID: n26778). He has provided more than 23 ASIST trainings for more than 130 K-12 school counselors, 200 counselor trainees, and 60 university faculty and staff. Dr. Lin's meta-analytic study on child-centered play therapy was selected as the 2016 ACA Best Practice Faculty Award, and the suicide intervention study by Dr. Lin and his colleagues was selected as the 2019 Outstanding Counselor Education and Supervision Journal-Article of the Year and 2019 Chi Sigma Iota (CSI) Outstanding Research Award.

Yumiko Ogawa, Ph.D., LPC, ACS, BC-TMH, NCC, RPT-S™, Certified CCPT-S, Certified CPRT-S

Dr. Ogawa is an Associate Professor of the Department of Psychology and Director of the Clinical Mental Health Counseling Program at Marist College. Yumi has been a counselor educator for the last 12 years. She also has over 25 years of experience providing mental health services to young children and their families in various settings, including schools, agencies, private practices, and disaster response sites. She is dedicated to making high-quality and culturally inclusive mental health services more accessible to minoritized populations, and she has been collaborating with local school districts and a nonprofit immigration law firm to actualize these efforts. Her current research interest includes play therapy outcome studies with children with minoritized backgrounds, play therapists' therapeutic characteristics, and the effective use of rhythms in child therapy. She is a past president of the New Jersey Association for Play Therapy and is one of the founders of Play Therapy in Asia Summit.

Matthew Nicholas Schramm, MA, PLCC

Matthew Nicholas Schramm (he/him) is a doctoral student in counseling education and supervision at the University of Montana. He previously worked as a high school counselor and is currently practicing as a mental health clinician for adolescents and young adults in Missoula. Matthew earned his Master's in Counseling and Human Services from the University of Colorado, Colorado Springs. His research has focused on group processing interventions for individuals with multiple sclerosis and the effects of interabled relationships when one partner acquires a disability. Additionally, he has been a presenter at regional and national conferences, sharing his insights on addressing ableism in counseling practice and intimate partner violence.

Althea T. Simpson, LCSW, RPT-S™

Althea is a licensed Clinical Social Worker and Registered Play Therapist-Supervisor™ who founded Brighter Day Therapeutic Solutions, Unicorn Life Play Therapy, and the Black Play Therapy Society. Althea has many years of experience in research, diagnosis, and treatment provision in the mental health field and specializes in guiding individuals and families toward building resiliency skills to overcome trauma. She is also certified in LEGO® SERIOUS PLAY® and Playmobil ProPlay and provides employee assistance program services and mental health consulting services. As a trainer, speaker, and author, Althea is committed to sharing her knowledge and creative expertise to help others.

Jessica Stone, Ph.D., RPT-S™

Dr. Stone is a licensed psychologist with over 30 years of diverse experience spanning private practice, academia, mentorship, and authorship. Dr. Stone has pioneered the integration of digital tools in therapeutic settings, with a particular emphasis on virtual reality, tablets, and consoles. Her groundbreaking work includes founding the MHVR International Coalition and co-creating the Virtual Sandtray App for iPad (VSA) and its virtual reality counterpart, the VSA-VR. Recently serving as the Chief Psychology Officer for AscendantVR, Dr. Stone is also an affiliate of the East Carolina University College of Education Neurocognition Science Laboratory and holds positions on several prominent boards in the field.

Jose Luis Tapia-Fuselier, Jr., Ph.D., CRC, LPC, RPT™, NCC

Dr. Tapia-Fuselier, Jr. (he, him) is currently an Assistant Professor at the University of Colorado, Colorado Springs. He graduated with his Ph.D. in counseling at the University of North Texas. His research is focused on disability-responsive care across the lifespan. Dr. Tapia has published in peer-reviewed journals on serving children with disabilities using play therapy, trauma-informed ethical decision-making, and serving interabled relationships in counseling. He has served the community in public and private rehabilitation settings as well as in private and community practice for eight years. He has provided individual, relationship, play, and family therapy with a special focus on serving people with disabilities in three languages (English, Spanish, and American Sign Language). He is a Certified Rehabilitation Counselor, Licensed Professional Counselor, Registered Play Therapist, and National Certified Counselor. Additionally, he is a Certified Child-Centered Play Therapist-Supervisor, a Certified Child-Parent Relationship Therapy-Supervisor, and has advanced training in Emotionally Focused Therapy. Dr. Tapia has led trainings and workshops centered around ableism and its impact on service delivery and disability-responsive practices for helping professionals.

Kim Vander Dussen, Psy.D., RPT-S™

Dr. Vander Dussen is a Professor at the Chicago School in Anaheim. She is the coordinator of the Child and Adolescent Concentration in the Clinical Psy.D. Program and teaches various child and adolescent courses. She is also a Licensed Psychologist in private practice in Placentia, Orange County, CA, specializing in the treatment of children and their families. She holds certificates in Infant and Toddler Mental Health and Play Therapy. Dr. Vander Dussen is a Registered Play Therapist and Supervisor™ and is certified in EMDR, the Neurosequential Model of Therapeutics, and the Circle of Security Parenting Program. She is a member of the Board of Directors for the Association for Play Therapy. She serves on the Play Therapy Certificate Program faculty at UCSD Extension. Dr. Vander Dussen's area of expertise includes the treatment of trauma, attachment, and the mental health needs of neurodivergent youth. She is an international speaker presenting on various child and adolescent topics.

Nichole Vernon, Ph.D., SB– RPT™

Dr. Vernon earned her BS degree in Psychology from Lander University in Greenwood, SC, and her MS degree in Education in Special Education from Tennessee State University; Dr. Vernon received her doctoral degree in Psychology from Tennessee State University. She has worked as a certified School Psychologist in Illinois and Maryland. Dr. Vernon began working as an Associate Adjunct Professor with the University of Maryland Global Campus, and she currently is a full-time Adjunct Professor. Dr. Vernon completed her credential to become a School-Based Registered Play Therapist™. Dr. Vernon currently works for the District of Columbia Public Schools as a certified School Psychologist and School-Based Registered Play Therapist. Dr. Vernon has worked in the field of education for 19 years (eight years as a Special Education teacher and 11 years as a School Psychologist).

PREFACE
PERSPECTIVES ON SUICIDE

Suicide is a worldwide phenomenon. Current research demonstrates a persistent upward trend of incidences among youth globally and in the United States, which needs to be addressed to improve prevention efforts. Suicide is a problem that is woefully misunderstood, especially regarding children and adolescents. This book seeks to break down the barriers to increase awareness and show how compassion for youth who seek to harm themselves can dramatically improve their emotional stability. Children and adolescents may ask for help and need connection but instead receive judgment and anger. Those responses close off rather than open channels of communication. Play therapy interventions can bridge youth communication gaps when words are not enough. This book asks mental health professionals to look at themselves and reflect, to grow in their capacity to assess, treat, and prevent suicidal ideation in their young clients. Using evidence-based theories and interventions will improve the competency and capability of mental health professionals. Families, caregivers, schools, and allied professionals must be part of the solution. Without them, we cannot initiate the familial and social changes necessary to remedy this deadly problem. With care and compassion, we can establish relationships that give support and understanding towards coping with suicide. We thank you for your commitment to learning, growing, and playing to impact the lives of children and adolescents who cope with suicide. You are their light in the darkness.

Leslie W. Baker and Mary Ruth Cross

PART 1

UNDERSTANDING YOUTH SUICIDE

CHAPTER 1

INTRODUCTION

Suicide Assessment, Treatment, and Prevention for Youth

Mary Ruth Cross and Leslie W. Baker

THE PROBLEM

Suicidal thinking and behaviors (STB) may present as dichotomous. On the one hand, they can seem mysterious and unseen to family and friends. Conversely, a child or adolescent may talk, write, or announce to their friends, teachers, family, and caregivers that they do not want to live. It is difficult for many even to fathom that a child or adolescent is thinking about dying. Denial that young children and adolescents experience real and intense suicidal ideation is not an uncommon response to thoughts and feelings about suicide from those closest to them. Even when a parent or other adult hears statements like "I do not want to be here anymore" or "Everyone would be better off without me," many adults respond with comments like "Oh, you do not feel that way" or "Of course, you do not mean that." This type of interaction demonstrates the vital need for all adults, caregivers, educators, and mental health professionals to truly understand not only the critical dynamics of suicidal thinking and behavior but also the truth about the genuine danger youth are in when thinking about self-harm to escape their pain. This danger is real and very present. Suicide is the second leading cause of death for people ages 10–14 (*Centers for Disease Control and Prevention, National Center for Health Statistics. National Vital Statistics System, Mortality 2018–2021 on CDC WONDER Online Database*, 2023).

Parents, caregivers, and family members concerned for their children and adolescents rely on mental health professionals for guidance. However, many mental health professionals do not address or cannot identify critical aspects of suicidal ideation (SI) or self-harm in children and adolescents. Unfortunately, many in authority minimize the risk of suicide in children. Hennefield et al. (2019) stated that these novel findings shed light on the connection between depression, suicidality, and death in early childhood, offering valuable insights for play therapists. They underscore the significance of addressing suicidal thoughts and behaviors during clinical interviews with young children affected by depression. Healthcare professionals must recognize the gravity of these issues, implement necessary safety precautions, and work towards fostering healthier coping strategies.

Many family members and professionals ascribe child suicide as a tragic death, often resulting from children's normal risk-taking behavior. For example, a child rides their bike out into the street and gets hit by a car, takes unusual physical risks while playing, or eats a detergent pod and medicines (Farah et al., 2023) – the behaviors of accidental or overly energetic play. However, a deeper examination could uncover signs of suicidal ideation. Play therapists, other mental health professionals, and educators need to be more attuned

DOI: 10.4324/9781003358565-2

to the signs and symptoms of suicidality and how to address suicidal thoughts and feelings directly. When children feel heard and seen, they do not feel the need to act out negative impulses. In their research, Ruch et al. (2021) noted that according to the Centers for Disease Control and Prevention (CDC), rates of suicide attempts and deaths among children have increased in the U.S. over the past decade, and suicide is now the eighth leading cause of death in children age 5–11. Factors such as attention-deficit disorder, family-related problems, school, trauma, and peer-related issues contribute to children's and adolescents' impulsive suicidal actions.

Can children possibly understand the concept of dying and suicide? Children with depression and suicidal ideation have a more advanced understanding of death than their peers, dispelling the myth that these ideations arise from a poor understanding of death (Hennefield et al., 2019). This topic is among the most challenging issues facing parents, play therapists, caregivers, social workers, and others in authority. Who wants to admit that a young child or adolescent can hurt so much that they long to be free of emotional pain by dying? At an age that we would expect feelings of joy and curiosity, wonderment and adventure, a magical time we call childhood, we may instead find a yearning for release from suffering. It challenges our fundamental beliefs about youth, making it difficult to make sense of their intense emotional pain (Miller, 2021).

Mental health professionals are entrusted with clinical assessment and intervention tasks. It is our responsibility to break through the widespread reluctance to accept the possibility of youth suicide. As mental health professionals, educators, parents, and caregivers, we cannot afford to avoid examining, understanding, discussing, and taking action as needed on suicidality in youth. Recent research by Whalen et al. (2022) noted that although suicide is relatively uncommon before age 10, about half of the children who experienced STBs in adolescence first displayed STBs in early childhood. It is imperative to recognize these behaviors to provide early and effective treatment.

In a stark statistic, the Center for Disease Control data on child, adolescent, and adult suicide indicate that suicide among 10–34-year-olds is the second leading cause of death and the tenth leading cause of death in the United States (2021). The CDC states that suicide causes more deaths in adolescents and young adults than combined cancer, heart disease, AIDS, congenital disabilities, stroke, pneumonia, influenza, and chronic lung disease. According to research, suicide rates and self-injury hospitalizations are rising in this age group (Ruch et al., 2019; Ballesteros et al., 2018).

Finally, the American Academy of Child & Adolescent Psychiatry (AACAP) reported in 2018 that attempts at suicide in children under the age of 10 tend to be impulsive and associated with feelings of sadness, confusion, anger, or issues with attention or hyperactivity. There is a scarcity of information available to address this very young population. Spears et al. found that despite the generally acknowledged urgency in managing the risk of youth suicide, efforts to understand and assist suicidal youth have been slow but steady (2022). A critical step is for play therapists to work through many defensive layers to engage children, help them develop comfort, and encourage them to share their inner thoughts and feelings. In this book, we will examine these unique risk factors and vulnerabilities to provide substantial assistance to those working with and supporting children and adolescents with good mental health. We will handle how making a psychiatric referral can further a youth's suicidal assessment and treatment through a coordinated effort between the clinician and the psychiatrist.

CARING FOR PLAY THERAPISTS AND EDUCATORS

Given the complexities of treating and assessing suicidality in children and adolescents, we must also consider the impact work of this nature may have on individual play therapists and caregivers. We will look at countertransference and appropriate models for self-care, particularly when the client dies due to suicide. The book will provide some suggestions regarding coping with grief and loss should a play therapist face a loss in their practice or assist a family in dealing with the loss of a child or adolescent. We will utilize expressive play-based interventions to provide opportunities to address grief and loss experienced by play therapists, teachers, parents, and caregivers. Case studies within this book will demonstrate vital concepts. Play therapists need to have appropriate high-level self-care. When a client dies by suicide, we must be able to examine our response to loss. Play therapists need effective coping strategies to continue delivering appropriate treatment. Combining proper self-care with consultation will allow play therapists to stay present through all the complexities of assessing and treating suicidality. According to Aasan et al., cultivating well-being and dealing with unresolved inner conflicts using Self-Guided Imagery in meditation has been shown to assist play therapists, school play therapists, and clinicians in managing their countertransference (2022).

Important Factors of Suicide

It used to be rare for mental health professionals to see a suicidal client under the age of ten before the pandemic. Statistics do show an increase in suicide, especially in black youth. There has been a steady increase in suicidal ideation due to the pandemic (CDC, 2023). According to Yard et al. in their 2021 research on the number of emergency room visits for suspected suicide attempts in children, adolescents, and young adults aged 12 to 25 before and during the pandemic in the United States (January 2019 through May 2020), demonstrated that the pandemic had worsened suicidal ideation in children and adolescents. The most significant increase was found in teen girls ages 12 to 17 beginning in the summer of 2020. The statistics show that in the summer of 2020, adolescent girls had a 26.2% higher rate of suicidal ideation. In the winter of 2021, there was a 50.6% higher rate of suicidal ideation in this same demographic. *The State of the World's Children 2021* noted in their research that the impact of the pandemic on teen boys and suicidal ideation remained stable over the years before and during the pandemic. Given the socialization patterns of females with a focus on relationship-building, the pandemic seems to have created a 'crisis of disconnection' (*The State of the World's Children 2021*, 2021). Although there has not been an increase in suicide deaths due to the pandemic, there has been evidence of children reporting more global distress, including social isolation, lack of participation in group activities, and a sense of generalized anxiety (*The State of the World's Children 2021*, 2021).

ASSESSMENT AND TREATMENT OF YOUTH SUICIDE

Assessing suicidality needs a multi-faceted approach. A thorough assessment includes gathering information from multiple sources. Starting with a comprehensive developmental history of youth, family history, specifically suicidal risk factors, warning signs, cultural factors, and protective factors. From this assessment, the clinician determines the level of suicidal risk as severe, moderate, or low to determine the appropriate course of action to ensure client safety and address treatment goals. Our approach explores and examines screening tools to help identify risk levels and seriousness of intent. We will explore the kind of support needed during and after the crisis. Once a child or adolescent demonstrates the intent to attempt suicide, all avenues are explored to keep the child or adolescent safe. Safety for children and adolescents may include contacting law enforcement to ensure a child or adolescent is safe if a parent is unwilling to ensure safety. Assessment of aftercare will provide additional strategies for the play therapist to help the transition back home. Parents and caregivers have essential roles throughout the process, especially in post-hospitalization. The most effective treatment comes from a sound theoretical approach.

We will show how the therapeutic powers of play are transformative for these distressed children and adolescents. Schaefer and Drewes have provided a comprehensive framework for understanding how therapeutic space can be transformative by identifying the 20 core agents of change (2014). These include facilitating communication, fostering emotional wellness, enhancing social relationships, and increasing personal strengths. The therapeutic powers of play discussed and demonstrated throughout this book show the direct therapeutic role that play therapy can provide when working with suicidal children and adolescents. When addressing suicide, play therapists must develop a multi-faceted treatment plan incorporating play's therapeutic powers, which engenders change. Schaefer and Drewes clarified that play therapy is "not just a medium for applying other change agents" but a central system of achieving therapeutic change (Schaefer & Drewes, 2014, p. 2).

The overriding goal of this book is to bridge evidence-based practice models for treating suicidality – such as Child-Centered Play Therapy (CCPT), an evidence-based intervention rooted in the theory that the therapeutic relationship between the therapist and the child can be a primary source of healing for children facing emotional and behavioral difficulties. Axline (1947) initially formulated CCPT and adapted Rogers's (1951) person-centered counseling approach for children. Known originally as nondirective play therapy, CCPT has been further refined and expanded upon by experts such as Landreth (2012) and Ray (2011). Cognitive Behavioral Play Therapy (CBPT) is rooted in the underlying theory of Cognitive Behavioral Therapy (CBT). Drawing from principles of classical and operant conditioning and social learning, CBPT aims to bring about positive changes in behavior (Knell, 1990). Dialectical Behavior Therapy for children is not a formal adaptation, however it preserves the theoretical foundation, principles, and therapeutic strategies of standard DBT while adapting them to suit the developmental and cognitive levels of pre-adolescent children. There is a formal adaptation for adolescents called DBT-A for adolescents (Fleischhaker et al., 2011).

Additionally, DBT with children and adolescents includes an extensive parent training component. DBT with children explains to parents how their child learns, including coping skills, problem-solving techniques, and emotional information (Tech, 2016). Expressive play-based therapies are also essential when working with children and adolescents dealing with suicidal thoughts and behaviors. Morison et al., in 2021, noted that their meta-analyses suggested a beneficial effect of creative arts-based interventions on negative moods. The general benefit of creative arts-based interventions is enhancing self-worth through self-expression (Malchiodi, 2015; Morison et al., 2021). Prescriptive Play Therapy (PPT), developed by Charles Schaefer in 2001, is an approach in which the practitioner relies on their expertise to select and apply specific play therapy theories and methods that match the child's or adolescent's needs. Research suggests this is effective for addressing a particular problem or symptom. Schaefer based this approach on the core belief that every child can benefit significantly from various play therapy approaches. However, only some universally applicable methods suit every child's needs. The reach of the therapist is limited; in the mission to care for at-risk youth, the participation of caretakers beyond the clinician's office is necessary. Play therapists must include parents and caregivers in the treatment process and provide appropriate resources to assist their child or adolescent in non-office settings such as home and school. In addition, the authors will discuss and bridge evidence-based practice by applying expressive play therapy and neuroscience to treating suicide. These theories in a PPT framework allow play therapists to create a treatment model that fits a client's specific needs alongside the Neurosequential Model of Therapeutics (NMT), which also allows for matching treatment with brain developmental stages (Perry, 2009).

Understanding the brain and suicide treatment through the Neurosequential model will help readers understand basic treatment ideas from a brain-based perspective. A firm conceptual understanding of the brain's workings gives play therapists more effective treatment outcomes (Perry & Szalavitz, 2017). Luby et al. noted that brain research assists play therapists with a further understanding of children's brain development and how they are affected by toxic stress (2017). Post-study, Dr. Luby notes the value of parents and caregivers providing emotional support to children and adolescents, making them less vulnerable to the effects of toxic stress and thus improving their emotional and developmental trajectories.

In addition to providing theoretical approaches to expressive play-based interventions designed to help move the child and adolescent clients through the treatment process, it is crucial to establish and maintain a solid therapeutic alliance with the youth. Suppose the crisis does not demand immediate emergency assessment by a qualified crisis team. In that case, the clinician can create a safety plan with the youth and their family, including prevention ideas and a focus on hope. Understanding the need for psychiatric medication evaluation when necessary, will also be reviewed by both play therapists and educators. As hard as it is to imagine that a child may long to die, underlying this perception for many youths is a need to escape their deep emotional pain. Through denial and minimization, adults convince themselves that children and adolescents are safe. This attitude makes the risk to children and adolescents much higher. Schools can help identify at-risk children and provide support so school counselors or a crisis team can treat suicidal ideation. The role of schools in suicide prevention will help us see how to respond and give resources to at-risk children and adolescents.

Suicide prevention in schools must have the following components to be successful: a systemic approach, education of teachers and counselors, peer education, training for all school personnel, accessibility to mental health resources, and acceptance of the need for help (Miller, 2021). "Effective social and emotional learning in schools improves problem-solving, aids in strengthening self-control, increases trust, and decreases self-destructive behaviors" (Durlak et al., 2011, p. 10). Many children of all ages would love to be seen and heard. We present expressive play-based interventions that help provide ways to increase trust and safety, which in turn support and improve social-emotional functioning. Teachers are the gatekeepers. Administrators need to help school personnel develop suicide prevention policies and procedures. Once in place, policies and practices will include staff training, student education, awareness, screening–prevention, and response (Singer et al., 2019).

RACISM, SOCIAL OPPRESSION, AND DISPARITIES IN SUICIDE

Recently, the true impact of racism and social oppression of Black Indigenous People of Color (BIPOC) has put issues of diversity, inclusiveness, and acceptance at the forefront of community awareness, including the cases of youth suicide. For example, statistical records concerning people affected by suicide exhibit racially – and gender-based disparities. (*Disparities in Suicide | CDC*, 2023). This book will deal with suicide assessment and prevention for children and adolescents, Black, Hispanic/Latino Native American and Alaskan Native, Asian American, Pacific Islander populations, LGBTQIA+ youth, and autistic and neurodiverse children and adolescents. Culturally specific protective factors on suicide risk will be examined, with inclusiveness and understanding of diversity as the central theme.

NEW APPROACHES

Digital Play Therapy™ (Stone, 2019, 2022, 2023) and its role in treating children and adolescents is essential for a deeper understanding of digital tools and their role in treating and preventing suicide for children and adolescents. Play therapists can explore digital options for assessment, treatment, and prevention through the lens of digital play. Today, children and adolescents are versed in technology, enabling play therapists to use digital assessments and Digital Play Therapy™ (Stone, 2019, 2022, 2023) and prevention in their treatment rooms. Play therapists gaining experience with digital play may experience an increase in engagement with digital natives as people born or brought up during the age of technology and, therefore, familiar with computers and the internet from an early age (Cambridge et al., n.d.) will react favorably to what could be called a 21st-century approach.

CONCLUSION

As play therapists, we hold a container of hope for all the children and families who come to us for care and help. The complexity of assessment and treatment of suicidality is a multi-faceted process. Sound theoretical models that integrate and understand the true therapeutic powers of play and how to utilize the core agents of change contribute to successful treatment outcomes. We cannot do this work alone. Collaboration with parents, caregivers, schools, and community outreach provides a unified treatment team for the health and safety of all children, especially those who cope with suicidality. A six-year-old child client asked, "Why do so many people care about me?" This child had been struggling with suicidal ideation and had attempted self-harm at school. He could not understand why so many people were working hard to keep him safe. We can only answer this question: "Because you are worth caring about." Through expressive play therapy, we can transform darkness into light. Mental health professionals, educators, and parents/caregivers can be the beacon of hope through assessment, treatment, and prevention for children and their families so that not even one more child or adolescent has suicidal thoughts or suicidal behaviors.

REFERENCES

Aasan, O. J., Brataas, H. V., & Nordtug, B. (2022). Experience of managing countertransference through self-guided imagery in meditation among healthcare professionals. *Frontiers in Psychiatry*, *13*. https://doi.org/10.3389/fpsyt.2022.793784
Axline, V. (1947). *Play therapy*. Ballantine.

Ballesteros, M. F., Williams, D. D., Mack, K. A., Simon, T. R., & Sleet, D. A. (2018). The epidemiology of unintentional and violence-related injury morbidity and mortality among children and adolescents in the United States. *International Journal of Environmental Research and Public Health, 15*(4), 616. https://doi.org/10.3390/ijerph15040616

Cambridge University Press. (n.d.). Digital native. In *Cambridge dictionary*. Retrieved May 13, 2023, from https://dictionary.cambridge.org/us/dictionary/english/digital-native

Centers for Disease Control and Prevention, National Center for Health Statistics. National Vital (By Centers for Disease Control and Prevention). (2023, May 9). *Disparities in suicide.* Centers for Disease Control and Prevention. Retrieved October 7, 2023, from www.cdc.gov/suicide/facts/disparities-in-suicide.html

Durlak, J. A., Weissberg, R. P., Dymnicki, A. B., Taylor, R. D., & Schellinger, K. B. (2011). The impact of enhancing students' social and emotional learning: A meta-analysis of school-based universal interventions. *Child Development, 82*(1), 405–432. https://doi.org/10.1111/j.1467-8624.2010.01564.x

Hennefield, L., Whalen, D. J., Wood, G., Chavarria, M., & Luby, J. L. (2019). Changing conceptions of death as a function of depression status, suicidal ideation, and media exposure in early childhood. *Journal of the American Academy of Child and Adolescent Psychiatry, 58*(3), 339–349. https://doi.org/10.1016/j.jaac.2018.07.909

Knell, S. M. (1990). Cognitive-behavioral play therapy [Dataset]. In *PsycEXTRA dataset.* https://doi.org/10.1037/e549312011-006

Landreth, G. (2012). *Play therapy: The art of the relationship* (3rd ed.). Routledge.

Luby, J. L., Barch, D., Whalen, D. J., Tillman, R., & Belden, A. C. (2017). Association between early life adversity and risk for poor emotional and physical health in adolescence. *JAMA Pediatrics, 171*(12), 1168. https://doi.org/10.1001/jamapediatrics.2017.3009

Malchiodi, C. A. (2015). Neurobiology, creative interventions, and childhood trauma. In C. A. Malchiodi (Ed.), *Creative arts and play therapy. Creative interventions with traumatized children* (pp. 3–23). The Guilford Press.

Miller, D. N. (2021). *Child and adolescent suicidal behavior: School-based prevention, assessment, and intervention.* Guilford Publications.

Morison, L., Simonds, L. M., & Stewart, S. F. (2021). Effectiveness of creative arts-based interventions for treating children and adolescents exposed to traumatic events: A systematic review of the quantitative evidence and meta-analysis. *Arts & Health: An International Journal for Research, Policy, and Practice, 14*(3), 237–262. https://doi.org/10.1080/17533015.2021.2009529

Perry, B. D. (2009). Examining child maltreatment through a neurodevelopmental lens: Clinical applications of the neurosequential model of therapeutics. *Journal of Loss & Trauma, 14*(4), 240–255. https://doi.org/10.1080/15325020903004350

Perry, B. D., & Szalavitz, M. (2017). *The boy who was raised as a dog: And other stories from a child psychiatrist's notebook* (Rev. and Updated ed.). Basic Books.

Ray, D. (2011). *Advanced play therapy: Essential conditions, knowledge, and skills for child practice.* Routledge.

Rogers, C. (1951). *Client-centered therapy: Its current practice, implications, and theory.* Houghton Mifflin

Ruch, D., Heck, K. M., Sheftall, A. H., Fontanella, C. A., Stevens, J., Zhu, M., Horowitz, L. M., Campo, J. V., & Bridge, J. A. (2021). Characteristics and precipitating circumstances of suicide among children aged 5 to 11 years in the United States, 2013–2017. *JAMA Network Open, 4*(7), e2115683. https://doi.org/10.1001/jamanetworkopen.2021.15683

Ruch, D., Sheftall, A. H., Schlagbaum, P., Rausch, J., Campo, J. V., & Bridge, J. A. (2019). Trends in suicide among youth aged 10 to 19 years in the United States, 1975 to 2016. *JAMA Network Open, 2*(5), e193886. https://doi.org/10.1001/jamanetworkopen.2019.3886

Schaefer, C. E. (2001). Prescriptive play therapy. *International Journal of Play Therapy, 10*(2), 57–73. https://doi.org/10.1037/h0089480

Schaefer, C. E., & Drewes, A. A. (2014). *The therapeutic powers of play: 20 core agents of change* (2nd ed.). Wiley.

Singer, J. P., Erbacher, T. A., & Rosen, P. (2019). School-based suicide prevention: A framework for evidence-based practice. *School Mental Health, 11*(1), 54–71. https://doi.org/10.1007/s12310-018-9245-8

Statistics System, Mortality 2018–2021 on CDC WONDER Online Database. (2023). CDC WONDER online database. Retrieved May 13, 2023, from http://wonder.cdc.gov/mcd-icd10-expanded.html

Stone, J. (2019). *Digital play therapy: A clinician's guide to comfort and competence* (1st ed.). Routledge.

Stone, J. (2022). *Digital play therapy: A clinician's guide to comfort and competence* (2nd ed.). Routledge.

Stone, J. (2023). *Technology in mental health: Foundations of clinical use.* Routledge.

Tech, B. (2016). Dialectical behavior therapy for children. *Behavioral Tech.* https://behavioraltech.org/dbt-for-children/

The State of the World's Children 2021. (2021, October 1). UNICEF. www.unicef.org/reports/state-worlds-children-2021

Whalen, D. J., Hennefield, L., Elsayed, N. M., Tillman, R., Deanna, M., & Luby, J. L. (2022). Trajectories of suicidal thoughts and behaviors from preschool through late adolescence. *Journal of the American Academy of Child and Adolescent Psychiatry, 61*(5), 676–685. https://doi.org/10.1016/j.jaac.2021.08.020

Yard, E. E., Radhakrishnan, L., Ballesteros, M. F., Sheppard, M. C., Gates, A., Stein, Z., Hartnett, K. P., Kite-Powell, A., Rodgers, L., Adjemian, J., Ehlman, D. C., Holland, K. M., Idaikkadar, N., Ivey-Stephenson, A. Z., Martinez, P. F., Law, M., & Stone, D. L. (2021). Emergency department visits for suspected suicide attempts among persons aged 12–25 years before and during the COVID-19 pandemic – United States, January 2019–May 2021. *Morbidity and Mortality Weekly Report, 70*(24), 888–894. https://doi.org/10.15585/mmwr.mm7024e1

CHAPTER 2

LAW AND ETHICS, RESEARCH, MEDIA, AND LOOKING FORWARD TOWARD ZERO SUICIDE

Leslie W. Baker and Mary Ruth Cross

SOCIETY AND SUICIDE

Throughout history, societies have sought to establish legal authority over suicide. For example, in ancient Athens, funeral rites and burial were denied for suicides. The body might be buried on the city's outskirts without any marker (Retterstol, 1998). In 1670, Louis XIV of France mandated the mutilation of a suicide victim's body by dragging it through the streets and dumping it on a garbage pile (Spaulding et al., 1997). Each country has its laws and ways of managing suicide. And one still faced difficulties if the attempt was unsuccessful– one could be fined or sent to jail (Weaver & Wright, 2008).

In the United States, the federal government has authorized chiefly states to enact their laws concerning suicide. Historically, many states saw the act of suicide as a felony. But by the late 1980s, more than half no longer had laws prohibiting suicide or suicide attempts. Currently, no states list suicide as a crime (Litman, n.d.). 2004, Congress passed the Garrett Lee Smith Memorial Act (GLSMA). This act made provisions for federal funding to states, tribes, and colleges throughout the U.S. to create and implement suicide prevention programs for youth and adults via community-based agencies. It is important to note that many programs already in place had goals based on the National Strategy for Suicide Prevention designed in 2001. A great need in suicide prevention was accessed to support in times of crisis. The National Suicide Hotline Act of 2020 created an easy-to-remember 3-digit universal number, 988, to be answered 24/7 to increase suicide prevention (Gardner, 2020). This bill was successfully passed and is currently law in the US.

Further efforts have been made to pass legislation in support of suicide prevention. The following year, the Suicide Prevention Act was passed by the House of Representatives. The bill was then forwarded to the Senate for consideration. If enacted, it would create a pilot program to increase and intensify self-harm surveillance and establish a grant program that could provide funding for more prevention services throughout the United States. This bill was initially introduced in the 116th Congress, reintroduced in the 117th Congress, and referred to a committee (Actions – S.4448–117th Congress, 2021–2022).

Laws prohibiting suicide were based on the presumption that all adults are competent and responsible for their actions (Stefan, 2016). A defendant in a criminal trial can be declared mentally unfit (incompetent) to stand trial (Lewis, 2016). Still, there is no current legal test for assessing the competency of a suicidal patient to self-determine (Mishara & Weisstub, 2016). Laws intended to prohibit certain behaviors are quite common, but laws that require a legal obligation to act are rare. (A notable exception is the Mandated Reporter law.) Many countries prohibit aiding, abetting, and even encouraging suicide. Still, when it comes to the rights and responsibilities of clinicians (and anyone, really) who actively seeks to

DOI: 10.4324/9781003358565-3

prevent suicide, the law becomes nebulous. In the United States, no federal law mandates the report of suicide risk. The obligation to report a potential suicide comes from professional ethics and clinical protocols set by individual states. To feel confident about their actions, clinicians need to know what local governing body determines the protocol for dealing with a potential suicide and what those guidelines are (Kalb et al., 2019). As noted, societies have long sought to respond to self-harm by legislating against it. Though the intentions may have been positive, the effects were adverse. Research has shown that it is the decriminalization of suicide that leads to lower rates of attempts (Mishara & Weisstub, 2016). The first modern examination of the subject was found in *Suicide: A Study in Sociology* by Émile Durkheim in 1897. He postulated that there were contributing factors at the root of suicidal ideation, namely societal stressors. Later, Freud proposed that psychosis or other mental health problems contributed to suicidality and that the subject should be seen through the lens of a psychiatrist (Behere et al., 2015). Some researchers (Pal & Ramanathan, 2023) suggest that suicide should be a separate diagnosis because data shows that half of those who die by suicide have no history of mental health issues.

Decriminalization has been shown to lessen the stigma of suicide by allowing patients to be more honest and forthcoming about their thoughts and feelings (Behere et al., 2015). With greater openness and trust comes a greater capacity to heal. Dispelling myths about suicide, raising awareness about suicide prevention, and using accurate language when talking about suicide (i.e., "died by suicide" instead of "committed suicide") are implicit ethical responsibilities (Bernert & Roberts, 2012). Please refer to Appendix 1 for more definitions of suicide.

ETHICAL CHALLENGES

In assessing and treating suicide, clinicians face many ethical challenges. Saigle and Racine (2018) found three main areas of ethical challenges: clinical decisions, issues with the therapeutic relationship, and organizational factors. In addition, they noted overarching themes of stigma, problems with risk-benefit assessments, and fear of being held liable for a patient's death by suicide. One of the essential precepts in counseling is "do no harm," a component of the ethical principle of beneficence and maleficence. Inherent in the freedoms of the individual is the right to privacy, confidentiality, and self-determination. These ethical challenges can challenge the clinician to balance a possible conflict of ethical responsibilities where the patient's rights are balanced with efforts to minimize their risk of self-harm (Andrews, 2020). Patients have the right to choose what type of care to receive (autonomy) and expect it to remain confidential (privacy). Managing suicidality requires making challenging decisions that minimize risk and maintain the dignity and respect of the patient. Autonomy versus the "best interest" of the client requires clinicians to take a longitudinal view of the patient's capacity. An individual's capacity may fluctuate, so care must be taken throughout the risk assessment to ensure an accurate diagnosis. Capacity decisions are determined through a combined examination of the decision's complexity and the outcome's consequences (Paul, 2004). To estimate a patient's capacity, the clinician must know sufficiently about the client and balance their immediate desires with their long-term welfare. Pal and Ramanathan (2023) identified ethical principles that impact suicidality management as non-maleficence, beneficence, autonomy, justice, respect, and privacy. Addressing these issues within the treatment of suicide can point to conflicts between what is in the patient's best interest and the patient's right to make decisions about their own body.

When treating suicidality and identifying ethical challenges, the clinician is not only assessing the risk of suicide but focusing on risk management. Participants in a notable study noted that they assumed that a clinician was sufficiently addressing ethical issues by simply questioning whether they were doing the right thing. It is misguided to follow this approach, as it limits relevant information to what the clinician already knows and does not examine the ethical dilemmas that a deeper dive into the subject will reveal. Other participants in the study noted that they need to pay more attention to ethical challenges (Jobes et al., 2008). Professional associations such as the American Psychological Association (APA) and the Association for Marriage and Family Therapy (AAMFT) have their own Code of Ethics. Members must refer to it as a basis for their conduct. Ethical decision-making involves integrity, truthfulness, fairness, and non-discrimination, as well as awareness of historical and social prejudice, misdiagnosing and over-pathologizing, treatment disruption, termination, abandonment, client autonomy, dual relationships, and the clinician's values and beliefs (*Attorney Articles: Working with Suicidal Clients*, n.d.). This is a lot of information for the clinician to remain aware of and integrate into the overall assessment and treatment of suicidality.

However, reasonable or appropriate steps should be taken as part of the duty to care, but what is considered reasonable? In Bella v. Greeson, a case that involved the family of a person who died by suicide, the treating psychologist neither took sufficient measures to prevent the suicide nor alerted the family to the seriousness of her condition (*Justia Law*, n.d.). It was found that there is no uniformity of interventions that can be applied to all suicidal clients in all circumstances. Clinicians are not required to be correct in their assessment of suicide. Still, there is an expectation that all reasonable steps will be taken to get sufficient information from the patient to assess and determine the risk of suicide fully (*Attorney Articles: Working with Suicidal Clients*, n.d.).

For many, facing ethical challenges can feel exhausting and burdensome. Jobes et al. (2008) recommend a multi-tiered approach to managing ethical challenges. First, it is recommended to reach out to trusted colleagues to enable deeper individual reflection by the clinician. Use ad hoc or regular meetings with peers and an explicit ethics meeting to examine thoughts and feelings about the present challenge. When confronted with ethical issues, Paul (2004) suggests three aspects of decision-making when treating suicidal patients: empirical challenges when assessing risk, balancing autonomy and exercising healthy paternalism. Medical paternalism occurs when a clinician decides that contrary to the patient's wishes, it is appropriate to prevent any attempt to damage one's body significantly.

The clinician overrides the patient's wishes, in this case, the want to self-harm. Bear in mind that, when assessing the risk of suicide, it is essential to differentiate self-harm behaviors from suicidality. Clinicians must ask and answer where to put their focus. Should it be on long-term therapy for self-harm or immediate hospitalization to prevent suicide? Andrews (2020) offers a framework. Instead of asking who their client is when sorting out conflicting interests, such as those between parent and child, the clinician can ask about the ethical responsibilities of all concerned parties. The treatment plan's *what, when,* and *how* are essential to disseminate for *all* those affected by treatment.

CLINICAL DECISION MAKING

Jobes et al. (2008) noted that ethical challenges in the treatment of suicide exist in these four key areas:

1. Sufficient Informed Consent

In the treatment room, clinicians work to establish a therapeutic alliance that garners trust so that the patient can freely discuss all issues. In treating suicide, honest answers and truthful disclosures are necessary to assess risk and apply risk management techniques accurately. Like evidence-based psychosocial interventions for suicidal behaviors, this process should be highly transparent, collaborative, and initiated at the beginning of treatment to ensure that the patient understands all ethical and legal responsibilities incurred by the clinician. Informed consent to treatment is a necessary part of risk management. It may be defined as explaining to the patient all procedures used in evaluating and managing suicide risk, clinical decision-making, and emergency assessment and referral practices (Bernert & Roberts, 2012). Using developmentally appropriate language when explaining informed consent to children and adolescents is crucial. Research shows that informed consent maximizes benefits while minimizing risk as much as possible. Informed consent should be revisited throughout treatment as clinical issues arise or change (Lambert, 2017).

2. Competent Assessment for Suicide Risk

Lambert (2017) found that the courts focus on causation and feasibility when evaluating the standard of care and whether confidentiality has been breached. Could the clinician have predicted that this patient would attempt suicide? They also asked if there was sufficient evidence of risk factors so the clinician could accurately identify risks and protect the client. Focusing on youth risk factors, warning signs, and protective factors is crucial in assessing suicide to determine clients' risk levels.

3. Use of Empirically Informed Treatments and Interventions

Competency relates to having the appropriate standard of care. Clinician competency in assessing and treating suicide is typically acquired through initial coursework in graduate school. Research has shown that more than this is needed to maintain competency. Clinicians must stay updated with training and analysis for the population they want to work with to maintain competency (Kalb et al., 2019). Strategies for maintaining the standard of care when managing suicide risk include regular consultation with peers and experts in the field. Careful and typical documentation of risk level, actions taken, safety planning, and continued education in suicidology. Continuing education requirements vary from state to state. For example, California only requires one 6-hour training, yet Washington State needs to update suicide education every two years. A clinician must be aware of their state's requirements.

4. Use of Proper Risk Management Techniques

Safety planning is a part of maintaining the standard of care for the patient. Ethical ways to protect patients who are suicidal are found in safety planning with the patient. According to Bernert and Roberts (2012), Safety Planning should:

- Be comprehensive.
- Be tailored to the patient.

- Be concise.
- Be easily accessible.
- Stress agency on the part of the patient.
- Honor the patient's autonomy, respect others, and maintain non-maleficence by protecting the patient from harm.

(Bernert & Roberts, 2012)

CLINICIAN RESPONSE TO MANAGING SUICIDE RISK

Clinicians often have heightened fears regarding malpractice when managing suicide risk. Research by Bernert and Roberts (2012) noted that this results in two possible responses by the clinician. The "Better Safe Than Sorry" approach overestimates risk. When suicide risk is overestimated, the patient's rights can be trampled, and clinical resources may be misused. The "Avoidant and Dismissive" approach underestimates suicide risk, potentially jeopardizing patient safety while increasing the therapist's liability concerns. Current studies continually provide new information for therapists to work with while challenging commonly held misconceptions. For example, a clinician taking the "Better Safe" approach may be surprised to find that evidence provided by Bernet & Roberts indicates hospitalization is not the optimal manner to achieve patient safety. Quantitatively measuring risk has been linked to hindsight bias. Hindsight bias refers to the inclination after an event to overstate the excessively predictable outcome.

MNEMONICS – ARE THEY HELPFUL?

Many clinicians would like a simplified system to assess a client's warning signs. Researchers on identifying warning signs for suicide in children show that a mnemonic can aid counselors' assessment. The SAD PERSONS scale (SPS) (Patterson et al., 1983) and the Adapted SAD PERSONS Scale (A-SPS) (Juhnke, 1996) have been used for many years. However, the American Association of Suicidology in 2006 recommended using a simpler mnemonic in the form of a question: IS PATH WARM? Each letter points the counselor toward a warning sign for suicide. In a 2011 study by Lester and his team, the 10 warning signs in IS PATH WARM for suicide could not differentiate between genuine suicide letters and those written by people pretending to be in a suicidal crisis. Additionally, the criteria could not separate notes written by those who died by suicide from those who made an attempt but lived (Lester et al., 2011). It's essential to consider a Mnemonic may be helpful but may not tell the whole story.

Identifying warning signs in children and adolescents is complicated because the warning signs may be more subtle and challenging to identify. It is easy to think that a child with crying spells is having a difficult time rather than being a warning sign of potential suicide. Another example of adolescent behavior might be isolation when a preadolescent or adolescent begins to resist family activities instead of staying in their room, not coming to family dinners and movies, or avoiding family time altogether. How might the play therapist or school counselor assess the difference between this as a developmental stage of adolescent individuation versus avoidance due to depression as a potential warning sign? We must look at the youth's development stage and consider any pre-existing problems that might impact how the child or adolescent thinks and behaves, like a child with ADHD or depression. Before a diagnosis, play therapists and school counselors must consider many aspects of the youth's life history and medical and developmental stages.

Global Suicide Rates

Although the existing research is mainly concerned with the United States (US), a look at the global statistics reveals suicide to be the number one cause of death among young people worldwide. It is Europe's second most frequent cause in the 10–19 age group (Bilsen, 2018). The rates of deaths from suicides, accidents, and other 'external causes' tend to rise steeply from childhood until adulthood (Dattani et al., 2023).

Suicide estimates are derived from death certificate data, specifically from deaths categorized as "intentional self-harm" according to the International Classification of Diseases (ICD). It's important to note that this category includes individuals who engaged in self-harm but did not intend to die, and they may not meet the legal definition of suicide in certain countries (Dattani et al., 2023). In many countries, deaths resulting from self-harm can be significantly underreported due to various factors such as social stigma, cultural norms, and legal considerations. As a result, these deaths are often misclassified in reported data, categorized as "events of undetermined intent and accidents, homicides, or unknown causes" (Dattani et al., 2023, para. 6). To address this issue, the World Health Organization's Global Health Observatory adjusts a portion of reported deaths with these causes and reclassifies them as suicides based on estimated proportions. This report helps provide a more accurate estimation of the number of people who die from suicide. However, even with this adjustment, suicides may still be underestimated, mainly if mistakenly classified as other types of deaths. Inaccurate data can also lead to rising suicide rates in certain countries if the rates of misclassification decrease. The variation in suicide rates across different countries can be attributed to many factors. These factors include variations in mental health conditions and access to treatment, individual and economic stress levels, limitations on methods of suicide, levels of recognition and awareness regarding suicide, and various other contributing factors (Dattani et al., 2023). For readers interested in suicide prevention globally, the World Health Organization published LIVE LIFE: An Implementation Guide for suicide prevention in Countries (Mental Health and Substance Use, 2021). The World Health Organization (WHO) encourages countries to proactively address suicide prevention by implementing a comprehensive national strategy to prevent suicides. LIVE LIFE is the World Health Organization's approach to initiating suicide prevention efforts, serving as a foundation for countries to develop further and establish a comprehensive national strategy for suicide prevention.

US Suicide Rates and Concerns

In 2021, suicide was among the top 9 leading causes of death for people ages 10–64. Suicide was the second leading cause of death for people ages 10–14 (*Centers for Disease Control and Prevention, National Center for Health Statistics. National Vital Statistics System, Mortality 2018–2021 on CDC WONDER Online Database*, 2023). Most children and adolescents who attempt suicide suffer from significant mental health disorders, most commonly depression.

Suicide attempts in younger children often occur impulsively and are associated with emotions like sadness, confusion, anger, and attention/hyperactivity issues. On the other hand, adolescents are driven to attempt suicide due to stress, self-doubt, pressure to succeed, financial uncertainty, disappointment, or loss. From 2020 to 2021, suicide rates increased for females in age groups 10–14 and 15–24 increased, but not significantly yet for males in age groups 15–24; suicide rates increased substantially in that one year. It is often difficult to track the statistics for very young children, as assessing intentional and accidental is challenging to discern; however, according to the Centers for Disease Control and Prevention National Center for Health Statistics, there were 54 suicides among California children ages 5–14 (Centers for Disease Control and Prevention National Center for Health Statistics, Multiple Causes of Death, 2018–2021, Single Race Request).

According to research, young children who make suicide attempts have a six-fold higher likelihood of attempting suicide again during adolescence than their peers. If children can be treated young, this will prevent child deaths and subsequent suicide attempts during the teenage years; it is crucial to intervene as early as possible to assist at-risk children. These findings highlight the importance of implementing strategies that involve comprehensive mental health and suicide risk screening in primary care settings. Additionally, counseling on safe firearm storage and implementing family-based interventions could reduce suicide risk in this age group. Although further research is necessary, this study serves as an initial step in identifying suicide risk factors in children and determining effective prevention measures to safeguard children's lives.

Among the suicide deaths examined, the most prevalent diagnoses were attention-deficit/hyperactivity disorder (ADHD) or depression. Many of these children showed signs of trauma, including suspected or confirmed cases of abuse, neglect, and domestic violence. Among the children who experienced trauma, almost half had gone through multiple traumatic events (Ruch et al., 2021). Family-related issues, such as divorce, custody disputes, parental substance use, or a family history of suicide or mental health concerns, were present in over a third of the children who died by suicide. School-related problems, including expulsion, changing schools, or suspension, were also reported in nearly one-third of the children who died by suicide (Ruch et al., 2021). Risk factors indicate that someone is at heightened risk for suicide but shows little about immediate suicidality. Depression is linked with suicidal thoughts with additional risk factors, including a family history of suicide attempts, exposure to violence, impulsivity, aggressive behavior, access to firearms, bullying, feelings of hopelessness or helplessness, and acute loss or rejection.

Cultural Research on Deaths by Suicide

Being vigilant as play therapists, school counselors, and clinicians is vital in identifying, assessing, and preventing these tragedies. Research findings contribute additional evidence to support the existence of a substantial racial disparity in childhood suicide rates that varies with age, challenging the previous notion that suicide rates are consistently higher among white individuals compared to black individuals in the United States. Our analyses demonstrated that the suicide rate among children under 13 is approximately twice as high for black children compared to white children, with this pattern observed in both boys and girls (Bridge et al., 2018).

Statistics are invaluable. The statistics focus our attention on existing situations that might otherwise go unnoticed. They cause us to delve deeper, to look beyond the whole and see what's going on with the parts. And they challenge beliefs that can be rooted in bias. It was once commonly held that suicide rates in the US are consistently higher among white individuals than Blacks. Recent age-based research shows a different story. The rate of occurrence within various ethnic groups differs according to age. We now know that the suicide rate among children under 13 is approximately twice as high for Black children compared to White children, with this pattern observed in both boys and girls (Bridge et al., 2018). Specific information related to culture, diversity, equity, and inclusion in child and adolescent suicidality is explored further in Chapter 8.

Pandemic Impact on Suicidality

The incidence of suicide deaths among youth increased before the onset of the COVID-19 pandemic; thus, it's crucial to comprehend how this public health emergency influenced this already escalating crisis. Bridge et al. (2023) scrutinized national suicide data from the Centers for Disease Control and Prevention. Initially, they identified all U.S. youth aged between 5 and 24 years who were registered as having suicide as the cause of death during the first ten months of the pandemic from March 1, 2020, to December 31, 2020. They estimated the overall and monthly suicide deaths by categorizing them by sex, age, race and ethnicity, and method of suicide. Subsequently, they examined the number of young people who died by suicide during the initial ten months of the pandemic and contrasted this with an estimated number of suicide deaths that might have occurred during the same timeframe had the pandemic not taken place (the estimate calculated using data from the preceding five years) (Bridge et al., 2023).

This research demonstrates that the pandemic affected youth suicide rates; however, the impact varied across sex, age, race, and ethnicity. As a result, the authors propose that it could be beneficial to employ widespread suicide prevention measures in places that cater to the youth while also customizing these efforts to tackle the disparities encountered by particular groups. Furthermore, considering the prolonged span of the pandemic and its continuous influence on young people in the United States, it's crucial to observe long-term trends in suicide rates linked to COVID-19 and pinpoint factors contributing to the heightened suicide risk among specific individuals (Bridge et al., 2023).

Since the pandemic, according to a Morbidity and Mortality Weekly Report (MMWR) published by the CDC, there was a 30% rise in suspected suicide attempts through self-poisoning among children aged 10 to 19 years in 2021 when compared to the rates before the COVID-19 pandemic in 2019. The National Poison Data System (NPDS) examined suspected suicide attempts through self-poisoning among individuals aged 10 to 19 (Farah et al., 2023). The substances most commonly involved in these overdoses were acetaminophen, ibuprofen, sertraline, fluoxetine, and diphenhydramine (Farah et al., 2023). Understanding the statistics highlights the importance for parents and caregivers to lock up medications. Many do not consider headache medicine a problem or other drugs; however, prevention is always the best practice.

During the COVID-19 pandemic, anxiety was prevalent in 35.12% of the population, with significant disparities identified through the anxiety measurement scale (Delpino et al., 2022). In 2022, the U.S. Department of Health and Human Services & Centers for Disease Control and Prevention provided new insights into the mental health of U.S. high school students during the COVID-19 pandemic, highlighting the disproportionate strain some students had to endure. The updated data revealed that in 2021(U.S. Department of Health and Human Services & Centers for Disease Control and Prevention, 2022), over a third of high school students admitted to dealing with mental health problems triggered by the COVID-19 pandemic, and almost half reported consistent feelings of sadness or hopelessness throughout the year. This analysis further emphasized the severe challenges faced by adolescents during the pandemic. Over half of the students confessed that they suffered emotional abuse from a parent or another adult in their home, including verbal mistreatment, insults, or derogatory remarks (U.S. Department of Health and Human Services & Centers for Disease Control and Prevention, 2022). Roughly over 10% stated they were subjected to physical violence, such as being hit, beaten, or kicked by an adult in their home. Lesbian, gay, and bisexual adolescents and female teenagers disclosed higher mental health struggles and emotional maltreatment by a parent or caregiver (U.S. Department of Health and Human Services & Centers for Disease Control and Prevention, 2022). They attempted suicides compared to their peers. During the pandemic, more unemployed parents subjected their children to psychological and physical harm than was anticipated. (Lawson et al., 2020).

This research demonstrates that the pandemic affected youth suicide rates; however, the impact varied across sex, age, race, and ethnicity. As a result, the authors propose that it could be beneficial to employ widespread suicide prevention measures, such as training for both parents and experts should emphasize imparting and improving resilience skills like positive cognitive reframing (Lawson et al., 2020) can be integrated into play therapy and school-based play therapy as a buffer against child and adolescent maltreatment in challenging times. Organizations catering to the youth, like youth clubs, afterschool programs, and other group care, customize these efforts to tackle the disparities particular groups encounter is crucial. Furthermore, considering the prolonged span of the pandemic and its continuous influence on young people in the United States, it's critical to observe long-term trends in suicide rates linked to COVID-19 and pinpoint factors contributing to the heightened suicide risk among specific individuals (Lawson et al., 2020).

Statistics Regarding Children and Teens: Death Rates

Donna Ruch, Ph.D., Jeffrey Bridge, Ph.D., Lisa Horowitz, Ph.D., M.P.H., and their colleagues conducted a study analyzing data from 134 children aged 5 to 11 who died by suicide between 2013 and 2017. The average age of the children was 10.6 years, and most were white and male (2016). The researchers examined various factors, such as the technique and place of the self-inflicted death, mental wellness, and drug abuse issues, challenges related to family, academics, and friends, and incidents that took place on the day of the suicide (Ruch et al., 2016). This study builds upon a previous NIMH-funded study from 2016 led by Arielle Sheftall, Ph.D., which found that younger children who died by suicide were more inclined to be male, of Black ethnicity, and pass away at home due to hanging, strangulation, or suffocation, in contrast to older teenagers who died by suicide compared to older adolescents who died by suicide. According to Ruch et al., most child suicide deaths occurred within the family home, precisely over half in the child's bedroom (2021). Hanging was the most common method of suicide among children, but a significant portion of deaths involved using firearms (Ruch et al., 2021). In cases involving firearms, over half of the deaths were related to handguns, and when gun access was known, firearms were not stored safely (Ruch et al., 2021). For example, over half of the guns seen unlocked on nightstands or loaded guns stored in a common living area; in more than half of the cases, a parent was at home when the child died.

Factors Contributing to Suicide

Hinduja and Patchin (2010, 2018) coined Cyberbullicide to describe suicides directly or indirectly influenced by online aggression or cyberbullying. Bullying is any unwanted aggressive behavior(s) by another youth or group of children and adolescents who are not siblings or current dating partners that involves an observed or perceived power imbalance and is repeated multiple times or is highly likely to be repeated (Patchin & Hinduja, 2015).

The continuous cycle of bullying establishes a situation where the victim constantly fears the bully's next move (Patchin & Hinduja, 2015). Bullying may inflict damage or distress on the targeted youth, including physical, psychological, social, or educational harm (Gladden et al., 2014). Many issues contribute to STB in children and adolescents, including social media, sexting, and child pornography and concerns within families. Adolescents aged 12–17 years old are more likely to report suicidal ideation if they experience either school-based bullying or online bullying, but either one alone does not increase suicidal attempts (Hinduja & Patchin, 2018). Although there is an associative relationship between cyberbullying, school-based bullying, and taking one's life, there is no purely causal link. Multiple factors contribute to a death by suicide, including depression, substance use, home stress, and other factors.

Parents and caregivers often need more preparation to manage the challenges children and adolescents are exposed to by the internet of the 21st century. The increased use of social media has provided connections to peers but also increased conflicts with parents. The explosion of access to information and social contact via social media sites Pew Research indicates adolescents' most popular social media in 2022. Among the five leading platforms – YouTube, TikTok, Instagram, Snapchat, and Facebook – about 35% of teenagers report using at least one of these platforms almost incessantly. Users of TikTok and Snapchat are the most active on their respective platforms, with teen YouTube users following closely behind in terms of engagement (Atske, 2022).

Today's youth and families are coping with how to use media safely. Bullying over the past decade has a more public arena to work in. Cyberbullying has become a significant issue for all youth. A UK study 2018 found that youth and young adults under 25 were more than twice as likely to self-harm and enact suicidal behavior.

Interestingly, perpetrators or the bully were also at higher risk for suicidal thoughts and behaviors (John et al., 2018). There are disturbing trends that were identified from a study in 2022 where it was found that nearly half of the adolescents, ages 13–17, have had some form of bullying or online harassment and that it is most often associated with one's appearance (Atske, 2022). Contributing factors for suicidal thinking or behavior were associated with youth sharing sexual content or images of cyberbullying or violence at a 50% higher risk for STB (Sumner et al., 2021). Massing-Schaffer and Nesi (2019) noted in their research that there needs to be a synthesis between traditional suicide research, where the factors that contribute to suicide are examined with contemporary social media research that has focused on computer-mediated communication to gain an understanding of the impact of social media on peer processes. This new model is called An Integrative Model of Cyber Victimization and Adolescent Suicide Risk (Massing-Schaffer & Nesi, 2019). The researchers noted that the biological changes during adolescence increase the youth's need for peer connection. The lack of increased feedback from peers and social rewards can lead to adolescents having a decreased capacity to manage stressors such as cyberbullying and heightened suicide risk (Massing-Schaffer & Nesi, 2019). For many adolescents, the online experience via social media gives them a sense of having an imaginary audience. It can feel "more real" as they monitor how many friends or followers they have (Massing-Schaffer & Nesi, 2019). Having peers online can equate to a feeling of popularity and acceptance. Jobes and Joiner (2019) discussed interrelated factors contributing to a heightened risk of STB in the Theory of Suicide, including perceived burdensomeness, thwarted belonging, and acquired capability for suicide. Acquired capability for suicide is present when there is not only an increased tolerance for pain but a reduction in fear of death. With the adolescent's increased need for social rewards and peer feedback, negative or harmful online experiences can lead to social pain (Massing-Schaffer & Nesi, 2019). When there have been feelings of social rejection, ostracism, or exclusion, the youth faces a negative social appraisal. The negative impact of this negative social appraisal can lead children and adolescents to feel as though they do not belong or are a burden to others, which has been shown to increase the possibility of STB (Jobes & Joiner, 2019). By comparison, online media has some preventive features in which youth can find peer support groups, blogs, and chats to work stressors and improve coping. Play therapists can leverage social media accessibility to guide adolescents to online supportive features. As understanding the elements of social media influence and known risk factors for suicide increases, the play therapist and school counselor can improve assessment, prevention, and interventions. For example, assessing the youth's exposure to online behaviors such as "flaming" or "trolling" is essential. With the former, another term is "roasting'. Roasting involves posting profanity, offensive language and insults online, whereas trolling is a term that involves deliberately and intentionally causing discord online or in person (Zhang et al., 2022). These online behaviors and others can harm a youth's self-esteem and self-worth, possibly increasing thwarted belongingness and STB. As noted previously, cyberbullying and social media affect children and adolescents. Other vital concerns that raise STBs are school bullying, sexting, pornography, youth as pornographers, and gaming addiction.

Sexting is slang for using a cell phone or other electronic device to distribute pictures or videos of sexually explicit images. It also refers to text messages of a sexually charged nature. Sexting builds secrets, shame, and risk for cyberbullying and cyber-harassment, victimization, and youth as pornographers. Pornography depicts erotic behavior intended to cause sexual excitement (Merriam-Webster, n.d.). Child pornography is almost universally prohibited. Child pornography is illegal federally and, in some states, often a part of cyberbullying and victimization, and creates youth as pornographers. These crimes lead to shame and sexual, physical, and emotional abuse, including dating violence and sexual exploitation of children and adolescents; these crimes, especially human trafficking, are defined as

> the recruitment, harboring, transportation, provision, obtaining, patronizing, or soliciting of a person for a commercial sex act, in which the commercial sex act is induced by force, fraud, or coercion, or in which the person induced to perform such an act has not attained 18 years of age (22 U.S.C. § 7102(11)(A).
>
> (*Human Trafficking*, 2023)

Child pornography cuts across all ethnicities, economic statuses, demographics, and genders (Toney-Butler et al., 2023). Federal legislation bans the creation, promotion, transfer, distribution, acquisition, selling, intent to view, and possession of child sexual abuse material (CSAM). Each explicit image or video depicting a child signifies abuse, rape, mistreatment, and exploitation, creating CSAM. Empowering children, their parents, and caregivers to prevent online sexual exploitation is crucial in tracking the exploitation on the CyberTipline®, part of The National Center for Missing and Exploited Children (NCMEC) (*National Center for Missing and Exploited Children*, 2024).

Helping parents with what to do in responding to sexual exploitation is essential to stop human exploitation and prevent suicidal thoughts and behaviors in children and adolescents. Contacting law enforcement so they can assist in tracking down the CSAM can help stop child exploitation (*National Center for Missing and Exploited Children*, 2024).

THEORIES OF SUICIDE: AN EFFORT TO GAIN UNDERSTANDING

Interpersonal Theory of Suicide

In 2012, Van Orden et al. posited the Interpersonal Theory of Suicide in their research on suicide and adolescents. Their study found two key concepts that drive suicidal ideation: thwarted belongingness and perceived burdensomeness. When the basic need for connection is not satisfied, a psychologically painful mental state known as thwarted belongingness results, whereas a mental state known as perceived burdensomeness is characterized by the perception that others would be "better off if I were gone" (Van Orden et al., 2012). The research further indicates that thwarted belongingness and perceived burdensomeness could indicate unmet psychological needs pushing suicidal desires forward. These two constructs have demonstrated "significant predictors of the presence of suicidal ideation one month later" (Van Orden et al., 2012, para. 69).

There is a third contributor to suicidal behavior noted in the Interpersonal Theory of Suicide capability. Suicide capability means that people will not act upon their wish to die unless they have acquired the capacity to do so. This acquired capacity is believed to develop through repeated exposure to distressing or terrifying experiences, leading to habituation. According to this theory, this acquired capacity is crucial for overcoming strong self-preservation instincts (Joiner et al., 2009). Despite being prevalent in suicide research, suicidal capability lacks empirical backing. The ability to commit suicide does not seem to be a prerequisite for engaging in suicidal behaviors, as it does not effectively distinguish between individuals who have attempted suicide and those who haven't, both in the present and future (Huang et al., 2021). To assess the sequence of events in therapeutic interventions for suicidal behavior, a method with clinical significance involves exploring the mechanisms of change. One way to do this is by investigating interventions that address feelings of low belongingness and perceived burdensomeness in therapy to decrease suicidal thoughts. Cognitive Behavioral Play Therapy (CBPT) approaches used such interventions, specifically targeting cognitive distortions like the belief that one's death would be more valuable to family, friends, society, and so on (related to perceived burdensomeness). In a randomized controlled trial, Motto and Bostrom (2001) developed an intervention that effectively reduced suicide deaths. This intervention involved reaching out to high-risk individuals who declined further treatment after being discharged by sending them letters expressing concern and support. The purpose of this non-demanding contact was to provide a sense of connection without requiring ongoing communication with the treatment team. The letters were designed to be uncomplicated and direct and could incorporate symbols or words that held personal significance to the recipient. This research demonstrates the need for integrating expressive play-based interventions to assess feelings of belongingness and burdensomeness, help clients work through these complicated and painful issues, and increase personal safety (Joiner et al., 2009).

Cultural Theory of Suicide

An inductive approach synthesizes a diverse range of research, identifying four key factors that account for 95% of culturally specific risk data: cultural sanctions, idioms of distress, minority stress, and social discord. These four cultural factors are then incorporated into a theoretical framework called the Cultural Model of Suicide developed by Chu et al. (2010). From this framework, three theoretical principles emerge: (1) culture influences the types of stressors that contribute to suicidal tendencies, (2) cultural interpretations associated with stressors and suicide impact the development of suicidal tendencies, tolerance for psychological distress, and subsequent suicidal behaviors, and (3) culture influences how suicidal thoughts, intentions, plans, and attempts are expressed. The Cultural Model of Suicide offers a cohesive and empirically guided approach that can inform culturally sensitive suicide assessment and prevention efforts in both research and clinical practice (Chu et al., 2010).

To better understand the suicide risk among ethnic, gender, and sexual minority youth, the Cultural Theory and Model of Suicide (Chu et al., 2010) has been expanded. This expansion aims to identify cultural factors that are significant or exhibit stronger correlations with suicide risk in youth populations. Extending the Cultural Theory and Model of Suicide to minority youth is supported by research, which validates its applicability. The theoretical principles and four cultural factors of cultural sanctions, idioms of distress, minority stress, and social discord remain relevant in this extension. Specific risk factors associated with youth are identified within these factors, such as academic stress, family rejection, intergenerational conflict, and experiences of peer rejection, victimization, and bullying based on their minority identities. Integrating these crucial cultural factors is essential for developing culturally sensitive suicide prevention strategies and practices that cater to diverse youth populations (Chu et al., 2022). By including ethnic and sexual minorities in our investigations, we aim to advance our understanding from a perspective that considers multiple identities.

MEDIA AND SUICIDE

The two theories of the impact of media coverage reporting on suicidality are the Werther Effect (Phillips, 1974) and the Papageno Effect (Domaradzki, 2021). Werther's theory states that media coverage of suicide increases suicide in others, whereas Papageno's theory states that suicide rates would decrease (Domaradzki, 2021). Through comparison research, suicide rates increase or decrease depending on what suicide details the media reports (Domaradzki, 2021). Consider the Netflix series "13 Reasons Why," where the main character makes 13 audio tapes about her reasons for wanting to die by suicide. The series became controversial due to the contradiction between what the creators intended the show's message to be and the delivery of the message to the viewers; in examining the impact of the "13 Reasons Why" series, researchers found positive and negative effects on adolescents. On the one hand, a positive impact indicated a reduced stigma about suicide, which created a greater likelihood of adolescents discussing mental health concerns and getting help. Unfortunately, results show that there was a significantly higher rate of death by suicide, the number of admissions for suicidal ideation, and the prevalence and severity of suicidal ideation and self-harm behaviors (Guinovart et al., 2023; Cruikshank & Sevigny, 2020). Despite these findings, the research could not establish a causal relationship due to the limitations of the methodology used (Guinovart et al., 2023). It is suggested that the glamorization of suicide has significant adverse effects on viewers who have a mental illness, particularly those who have thought about suicide or used self-harm to cope with trauma, neglect, or even abuse (Da Rosa et al., 2019). In short, people who have attempted suicide, self-harmed, or had suicidal thoughts are more likely to be adversely affected by media (Grant et al., 2020).

In 2009, discussions between mental health researchers and journalism professionals in Canada led to the creation of a policy paper on the impact of suicide reporting on youth. It was noted that there is evidence from many countries examining the same issue that their recommendations and proposed guidelines were synchronous with the policies created in Canada. Many countries adopted some of these recommendations for their media outlets (*Media Guidelines – Canadian Association for Suicide Prevention*, 2023). The Canadian Journalism Forum on Violence and Terror introduced media guidelines called Mindset. The 12 recommendations in the Mindset guidelines state that *media suicide stories should not:* (1) romanticize the act, (2) jump to conclusions about causes because causes are complex, (3) suggest nothing can be done, (4) go into details about the method used, (5) say the person committed suicide, (6) call the suicide successful or attempted suicide unsuccessful, (7) use derogatory terms like "the coward's way out," and *media stories should:* (8) link to broader issues (9) respect the privacy and grief of family or other survivors, (10) include reference to their suffering, (11) tell others considering suicide that they should get help, and (12) use plain words – say "the person died by suicide, killed herself, or took his own life" (Stack, 2020). Most findings on the relationship between suicide stories and suicide rates do not support a suggestion or imitation effect, so urging the mass media to follow some media guidelines to make stories safer may not always be relevant in such cases. As a result, work on the media and suicide generally needs to be mindful of this inconvenient truth (Stack, 2020). The limited evidence indicates that media guidelines frequently do not function as predicted (Stack, 2020). It has been suggested that by providing sources for help when reporting on suicide and suicide attempts, there will be less contagion and imitation; however, once the amount of suicide coverage was controlled and managed, there weren't any significant rates of suicide. In addition, the rate of suicide increases when there are more details about suicide.

Call to Action – Zero Suicide

Changing how diverse communities come together to move forward to change the way society treats suicide for all ages is the ultimate call to action. Zero Suicide aims to apply a life-saving perspective in preventing suicide (*Zero Suicide*, 2022). It serves as a model for implementing a comprehensive commitment to providing safer care for individuals at risk of suicide throughout an entire system or organization. Zero Suicide recognizes that individuals grappling with suicidal thoughts and urges often slip through the cracks within a fragmented and distracted healthcare system. A significant percentage (over a third) of individuals who have attempted suicide have had contact with healthcare settings (such as primary care, emergency departments, specialty care, etc.) in the week leading up to their attempt (*Zero Suicide*, 2022).

Moreover, 95% had a healthcare visit within the year before their attempt (Ahmedani et al., 2015). While these figures may differ based on race and ethnicity, it is evident that missed opportunities to identify and provide care for individuals at risk of suicide. By adopting a system-wide approach, Zero Suicide seeks to enhance outcomes and address existing gaps. In healthcare systems regarding physical and mental well-being, Zero Suicide signifies a dedication to patient safety and establishing a supportive culture for care providers.

A significant advancement in this initiative was the development of a comprehensive online resource called the Zero Suicide ToolkitSM, which offers valuable guidance, resources, and multimedia materials to clarify further and define the model (*Zero Suicide*, 2022).

Incorporating a "zero-based" mindset involves regularly and consistently integrating evidence-based practices that prioritize patient safety and provide hope and support for individuals vulnerable to suicide. The Zero Suicide (2022) approach rejects the prevailing belief within the healthcare industry that little progress is made in addressing the outcomes for those at risk of suicide. Instead, it represents an inspiring yet achievable method for identifying and providing care to individuals in danger of suicide. Directly inquiring about suicide and responding appropriately should be as commonplace as measuring blood pressure, height, and weight during every healthcare visit. However, the normalization of this practice has largely been met with resistance thus far.

Organizations that Embrace the Zero Suicide (2022) Framework

- Integrate a comprehensive set of evidence-based elements to reduce suicide effectively.
- Gather data to assess the outcomes of these interventions and adherence to using them.
- Engage in ongoing efforts to enhance the quality of care by educating staff and addressing any areas of weakness in performance.
- Establish a culture where suicide prevention and care practices are seen as the norm for staff, individuals at risk, and their families, representing the expected standard of care.

(Zero Suicide, 2022)

The principles underlying Zero Suicide (2022) are as follows:

Core Values: Zero Suicide (2022) is rooted in the belief and dedication that suicide can be eradicated among the population under care. Suicide eradication is achieved by improving service access, enhancing service quality, and consistently implementing continuous quality improvement practices.

Systems Management: Zero Suicide (2022) takes a systematic approach across various care systems. It aims to foster a culture where suicide is no longer deemed acceptable. A systemic process involves setting ambitious yet attainable goals to eliminate suicide attempts and deaths. Service delivery and support are organized in alignment with this objective.

Evidence-Based Clinical Care Practices: Zero Suicide (2022) advocates are adopting clinical care practices substantiated by research to reduce suicide deaths and behaviors in youth and adults. These practices are implemented throughout the entire care system, emphasizing the importance of constructive interactions between patients and staff.

Impacts of Suicide on Parents and Caregivers

In a recent review of the currently available research about the effect of suicide crisis on parents and caregivers, Weissinger et al. (2023) found this to be a woefully under-researched topic and deserves far greater attention to support the whole family system. Whether there has been a suicide attempt or a suicide loss, the parents/caregivers are challenged on many different levels to manage the crisis. Five themes have been identified by Weissinger et al. (2023) as being present for parents/caregivers during suicide crises.

1) Trauma of the experience, especially feelings of failure.
2) Living in fear.
3) Alone and seeking connection.
4) Lasting impact.
5) A new normal, turning the pain into purpose.

Part of the traumatic impact is that self-esteem is damaged. Treatment recommendations suggest a need to support the parent as a person and as a caregiver. In addition, when a child or adolescent dies by suicide, it impacts the entire family system. Across cultures and systems, parents of adolescents with suicide risk may work to protect and get them to help, but they also experience significant distress and burden. Parents in this study reported feeling torn by responsibilities and cut off from those around them (Weissinger et al., 2023). In other research, participants described feelings of shame, guilt, and self-blame concerning their loved one's suicide; they felt awkward talking about the suicide; they found social interactions to be painful and difficult; this led to social withdrawal and self-isolation; participants also expressed hurt and anger at the way family and friends seemed embarrassed talking about the suicide and made comments that were perceived as being insensitive. Some survivors spoke of having arguments with family and friends, which led to ongoing estrangement (Ross et al., 2019). Survivors of suicide loss said of their feelings of rejection, loneliness, and isolation due to this loss of contact and social support from family and friends (Ross et al., 2019). Self-compassion has been identified by Zhang et al. (2023) as the foundation for individual and family processes that support bereavement adjustment. They propose that three aspects of self-compassion – mindfulness (as opposed to over-identification), self-kindness (as opposed to self-judgment), and common humanity (as opposed to isolation) – can facilitate loss-oriented coping, restoration-oriented coping, and the oscillation process between the two (Zhang et al., 2023).

Bereavement for suicide loss is complicated due to stigma, shame, and rejection. Ross et al. (2019) found a heightened risk for parents/caregivers and other familial survivors to develop depression, anxiety, or some other mental health disorder, as well as being at risk for suicide attempts and dying by suicide. Cerel et al. (2018) found that 135 people are directly affected by suicide death. The World Health Organization (2021) estimates that 703,000 people annually die by suicide, which means an estimated 94.9 million people were affected.

Common grief reactions of sadness, anxiety, depression, anger, and loneliness are compounded by the additional feelings of stigma, shame, responsibility, and rejection (Ross, 2019). Understanding what suicide loss survivors need is vital. Researchers recommend a bottom-up approach, which means designing services informed by the bereaves experiences instead of the top-up method where a mental health counselor's ideas and beliefs drive the treatment. The client's loss narrative is the starting place for designing services. Key areas to be aware of when working with bereaved by suicide is to have practical and proactive support in the early stages. Parents/caregivers are often in a state of confusion or numbness, so flexibility to allow survivors ample time to feel ready for support and flexibility in the approach to supporting the bereaved is needed (Ross, 2019). In the early stages of recovery, they must be guided through the services and systems such as funeral arrangements, insurance, legal, and financial issues.

Vatne et al. (2023) found that the first professional to encounter the family after a suicide loss can significantly influence what can alleviate the family's suffering and promote long-term health and well-being. The research also noted that the initial care with the family should include confirmation of the suffering, creating an encounter through dialogue, and providing consolation and reconciliation. Witnessing the grief of the bereaved led to mental health professionals having a strong sense of responsibility toward bringing healing and resolution to the suffering (Vatne et al., 2023).

CONCLUSION

Suicide is a worldwide phenomenon that impacts millions of people annually. Youth of all ages can have STB. Mental health professionals, educators, families, and communities must come together in a voice of compassion to understand the complexities of the scope of suicide and suicide prevention. Law and ethics are critical components of clinical work in suicide, including many ethical challenges and clinical decision-making. History has shown us the path taken toward decriminalizing suicide to develop a deeper understanding of suicide as emotional pain. Appropriate services and interventions for those with STB and families that have experienced loss by suicide can be appropriately applied. This chapter reviewed factors impacting suicide, including the pandemic, social media, cyberbullying, bullying, and sexual exploitation through the cyber victimization of minors. Understanding global, local, and cultural research statistics assists clinicians in this issue's scope. The COVID-19 pandemic and its impact on suicidality for youth is vital to assist in prevention efforts. Knowing the theories of suicidality facilitates clinician's case conceptualizations for optimal outcomes. The media's role in reporting suicide illustrates mixed results. Many complicating factors impact how the details and messages of suicide are received and by whom. Those with a prior mental health issue or previous suicide attempts are more vulnerable than those without. The overarching goal of Zero Suicide may seem impossible; however, it remains that effort by the world community is to reach this goal.

REFERENCES

Actions-S.4448-117th Congress (2021–2022): Suicide Prevention Act. (2022, June 22). www.congress.gov/bill/117th-congress/senate-bill/4448/actions

Administration (SAMHSA). Substance Abuse and Mental Health Services. (2022). U.S. transition to 988 suicide & crisis lifeline begins Saturday. *HHS.gov*

Ahmedani, B. K., Stewart, C. P., Simon, G. E., Lynch, F. L., Lu, C. Y., Waitzfelder, B. E., Solberg, L. I., Owen-Smith, A., Beck, A., Copeland, L. A., Hunkeler, E. M., Rossom, R. C., & Williams, L. K. (2015). Racial/ethnic differences in health care visits made before suicide attempt across the United States. *Medical Care, 53*(5), 430–435. https://doi.org/10.1097/mlr.0000000000000335

Andrews, J. R. (2020). Ethically uncharted territory: Providing psychological services to parents in pediatric settings. *Ethics & Behavior, 31*(2), 77–90. https://doi.org/10.1080/10508422.2020.1772063

Atske, S. (2022, December 15). Teens, social media and technology 2022 | Pew Research Center. *Pew Research Center: Internet, Science & Tech.* www.pewresearch.org/internet/2022/08/10/teens-social-media-and-technology

Attorney Articles | Working with Suicidal Clients. (n.d.). www.camft.org/Resources/Legal-Articles/Chronological-Article-List/working-wit h-suicidal-clients

Behere, P. B., Rao, T. S., & Mulmule, A. N. (2015). Decriminalization of attempted suicide law: Journey of fifteen decades. *Indian Journal of Psychiatry, 57*(2), 122. https://doi.org/10.4103/0019-5545.158131

Bernert, R. A., & Roberts, L. W. (2012). Ethics commentary: Suicide risk: Ethical considerations in the assessment and management of suicide risk. *Focus, 10*(4), 467–472. https://doi.org/10.1176/appi.focus.10.4.467

Bilsen, J. (2018). Suicide and youth: Risk factors. *Frontiers in Psychiatry, 9.* https://doi.org/10.3389/fpsyt.2018.00540

Bridge, J. A., Horowitz, L. M., Fontanella, C. A., Sheftall, A. H., Greenhouse, J. B., Kelleher, K. J., & Campo, J. V. (2018). Age-related racial disparity in suicide rates among US youths from 2001 through 2015. *JAMA Pediatrics, 172*(7), 697. https://doi.org/10.1001/jamapediatrics.2018.0399

Bridge, J. A., Ruch, D. A., Sheftall, A. H., Hahm, H. C., O'Keefe, V. M., Fontanella, C. A., Brock, G., Campo, J. V., & Horowitz, L. M. (2023). Youth suicide during the first year of the COVID-19 pandemic. *Pediatrics, 151*(3). https://doi.org/10.1542/peds.2022-058375

Centers for Disease Control and Prevention, National Center for Health Statistics. National Vital Statistics System, Mortality 2018–2021 on CDC WONDER Online Database. (2023). CDC WONDER Online Database. Retrieved May 13, 2023, from http://wonder.cdc.gov/mcd-icd10-expanded.html

Cerel, J., Brown, M., Maple, M., Singleton, M., Van De Venne, J., Moore, M., & Flaherty, C. (2018). How many people are exposed to suicide? Not six. *Suicide and Life Threatening Behavior, 49*(2), 529–534. https://doi.org/10.1111/sltb.12450

Chu, J., Goldblum, P., Floyd, R., & Bongar, B. (2010). The cultural theory and model of suicide. *Applied and Preventive Psychology, 14*(1–4), 25–40. https://doi.org/10.1016/j.appsy.2011.11.001

Chu, J., O'Neill, S. L., Ng, J., & Khoury, O. (2022). *The cultural theory and model of suicide for youth* (eBooks, pp. 99–106). Springer. https://doi.org/10.1007/978-3-031-06127-1_11

Cruikshank, E., & Sevigny, P. R. (2020). Reasons why not: A critical review of the television series 13 reasons why. *Canadian Journal of Counselling and Psychotherapy, 54*(4), 803–818. https://doi.org/10.47634/cjcp.v54i4.69046

Da Rosa, G. M., Andrades, G. S., Caye, A., Hidalgo, M. P. L., De Oliveira, M. A. B., & Pilz, L. K. (2019). Thirteen reasons why: The impact of suicide portrayal on adolescents' mental health. *Journal of Psychiatric Research, 108*, 2–6. https://doi.org/10.1016/j.jpsychires.2018.10.018

Dattani, S., Rodés-Guirao, L., Ritchie, H., Roser, M., & Ospina, E. (2023, April 2). Suicides. *Our World in Data.* Retrieved May 21, 2023, from https://ourworldindata.org/suicide

Delpino, F. M., Da Silva, C. N., Jerônimo, J. S., Mulling, E. S., Da Cunha, L., Weymar, M. K., Alt, R., Caputo, E. L., & Feter, N. (2022). Prevalence of anxiety during the COVID-19 pandemic: A systematic review and meta-analysis of over 2 million people. *Journal of Affective Disorders, 318*, 272–282. https://doi.org/10.1016/j.jad.2022.09.00

Domaradzki, J. (2021). The Werther effect, the Papageno effect or no effect? A literature review. *International Journal of Environmental Research and Public Health, 18*(5), 2396. https://doi.org/10.3390/ijerph18052396

Farah, R., Rege, S. V., Cole, R. J., & Holstege, C. P. (2023). Suspected suicide attempts by self-poisoning among persons aged 10–19 years during the COVID-19 pandemic – United States, 2020–2022. *Morbidity and Mortality Weekly Report, 72*(16), 426–430. https://doi.org/10.15585/mmwr.mm7216a3

Gardner, C. (2020). S 2661–116th congress (2019–2020): National Suicide Hotline Designation Act of 2020. *www.congress.gov.* Retrieved June 17, 2023, from www.congress.gov/bill/116th-congress/senate-bill/2661/text

Gladden, R. M., Vivolo-Kantor, A. M., Hamburger, M. E., & Lumpkin, C. D. (2014). Bullying surveillance among youth: Uniform definitions for public health and recommended data elements, version 1.0. *National Center for Injury Prevention and Control, Centers for Disease Control and Prevention, and U.S. Department of Education.* Retrieved September 9, 2023, from http://www.cdc.gov/violenceprevention/pdf/bullying-definitions-final-a.pdf

Grant, M., El-Agha, H., Ho, T., & Johnson, S. D. (2020). Commentary: Thirteen reasons why: The impact of suicide portrayal on adolescents' mental health. *Journal of Mental Health and Clinical Psychology, 4*(2), 45–48. https://doi.org/10.29245/2578-2959/2020/2.1193

Guinovart, M., Cobo, J., González-Rodríguez, A., Parra-Uribe, I., & Palao, D. (2023). Towards the influence of media on suicidality: A systematic review of Netflix's 'thirteen reasons why.'

International Journal of Environmental Research and Public Health, 20(7), 5270. https://doi.org/10.3390/ijerph20075270

Hinduja, S., & Patchin, J. W. (2010). Bullying, cyberbullying, and suicide. *Archives of Suicide Research, 14*(3), 206–221. https://doi.org/10.1080/13811118.2010.494133

Hinduja, S., & Patchin, J. W. (2018). Connecting adolescent suicide to the severity of bullying and cyberbullying. *Journal of School Violence, 18*(3), 333–346. https://doi.org/10.1080/15388220.2018.1492417

Huang, X., Funsch, K. M., Park, E., Conway, P., Franklin, J. C., & Ribeiro, J. D. (2021). Longitudinal studies support the safety and ethics of virtual reality suicide as a research method. *Scientific Reports, 11*(1). https://doi.org/10.1038/s41598-021-89152-0

Human trafficking. (2023, May 13). United States Department of Justice. www.justice.gov/humantrafficking#:~:text=%C2%A7%207102(11)

Jobes, D. A., & Joiner, T. E. (2019). Reflections on suicidal ideation. *Crisis-the Journal of Crisis Intervention and Suicide Prevention, 40*(4), 227–230. https://doi.org/10.1027/0227-5910/a000615

Jobes, D. A., Rudd, M. D., Overholser, J. C., & Joiner, T. E. (2008). Ethical and competent care of suicidal patients: Contemporary challenges, new developments, and considerations for clinical practice. *Professional Psychology: Research and Practice, 39*(4), 405–413. https://doi.org/10.1037/a0012896

John, A., Glendenning, A. C., Marchant, A., Montgomery, P., Stewart, A., Wood, S., Lloyd, K. E., & Hawton, K. (2018). Self-harm, suicidal behaviours, and cyberbullying in children and young people: Systematic review. *Journal of Medical Internet Research, 20*(4), e129. https://doi.org/10.2196/jmir.9044

Joiner, T. E., Van Orden, K. A., Witte, T. K., Selby, E. A., Ribeiro, J. D., Lewis, R., & Rudd, M. D. (2009). Main predictions of the interpersonal–psychological theory of suicidal behavior: Empirical tests in two samples of young adults. *Journal of Abnormal Psychology, 118*(3), 634–646. https://doi.org/10.1037/a0016500

Juhnke, G. A. (1996). The adapted SAD PERSONS: A suicide assessment scale designed for use with children. *Elementary School Guidance and Counseling, 30*(4). https://eric.ed.gov/?id=EJ531992

Justia law. (n.d.). https://law.justia.com/

Kalb, R., Feinstein, A., Rohrig, A., Sankary, L. R., & Willis, A. (2019). Depression and suicidality in multiple sclerosis: Red flags, management strategies, and ethical considerations. *Current Neurology and Neuroscience Reports, 19*(10). https://doi.org/10.1007/s11910-019-0992-1

Lambert, K. N. (2017). Risk management considerations when treating suicidal patients. *Psychiatric News, 52*(1), 1. https://doi.org/10.1176/appi.pn.2017.1a21

Lawson, M., Piel, M. H., & Simon, M. (2020). Child maltreatment during the COVID-19 pandemic: Consequences of parental job loss on psychological and physical abuse towards children. *Child Abuse & Neglect, 110*, 104709. https://doi.org/10.1016/j.chiabu.2020.104709

Lester, D., McSwain, S., & Gunn, J. (2011). A test of the validity of the *is path warm* warning signs for suicide. *Psychological Reports, 108*(2), 402–404. https://doi.org/10.2466/09.12.13.pr0.108.2.402-404

Lewis, S. (2016). *Legal and ethical issues for mental health clinicians: Best practices for avoiding litigation, complaints, and malpractice.* Pesi Publishing & Media.

Litman, R. E. (1966–1967). Medical-legal aspects of suicide. *Washburn Law Journal: Medical-Legal Aspects of Suicide, 6*, 395. https://heinonline.org/HOL/LandingPage?handle=hein.journals/wasbur6&div=41&id=& page=

Massing-Schaffer, M., & Nesi, J. (2019). Cybervictimization and suicide risk in adolescence: An integrative model of social media and suicide theories. *Adolescent Research Review, 5*(1), 49–65. https://doi.org/10.1007/s40894-019-00116-y

Media Guidelines – Canadian Association For Suicide Prevention. (2023, April 5). Canadian Association for Suicide Prevention. https://suicideprevention.ca/media/media-guidelines/

Merriam-Webster. (n.d.). Pornography. In *Merriam-Webster.com dictionary*. Retrieved September 9, 2023, from www.merriam-webster.com/dictionary/pornography

Mishara, B. L., & Weisstub, D. N. (2016). The legal status of suicide: A global review. *International Journal of Law and Psychiatry, 44*, 54–74. https://doi.org/10.1016/j.ijlp.2015.08.032

Motto, J. A., & Bostrom, A. (2001). A randomized controlled trial of postcrisis suicide prevention. *Psychiatric Services, 52*(6), 828–833. https://doi.org/10.1176/appi.ps.52.6.828

National Center for Missing and Exploited Children (By Office of Juvenile Justice and Delinquency Prevention & Office of Justice Programs, U.S. Department of Justice). (2024). Our 2022 impact. Retrieved March 29, 2024, from https://www.missingkids.org/ourwork/impact

Pal, S., & Ramanathan, S. (2023). Ethical consideration in dealing with suicide in different populations. *Focus, 21*(2), 173–177. https://doi.org/10.1176/appi.focus.20220082

Patchin, J. W., & Hinduja, S. (2015). Measuring cyberbullying: Implications for research. *Aggression and Violent Behavior, 23*, 69–74. https://doi.org/10.1016/j.avb.2015.05.013

Patterson, W. P., Dohn, H. H., Bird, J., & Patterson, G. (1983). Evaluation of suicidal patients: The SAD PERSONS scale. *Psychosomatics, 24*(4), 343–349. https://doi.org/10.1016/s0033-3182(83)73213-5

Paul, M. (2004). Decision-making about children's mental health care: Ethical challenges. *Advances in Psychiatric Treatment, 10*(4), 301–311. https://doi.org/10.1192/apt.10.4.301

Phillips, D. P. (1974). The influence of suggestion on suicide: Substantive and theoretical implications of the Werther effect. *American Sociological. Review, 39*, 340–354. doi: 10.2307/2094294

Retterstol, N. (1998). *Suicide in a cultural history perspective, part 1 Western culture; Attitudes to suicide up to the 19th century*. University of Oslo, the Suicide Research and Prevention Unit. Retrieved August 14, 2023, from www.med.uio.no/klinmed/english/research/centres/nssf/articles/culture/Retterstol1.pdf

Ross, V., Kõlves, K., & De Leo, D. (2019). Exploring the support needs of people bereaved by suicide: A qualitative study. *Omega – Journal of Death and Dying, 82*(4), 632–645. https://doi.org/10.1177/0030222819825775

Ruch, D., Heck, K. M., Sheftall, A. H., Fontanella, C. A., Stevens, J., Zhu, M., Horowitz, L. M., Campo, J. V., & Bridge, J. A. (2021). Characteristics and precipitating circumstances of suicide among children aged 5 to 11 years in the United States, 2013–2017. *JAMA Network Open, 4*(7), e2115683. https://doi.org/10.1001/jamanetworkopen.2021.15683

Saigle, V., & Racine, E. (2018). Ethical challenges faced by healthcare professionals who care for suicidal patients: A scoping review. *Monash Bioethics Review, 35*(1–4), 50–79. https://doi.org/10.1007/s40592-018-0076-z

Sheftall, A. H., Asti, L., Horowitz, L. M., Felts, A., Fontanella, C. A., Campo, J. V., & Bridge, J. A. (2016a). Suicide in Elementary School-Aged Children and Early Adolescents. Pediatrics, 138(4). https://doi.org/10.1542/peds.2016-0436

Spaulding, J. A., Simpson, G., & Durkheim, E. (1997). *Suicide*. Free Press.

Stack, S. (2020). Media guidelines and suicide: A critical review. *Social Science & Medicine, 262*, 112690. https://doi.org/10.1016/j.socscimed.2019.112690

Stefan, S. (2016). *Rational suicide, irrational laws: Examining current approaches to suicide in policy and law.* Oxford University Press.

Sumner, S. A., Ferguson, B., Bason, B., Dink, J., Yard, E. E., Hertz, M., Hilkert, B., Holland, K. M., Mercado-Crespo, M. C., Tang, S., & Jones, C. M. (2021). Association of online risk factors with subsequent youth suicide-related behaviors in the US. *JAMA Network Open, 4*(9), e2125860. https://doi.org/10.1001/jamanetworkopen.2021.25860

Toney-Butler, T. J., Ladd, M., & Mittel, O. (2023, June 11). *Human trafficking*. StatPearls Publishing. www.ncbi.nlm.nih.gov/books/NBK430910/

U.S. Department of Health and Human Services & Centers for Disease Control and Prevention. (2022). Adolescent behaviors and experiences survey – United States, January–June 2021. *Morbidity and Mortality Weekly Report, 71*(3), 1–40. www.cdc.gov/mmwr/volumes/71/su/pdfs/su7103a1-a5-H.pdf

Van Orden, K. A., Cukrowicz, K. C., Witte, T. K., & Joiner, T. E. (2012). Thwarted belongingness and perceived burdensomeness: Construct validity and psychometric properties of the Interpersonal Needs Questionnaire. *Psychological Assessment, 24*(1), 197–215. https://doi.org/10.1037/a0025358

Vatne, M., Nåden, D., & Lohne, V. (2023). Caring for family members following suicide: Professionals' experiences of responsibility. *Nursing Ethics, 30*(3), 394–407. https://doi.org/10.1177/09697330221136631

Weaver, J. B., & Wright, D. W. (2008). *Histories of suicide: International perspectives on self-destruction in the modern world.* http://ci.nii.ac.jp/ncid/BA88985217

Weissinger, G., Evans, L., Van Fossen, C., Winston-Lindeboom, P., Ruan-Iu, L., & Rivers, A. S. (2023). Parent experiences during and after adolescent suicide crisis: A qualitative study. *International Journal of Mental Health Nursing.* https://doi.org/10.1111/inm.13137

World Health Organization (WHO). (2021). *Suicide.* www.who.int/news-room/fact-sheets/detail/suicide

Zero suicide (By Education Development Center). (2022). *Zerosuicide.edc.org.* Retrieved August 13, 2023, from https://zerosuicide.edc.org/

Zhang, N., Sandler, I., Thieleman, K., Wolchik, S., & O'Hara, K. (2023). Self-compassion for caregivers of children in parentally bereaved families: A theoretical model and intervention example. *Clinical Child and Family Psychology Review.* https://doi.org/10.1007/s10567-023-00431-w

Zhang, W., Huang, S., Lam, L., Evans, R., & Zhu, C. (2022). Cyberbullying definitions and measurements in children and adolescents: Summarizing 20 years of global efforts. *Frontiers in Public Health, 10.* https://doi.org/10.3389/fpubh.2022.1000504

CHAPTER 3

INTEGRATING PSYCHIATRY INTO TREATMENT OF SUICIDAL YOUTH
Information for Clinicians

Daniel Jon Kostalnick

INTRODUCTION

Psychiatrists are medical doctors (M.D. or D.O.) who have completed medical school, internship, and residency – and, in some cases, have further fellowship training. They are uniquely qualified to diagnose, treat, monitor, prevent, and manage the clinical manifestations of psychiatric mental health disorders and promote mental health wellness and well-being (Liu, 2023). They can utilize the full spectrum of interventions, including psychotherapy and medical interventions, i.e., medications. Psychiatric physicians may focus on the medical part of the treatment plan and refer the patient for the psychotherapy part to colleagues such as psychologists, marriage and family play therapists, social workers, licensed professional counselors, school-based counselors, and play therapists.

Referral to Psychiatry

Clinicians may consider referring to a psychiatrist for further evaluation when the diagnosis is unclear or when a clinician becomes uncomfortable with the patient's symptom severity or complexity increases during treatment, for example, if a patient begins to exhibit signs or symptoms of mania, hypomania, psychosis (delusions or hallucinations), conduct, eating disorders, acute anxiety, and substance use (intoxication or withdrawal) (Shaffer & Pfeffer, 2001). A psychiatric evaluation may be necessary when there is functional impairment (school attendance, psychosocial decline) (Shaffer & Pfeffer, 2001) and unexpected changes, such as suicidal or homicidal thoughts. The patient and parents/guardians must understand that any referral to a psychiatrist is for assessment only and does not necessarily place the client on the road to medications. Once the clinicians, patient, and parents or guardians agree on this course, play therapists must offer the name and contact information of three psychiatrists they determine suitable for treatment services. It is the parents' and caregivers' choice to choose the psychiatrist that meets their child's or adolescent's needs, and a professional relationship of trust between doctor and patient is essential. That said, insurance often decides where a client receives treatment. Billing protocols vary between psychiatric services, with some accepting insurance while others bill the client directly, and insurance plans may also limit the client's options.

DOI: 10.4324/9781003358565-4

WORKING WITH PSYCHIATRISTS

A psychiatric clinical interview begins with an initial consultation, which usually takes 45 to 60 minutes. The pediatric client and their parents or caregivers provide history and essential information to the psychiatrist. The psychiatrist will conduct a mental status examination. The data collected is collated into collections of symptom clusters and evaluated for diagnosis. A proposed treatment plan may include laboratory evaluation and referral to other medical specialists. Psychotherapy and medications may be discussed at that time as well. In particular, appropriate laboratory tests are reviewed and completed to rule out any medical disorders contributing to or causing symptoms' psychiatric presentation. Medical examples can include issues with major organ systems, infections, epilepsy, brain tumors, or electrolyte disturbances.

Risk Factors for Suicidal Youth

Assessing risk factors, protective factors, and warning signs in children and youth is crucial. According to Carballo et al., children, adolescents, and young adults (10–24 years old) are subject to three main areas that can increase risk: Psychological factors (depression, anxiety, previous suicide attempts, drug and alcohol use, and other comorbid psychiatric disorders), stressful life events (family problems and peer conflicts), and personality traits (such as neuroticism and impulsivity) (Carballo et al., 2019). Of significant concern are suicidal ideation and suicide attempts (Shain, 2016). Risk factors increasing the likelihood of these conditions include (Rudd et al., 2006):

- mental conditions such as disorders of mood (depression, mania), thought (psychosis), and substance use (both intoxication and withdrawal)
- prior suicide attempt
- family history of death by suicide
- sexual orientation, transgender/gender, non-conforming identity
- history of physical or sexual abuse

Assessing for Medication

Psychiatrists select medication based on several factors driven by establishing a diagnosis and considering other medical complications and the potential for side effects and interactions with other medicines the patient may be taking (Bonin & Moreland, 2023). Personal history with a medication the patient may have taken or if a family member has benefitted from (or had a poor reaction to) medication for the diagnosis is an important consideration when choosing medications for a pediatric client. Many medication "groups" are organized by what the medication does and the conditions or diagnosis for which the medication is used. There are many factors in the choice of medication, and establishing a solid professional relationship with a physician who is a psychiatrist with training in neuropsychopharmacology is essential to foster the potential for positive treatment outcomes. Pharmaceutical options for the psychiatrist include:

- antianxiety medications (major tranquilizers, minor tranquilizers/benzodiazepines)
- antidepressant medications (i.e., selective serotonin reuptake inhibitors (SSRI), sero-tonin-norepinephrine reuptake inhibitors, tricyclic and tetracyclic antidepressants)
- mood stabilizing medications (anti-epileptic medications, neuroleptic medications)
- antipsychotic medications (also known as neuroleptic medications (both "typical" and "atypical")
- medications used to treat substance use disorders
- medications used to treat insomnia
- medications used to treat disorders of attention, focus, and concentration
- medications used to treat dementia

The choice of medication used to treat suicidal thoughts and behaviors (STB) depends mainly on the primary diagnosis – which is, in part, why a full assessment and consideration of the entire symptom cluster and diagnosis is essential for effective treatment. Effective treatment begins with an accurate diagnosis. Psychiatrists formulated and used the Diagnostic Statistics Manual TR, which was revised and updated regularly by large committees formed by universities and research centers (American Psychiatric Association, 2022). The DSM-5-TR provides a "common language" for evaluating symptoms that, when clustered together, allow for diagnostic conclusions (American Psychiatric Association, 2022).

SYMPTOM ASSESSMENT

It is interesting to note the important things to communicate to the psychiatrist when making a referral that will assist in the diagnostic process. Primary attention is given to signs (things the clinician observes) and symptoms (issues that the patient reports to the clinician) (Wintersteen et al., 2007). These can include the following and should note, as precisely as possible, the onset, duration, and intensity of the symptoms:

- mood changes
- anxiety
- sleep disturbance
- appetite
- interest
- enjoyment
- motivation
- energy
- irritability
- anger
- impulsivity
- attention and concentration
- agitation
- psychosis

- sexual function changes
- suicidal thoughts
- self-harm

While every aspect holds significance within the context of therapy, specific details may carry more weight in a diagnostic psychiatric evaluation. For instance, if an individual experiences nightmares, it is relevant for the review. However, the specific content of the nightmare itself may or may not be as crucial for diagnostic purposes, though it remains essential for play therapists involved in the patient's care.

Understanding Roles

Commonly, there are questions about what play therapists may want to discuss with the parents or pediatric patient regarding medications and their side effects and how to manage these in the therapy. The topic of medication can be very confusing to the pediatric patient and can innocently and unintentionally blur the roles of the clinician and psychiatrist. It is essential that, in the context of mental health treatment, the pediatric patient and their families clearly understand the positions of the members of the comprehensive treatment team.

Research shows in a meta-analysis researching random controlled studies by Lim et al. that positive case management is associated with fewer psychiatric symptoms and a positive quality of life in clients with severe mental illness (2022). Generally, when a patient brings up an issue related to medication, the best response is to assist the patient in communicating the issue to the psychiatrist, who may work with the patient to that end. Similarly, when a patient brings up a topic relevant to the therapy (given that the psychiatrist is not engaging in psychotherapy with the patient), the psychiatrist defers to the treating therapist and helps guide the patient to the therapist on the presenting issue or topic. With that understanding, the parents and pediatric patients identify whom best to talk to about their medication. There are times when a clinician may inadvertently share an anecdotal experience with their client (who is also the psychiatrist's patient) concerning a medication taken for "the same (or similar)" diagnosis, symptom, or concern. Such sharing is discouraged for several reasons, including the possibility of disclosing identifiable information about another client, but primarily because it may have the power to undermine medical treatment. It is best to bring anecdotal information to the psychiatrist rather than the patient. While it may be tempting to ask about medication out of genuine concern and care for the patient, such discussions are best conducted solely between the client and the psychiatrist.

Case Consultation

Conferring with the psychiatrist is essential when working with youth and families. Given that both clinician and psychiatrist may bill the patient for their time in conference with one another, it is beneficial to have a specific question or agenda for the meeting. If the psychiatrist is not the therapist's supervising clinician, it is crucial to share perspectives on a particular case that may be impacting the role of the professional counterpart. For example, a client may tell the clinician that they are not taking medication or are missing doses of the medication along with a reason (i.e., appetite, weight, and body changes) they may be reluctant to share with the psychiatrist. The therapist must help the client overcome this reluctance so that the psychiatrist can have the necessary information. Unhindered sharing of information enables comprehensive support to the client.

Case Example

The single mother of two children was referred to psychiatry by the family's pediatrician. The mother stated that she found her daughter, Sally, age 10, curled up in the bedroom closet, too fearful to come out. She was having anger outbursts, raging, and yelling over "nothing." The mother reported that her daughter had a history of sexual molestation by a babysitter at age 4. The case was reported to Child Protective Services but never prosecuted. The child was seen by a Registered Play Therapist™ for multiple sessions at ages 4–5 and continued therapy during a parental divorce when she was 7.

The mother provided a lengthy history of what led to the referral. She reports seeing her daughter struggle with mood swings, isolating, crying, refusing to eat with family, and raging with simple compliance requests. The daughter was hospitalized once at age 7 for stabbing a kitchen knife into her hand with no warning. The hospital began a medication regimen for her with Lexapro (Escitalopram). This medication seemed to help partially and was increased during the outpatient phase by the medical provider shortly after discharge from the hospital until recently when the school called after finding Sally being disruptive in class, putting her coat on like a cape, and jumping over lunch tables saying, "I am going to fly! I can kill myself!" The mother called the pediatrician, who discontinued the medication and recommended the patient for psychiatric evaluation with a child psychiatrist.

The evaluation process in psychiatry included a thorough interview with the mother and attempted to involve the father in the initial diagnostic interview process, completed over three appointments. Further, collaboration was sought with the child therapist for collateral information regarding the psychosocial aspect of the child and the family dynamics. The initial diagnostic interview in psychiatry involved a thorough intake evaluation of the family history, which revealed bipolar disorder presenting in the biological parent beginning in high school. During the evaluation of the patient, the child was calm, interactive, and appropriate to the context of the appointment. The mental status exam revealed an appropriately attired young girl with appropriate eye contact, well-nourished, and developed no acute distress. Collateral history with the child's therapist revealed family dynamics, which included a problematic relationship with the father, who had become increasingly disengaged with the family and precisely distant from his daughter, only responding to the child during times of disruption at school when the school would contact the father and inform him of difficulty with his daughter. The pediatrician appropriately diagnosed depression in the child consistent with DSM-5 criteria.

However, Lexapro (Escitalopram), a selective serotonin reuptake inhibitor (SSRI), was discontinued when suicidal behaviors increased consistently and simultaneously with medication-induced mood dysregulation. Consideration of pediatric bipolar disorder presentation remained within the differential diagnosis. In the context of pediatric presentation of bipolar disorder, evaluation was given to mood dysregulation, sleep habit changes, presentation of grandiosity and euphoria, hypersexual and hyperverbal symptoms, impulsivity, self-harm (threats and actions), as well as the presence of any psychosis. The patient threatened to harm herself at her school in the previously noted presentation and had a history of seemingly unprovoked self-harm. The appropriate medical investigation, which included lab work, revealed medically non-contributory data. The child continued play therapy, and care coordination appointments were set approximately four weeks and eight weeks after the initial psychiatric interview between the play therapist and psychiatrist. The patient's depression continued, and the play therapist elucidated information regarding the family dynamics that strongly influenced the child's mood reactivity and self-harm actions. The psychiatrist began the child on a low-dose antidepressant, but this time with a lower potency (though equally effective) medication, Zoloft (Sertraline), and titrated slowly over time. The patient's therapist and psychiatrist continued to contact each other. They reported their observations, which helped to determine which aspects of the child's symptoms were best targeted by medication and psychotherapy interventions – as apparent target symptoms were calling for both interventions. The child stabilized on the medication and, through play therapy, could work through challenging aspects of her relationship with her father and further work in the family play therapy context. The child's impulsivity and angry outbursts subsided over time with dose escalation, and her meaningful participation in play therapy improved.

CONCLUSION

In conclusion, healthcare providers should know the referral criteria for pediatric patients dealing with suicidal thoughts and behaviors (STB) when considering a psychiatrist's involvement. Effective communication and collaboration between the play therapist and psychiatrist are essential for providing the best possible care for pediatric patients. By understanding these criteria and employing effective communication strategies, healthcare providers can make informed decisions and support pediatric patients in achieving optimal mental health while managing STB and other mental health diagnoses.

REFERENCES

American Psychiatric Association. (2022). *Diagnostic and statistical manual of mental disorders* (5th ed., Text Rev., DSM-5). Author.

Bonin, L., & Moreland, C. S. (2023). Overview of prevention and treatment for pediatric depression. *www.uptodate.com/*. Retrieved February 3, 2023, from www.uptodate.com/contents/overview-of-prevention-and-treatment-for-pediatric-depression?search=Children%20referral%20to%20psychiatry&source=search_result&selectedTitle=2~150&usage_type=default&display_rank=2#

Carballo, J. J., Llorente, C., Kehrmann, L., Flamarique, I., Zuddas, A., Purper-Ouakil, D., Hoekstra, P. J., Coghill, D., Schulze, U. M. E., Dittmann, R. W., Buitelaar, J. K., Castro-Fornieles, J., Lievesley, K., Santosh, P., Arango, C., Sutcliffe, A., Curran, S., Selema, L., Flanagan, R., . . . Aitchison, K. (2019). Psychosocial risk factors for suicidality in children and adolescents. *European Child & Adolescent Psychiatry*, *29*(6), 759–776. https://doi.org/10.1007/s00787-018-01270-9

Lim, C. T., Caan, M. P., Kim, C. H., Chow, C. M., Leff, H. S., & Tepper, M. C. (2022). Care management for serious mental illness: A systematic review and meta-analysis. *Psychiatric Services*, *73*(2), 180–187. https://doi.org/10.1176/appi.ps.202000473

Liu, H. (2023, January). What is psychiatry? *Psychiatry.org*. www.psychiatry.org/patients-families/what-is-psychiatry

Rudd, M. D., Berman, A. L., Joiner, T. E., Nock, M. K., Silverman, M. M., Mandrusiak, M., Van Orden, K., & Witte, T. (2006). Warning signs for suicide: Theory, research, and clinical applications. *Suicide and Life-Threatening Behavior*, *36*(3), 255–262. https://doi.org/10.1521/suli.2006.36.3.255

Shaffer, D., & Pfeffer, C. R. (2001). Practice parameters for the assessment and treatment of children and adolescents with suicidal behavior. *Journal of the American Academy of Child & Adolescent Psychiatry*, *40*(7), 24S–51S. https://doi.org/10.1097/00004583-200107001-00003

Shain, B., Braverman, P. K., Adelman, W. P., Alderman, E. M., Breuner, C. C., Levine, D. A., Marcell, A. V., & O'Brien, R. F. (2016). Suicide and suicide attempts in adolescents. *Pediatrics, 138*(1). https://doi.org/10.1542/peds.2016-1420

Wintersteen, M. B., Diamond, G. S., & Fein, J. A. (2007). Screening for suicide risk in the pediatric emergency and acute care setting. *Current Opinion in Pediatrics, 19*(4), 398–404. https://doi.org/10.1097/mop.0b013e328220e997

CHAPTER 4

COUNTERTRANSFERENCE IN THE TREATMENT OF YOUTH SUICIDE AND INTERVENTIONS FOR PROVIDING INNER AND EXTERNAL SUPPORT

Leslie W. Baker and Mary Ruth Cross

COUNTERTRANSFERENCE

The play therapist's emotional response to what happens in treatment is countertransference (Hayes et al., 2018). The original concept of countertransference comes from Freud and his work with psychoanalysis (Gabbard, 2020). Initially, the therapist would examine their response to the client's transference of feelings or desires onto the therapist. A fuller understanding of the therapeutic relationship has since evolved. Countertransference occurs when a clinician's emotional experience is projected onto an existing client relationship (Hayes et al., 2018). For example, if a clinician experienced a traumatic loss in life and the client is talking about a traumatic loss experience, it could trigger emotionally unresolved matters within the therapist. A personal experience can lead the clinician to project their emotional response into the moment with the client rather than keep the focus on what the client is processing from their own experience. Awareness of personal feelings about the client and attention to our non-verbal clues, such as body movements and facial expressions, provide play therapists insight into their countertransference issues. Countertransference and transference exist together in the therapeutic relationship. According to Carl Jung, "transference therefore consists in a number of projections which act as a substitute for a real psychological relationship" (1956/1966, p.134). Originally seen as obstacles in psychotherapy are now regarded as co-existing processes that is if understood and reflected upon by the clinician can create an opportunity for deeper change in the therapeutic process (Aggarwal, 2015).

Countertransference reactions may be discussed with colleagues and supervisors so that the play therapist can better understand the dynamics at work. Evaluating one's response toward a client can help determine whether the clinician's countertransference inadvertently affects current treatment. In supervision and therapy, conceptualizing the issues from a theoretical orientation provides play therapists and students with a framework for successful exploration of the concepts of transference and counter transferential responses. In contrast, when there is a lack of containment, the experience of countertransference can be detrimental to the therapeutic relationship (Gait & Halewood, 2019). Understanding countertransference and transference, the interplay of these concepts in the therapeutic relationship and learning how awareness can assist the clinician to use these concepts to understand their client more deeply, can lead to a deeper understanding that the complex relationships suicidal clients bring to therapy.

It takes years of education and many more years of training to reach the goal of becoming a play therapist or educator. Play therapists confront challenging mental health concerns for the child or adolescent and their families. Helping to manage a suicide crisis can trigger many different responses in the play therapist. Possible responses could be questioning one's

DOI: 10.4324/9781003358565-5

abilities, feeling defeated, confusion, stress, grief, and loss. Other possible responses could be a feeling of burnout or compassion fatigue (Hayes et al., 2018; Prasko et al., 2010). There are as many responses as there are play therapists. Play therapists of all theoretical orientations must attend to their conflicts and monitor their reactions to children and adolescents as a routine part of effective clinical practice. Unresolved personal disputes can lead to responses that negatively affect the outcome of therapy, and successfully managing these reactions is an essential element in positive therapy outcomes (Hayes et al., 2018). The treatment focus must remain on the children and adolescents with STB.

Treating and managing STBs is a complex matter. A complete understanding of suicidality is necessary for effective intervention. For example, it is not uncommon for those with suicidal ideation to have a sense of resolve and determination when they perceive dying by suicide as the path to relief from the pain (Miller, 2021). Be aware that what seems to be an "accident" may have been a suicide attempt.

When we examine the countertransference issue, we have to look at it through the lens of what has been projected onto the play therapist by the client (transference) and then our reaction to it. An emotional response to something a child or adolescent said or demonstrated in the play can trigger countertransference from the therapist's background. Rosenberg and Hayes (2002) found that when client material touches upon a play therapist's unresolved issues, it may affect the working alliance, session impact, and the play therapist's perceptions of their social influence attributes. A client's perception of the operating partnership and the depth of the session may both be improved by effective countertransference management (Rosenberger & Hayes, 2002). In the case of child suicidality, the projection could be, "You are not helping me. You are supposed to keep me safe." It can feel like a parental response the child might be having: "Mommy, please keep me safe." A parent and child advocate will find that an emotionally challenging place to hold. With empathy and compassion, we can understand feeling so overwhelmed, unsafe, and desperate to feel safe that it would look like the only option was to die by suicide. Feelings of helplessness and frustration can arise when the community lacks support or understanding regarding how to help and support suicidal children and adolescents. It would be easy to feel disillusioned when seeking help from medical professionals or law enforcement and finding that help to be insufficient or non-existent. Inadequate (or total absence of) services bring feelings to the play therapist, such as hopelessness, helplessness, and despair. The play therapist could also respond by stepping more into a child advocacy role. For example, the efforts of the Zero Suicide initiative project across the nation bring awareness of suicide at all ages to diverse communities and people by working with public and private agencies to improve the overall response of care to children, adolescents, and adults who need not only well-trained but compassionate and understanding allies to prevent suicide (*Zero Suicide*, 2022).

COUNTERTRANSFERENCE INTERVENTION

This intervention is to help play therapists understand their possible countertransference responses, called *"What Jar Your Issues?" Intervention* (Baker & Cross, 2019b). One can use a jar template or an actual jar. If using the jar template, write on the jar template what thoughts and feelings you may have about suicidality in children and adolescents. If you choose to use the actual jar, write your thoughts and feelings regarding suicidality on paper strips. To aid further self-expression, decorate your paper jar or actual jar with paint, stickers, ribbon,

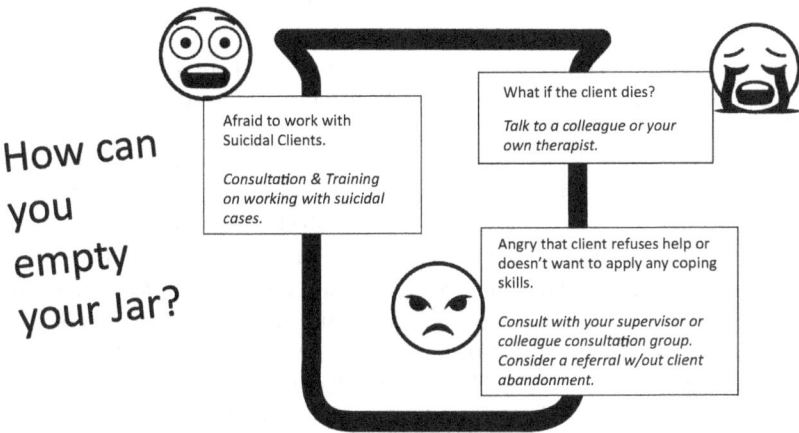

Figure 4.1 What Jar Your Issues?

glitter glue, or jewels that express your personality. Some questions to consider when utilizing the *"What Jar Your Issues?" Intervention* is:

- Am I afraid to deal with suicidal clients?
- What if the client dies by suicide?
- I may feel angry that the client does not want to get better.

These thoughts and reactions can fill a play therapist. Once completed, work on emptying the jar. Be open to input from others. Experienced play therapists will benefit by discussing countertransference with supervisors.

SELF-CARE AS TREATMENT

Research by Hayes et al. (2018) supports the need for the play therapist to work with a mentor or fellow therapist to ensure good mental health. The play therapist should be aware of applicable countertransference schemas (beliefs). They should monitor any feelings that indicate countertransference (Prasko et al., 2010; Prasko et al., 2022). The *"What Jar Your Issues?" Intervention* (Baker & Cross, 2019b) utilizes concepts from the expressive therapy technique and Cognitive Behavior Therapy (CBT) in that by examining what you think, you gain awareness of how you behave. CBT theorists have noted that countertransference reactions are likely to impact the quality of the therapeutic alliance, which is one of the fundamental principles of CBT (Ellis et al., 2018). CBT considers four aspects: thoughts, feelings, behaviors, and beliefs (schemas).

Each aspect influences the next. For example, suppose the play therapist believes suicidal clients are too risky to treat. In that case, fear, worry, and lack of self-confidence may cause a refusal to treat suicidal clients, reluctance to attend workshops about suicidality, and anxiety when a suicidal client appears in their practice. The best way to help a play therapist address these concerns is to evaluate beliefs or schemas about potentially suicidal children and adolescents. They must consider what suicidality means to them. For example, the therapist may equate suicidality with death or failure or possibly a sense of insufficiency when, in actuality, their intervention may result in successful treatment for youth. If they change their definition of or belief about suicide, they can change their relationship (thoughts, feelings, and behaviors) to suicidality. The final step in the intervention *"What Jar Your Issues?"* is to consider how to "empty the jar" to support the therapist's emotional health.

A multi-step approach is required for play therapists to understand their emotional responses to clinical work fully. They must recognize their thoughts and feelings to gain the insight needed to explore and manage "countertransference hate" (Maltsberger & Buie, 1974). This combination of aversion and malice may be unconscious, further obstructing the relationship (Rensko, 2017; Prasko et al., 2022). "Countertransference hate" is often demonstrated by clinicians experiencing negative feelings about their suicidal clients that may often impact treatment (Maltsberger & Buie, 1974). For example, an adolescent who is repeatedly suicidal and refusing help, hospitalized multiple times, and experiencing numerous suicidal attempts and self-harm can create an environment where a play therapist or school counselor could develop "countertransference hate," resulting in wanting to cancel sessions, being inadvertently rude or aggressive to the client, or having thoughts of terminating or abandoning the client's treatment (Maltsberger & Buie, 1974). Integrating self-awareness with clinical action can reduce countertransference hate from derailing the therapy. By focusing on empathy and managing possible anxiety about self-care, the play therapist or school counselor can improve their overall well-being and be fully present in the therapeutic process. Lastly, developing and maintaining skills in suicide assessment, intervention, and prevention (Rensko, 2017) to minimize or learn how to utilize countertransference through awareness to deepen the therapeutic relationship.

The best way to "empty your jar" is to have solid self-care strategies to rely on (*Compassion Fatigue and Self-care for Crisis Counselors*, n.d.). Some of the ways to look at self-care are through the following methods:

- Attend to your comfort
- Acceptance of emotions, feelings, and behaviors
- Awareness – be aware of your thoughts, feelings, and behaviors
- Mindfulness – being kind and gentle with yourself
- Getting enough support – including seeking professional support
- Good nutrition – eat well
- Sleep – sleep is critical to mental health
- Finding joy daily – personal to you
- Insight – recognize your thoughts and emotions
- Put self-awareness into action – integrate
- Exercise – walk, swim, treadmill, yoga, VR game
- Manage anxiety – self-care
- Focus on empathy
- Develop and maintain skills in suicide prevention, assessment, response, treatment, and recovery from grief and loss.

(*Compassion Fatigue and Self-care for Crisis Counselors*, n.d.)

CASE EXAMPLE

The play therapist feels drained and disappointed. The police had just left her office, saying they would not assist in hospitalizing the suicidal 7-year-old client, Selena, who has clear signs of depression and has been struggling with suicidal thinking for three months, after which her thoughts shifted to a clear intent of self-harm. Selena's mother is at the play therapy session and is expressing confusion and distress when Selena says, "I do not want to be here any-more." Selena's stepfather was emotionally abusive to her and her mother. Selena's mother, Roberta, is not sure how she should help her daughter. The play therapist provided a full suicide assessment, and Selena disclosed that she wanted to run into the street and get hit by a car. Selena also said that if she died, her mother would be sad, but she would be happy in heaven. Selena said she would "do it" that day if she went home. Selena was assessed, and it was determined that the suicide attempt was imminent, and that Selena intended to attempt suicide. The play therapist contacted the local police department to assess Selena for possible hospitalization. When the police officer arrived, the stepfather was waiting in the parking lot outside the play therapist's office and spoke with him before the officer entered the office. When the police officer interviewed Selena, it was clear that he had a preconceived idea of the problem. He used leading questions and tried to convince Selena that her stepfather was just disciplining her "as any dad is supposed to do." Selena became distressed and started to cry. The police officer then asked the play therapist what she wanted him to do. It was clear that Selena was a danger to herself and that possible hospitalization was needed to ensure her safety. The officer refused and said that the county does not hospitalize children this young.

Furthermore, no child hospitals were available for evaluation; it would be at the county hospital where "all the drunks and drug addicts are." The play therapist inquired about taking her to the Children's Hospital, but there was no contract with the Children's Hospital to allow this. No county Crisis Management Team could provide Selena with safety from self-harm. After the officer left, the play therapist worked with Selena's mother to get support and resources. Roberta was able to take Selena to her pediatrician later that day for evalua-tion, and the doctor recommended hospitalization.

Fortunately, Selena did go to a safe place where her suicidal ideation could be assessed and managed. For the play therapist, managing a suicidal crisis while impeded by police obstruction created intense anger, fear, and helplessness. The play therapist had grown up believing that the police were the "good guys" who would help her and make all well. Now, she distrusted law enforcement as an ally in preventing suicide. She felt distressed. She ques-tioned whom she could rely on for help in an urgent situation.

A week after this incident, the play therapist felt depressed and had trouble sleeping. She started to reduce the number of clients she saw for play therapy. Reluctant to go to work, she felt sluggish and tired there. She found entering the play in her play therapy sessions difficult. The play therapist empathized with Selena's mother and wanted to do more to help her. She thought about going out for coffee with her to provide support. She noticed that her feelings at home seemed much closer to the surface, and she would cry at a sentimental commercial or when see-ing a mother and child hugging each other. She began thinking about a childhood friend who died by suicide at age 13. She marveled that she had not considered this friend in over ten years.

The play therapist began to realize that she was struggling with countertransference and decided to contact a colleague to discuss what was happening. She explored her reactions to what happened to Selena and how she felt continuing as a play therapist. She loved her work with children and their families; however, she felt irritable and, at times, disengaged from the children. It just seemed too hard to care so much. She usually felt confident in her effectiveness as a play therapist, but not being able to get the expected help when Selena was suicidal had her questioning that effectiveness. With the help of her colleague, the play therapist made a Self-Care Plan. Her Self-Care Plan focused on increasing mindfulness practice during the day between sessions. The Self-Care Plan included deep breathing exercises and simple yoga movements (West et al., 2017). She also started taking a morning walk daily to start each day with exercise and quiet reflection.

The play therapist's Self-Care Plan included planning to be with friends and writing in her journal. She considered starting her therapy but decided to see if her plan would alleviate enough feelings that she could be more present in the playroom. The play therapist and her colleague decided to meet regularly to help her manage all of her countertransference responses effectively. She could maintain healthy boundaries with Selena's mother and enter effectively into the play with Selena. The play therapist also contacted the chief of police and the county mental health department to advocate and assist in creating a crisis management team that could respond more effectively to suicidal youth. The play therapist used her countertransference to learn and grow personally and professionally.

As play therapists and educators, we often talk about self-care. The research on this subject shows how necessary counselor self-care is for efficacious treatment and the prevention of counselor burnout and compassion fatigue. Thompson et al. (2014) found that with higher levels of mindfulness, there are lower levels of burnout and a decrease in compassion fatigue. Self-care starting with mindfulness processes has shown promise in reducing stress among play therapists, thereby improving the quality and effectiveness of treatment. Promoting self-care practices will benefit the play therapist, educators, and client relationships by reducing compassion fatigue and increasing professional satisfaction (Cuartero & Campos-Vidal, 2018).

PARENTS AND CAREGIVERS

Daily self-care is crucial for play therapists and educators, and these concepts also apply to parents and caregivers. Taking steps to improve physical well-being can contribute to holistic mental health support. When one's body is solid and resilient, positive mental habits are easier to maintain. Parents and caregivers who attend to their mental wellness can better support their child or adolescent in crisis and throughout treatment. Parents and caregivers cope with enormous stress, including vigilance, fear, worry, and the torment of "What if . . ." Supporting a child or adolescent who is suicidal may take all the energy a parent or caregiver has to give. Incorporating regular exercise into a daily routine is vital. It can involve simple activities like opting for stairs instead of escalators, walking or biking instead of driving, and even joining fitness classes to establish a consistent schedule. A healthy diet is essential for a strong body. Prioritizing unprocessed foods such as whole grains, fresh fruits, and vegetables helps reduce the risk of chronic diseases while promoting stable energy levels and mood. Sufficient sleep is crucial; most adults require seven to nine hours each night. Taking short naps, even as briefly as 15 minutes, can help restore daytime alertness. Incorporating relaxation exercises into a routine can help alleviate stress. Parents and caregivers can apply techniques such as deep breathing, meditation, and progressive muscle relaxation to offer quick and easy ways to unwind (*Taking Care of Yourself* | *NAMI: National Alliance on Mental Illness*, n.d.). Healthy habits provide us with tools to regain control over turbulent emotions and provide the mental space to manage family conflicts.

Parents and caregivers can seek support through individual therapy, a community support group, a church group, or meetings with religious-based groups, and clinics offer groups on meditation, mindfulness, yoga, dance, art, and other creative modalities to support mental health for adults. The National Alliance on Mental Illness (NAMI) recommends avoiding guilt, focusing on the positive, and gaining strength from those around us to assist in coping with stress (*Taking Care of Yourself | NAMI: National Alliance on Mental Illness*, n.d.).

THERAPIST PROTOCOL

Play therapists, school counselors, parents, and caregivers face the unthinkable: a child or adolescent dying by suicide. In some cases, it is an impulsive act. In other cases, it consists of a series of suicidal ideations and suicidal behaviors, such as gestures, threats to kill oneself, self-harm, or multiple non-completed attempts. It can happen even when it seems all the pieces were in place to prevent it. The clinical team has worked hard to assess, treat, and provide crisis care as needed. The psychiatrists may have offered multiple medications, and play therapists used interventions addressing the child's or adolescent's needs. The schools have played their role, diligently working with the youth and engaging the child or adolescent on multiple levels. Parents and caregivers also often work hard in treatment to address the needs of their child or adolescent at school and home. Despite everyone's best efforts, a child, or adolescent dies by suicide. What do we do now? How do we manage the traumatic loss and grief that inevitably follows? Shock is often a typical response for all involved. A treatment team may not find out about the loss immediately. However, shock is not uncommon when they do, and neither is grief, worry, guilt, and a mental review of all their assessment, treatment, and prevention procedures applied to the case. Parents and caregivers often call to learn about the last meeting with everyone involved. Checking in with a legal advisor before contacting the families is essential to protect confidentiality and other legal and ethical issues for the play therapist and the client.

Confidentiality issues remain, and although play therapists and educators want to connect, educators recommended getting advice and only then proceeding with a call if the family is requesting this. For further information, review the association ethics under which one practices as a play therapist. For example, NASW provides the following resource: Legal Considerations When a Client Dies by Suicide (Legal | NASW-IL, 2023). This article provides information on liability, speaking with family members, how to talk with family members, requests for the records of deceased clients, HIPAA concerns, NASW Codes of Ethics, and practice tips. Play therapists and educators must remember to seek the information applicable to their association.

TREATING SUICIDE LOSS SURVIVORS

The American Association of Suicidology (n.d.) proposes that a practical post-intervention framework should encompass activities that cater to the needs of all individuals affected by suicide. Specifically, schools need to develop a comprehensive plan that offers counseling services to students, parents, teachers, and other community members impacted by suicide. The aftermath of a suicide death profoundly affects those who have experienced loss, especially during the postvention bereavement period.

Experiencing a traumatic loss undermines an individual's fundamental beliefs about the world, such as its predictability, controllability, meaningfulness, fairness, justice, and personal safety and security. At the outset, the effects are particularly destabilizing and overwhelming, and those who have suffered such a loss exhibit distinct symptoms, including flashbacks, disrupted sleep patterns, and a tendency to avoid anything that reminds them of the loss. Efforts to remember the departed loved one are accompanied by distressing memories, images, and thoughts, leading to avoidance behaviors that hinder the grieving process and coming to terms with the loss. As a result, survivors often endure persistent and debilitating symptoms that show minimal signs of improvement as time goes on. These symptoms include a heightened risk of depression, a decreased quality of life, impaired job performance, increased conflicts with relatives and surviving children, and a higher mortality rate (Pearlman et al., 2014).

Understanding the cultural, religious, and societal attitudes toward suicide is crucial to postvention (Sheehan et al., 2016). Play therapists, educators, parents, and caregivers alike can suffer traumatic loss and grief after a suicide, but reactions can also vary widely. Suicide loss is unique for several reasons. According to research by Levi-Belz and Hamdan (2023), there is a strong link between shame and the development of Complicated Grief (CG) and depression after losing someone to suicide. Additionally, the influence of interpersonal relationships on the distress and mourning experienced by those who've lost someone to suicide is crucial, as these relationships can potentially mitigate the harmful effects of such a loss. Suicide carries a significant societal stigma and is taboo in many cultures. This stigma can make it challenging for those who have lost someone to suicide to discuss their grief and openly seek support (Sheehan et al., 2016). The unique circumstances surrounding suicide can intensify the survivors' feelings of shame, guilt, and isolation. Unlike other forms of loss, suicide is often sudden and unexpected. The abrupt nature of suicide can leave survivors in shock and disbelief, making it more challenging to process their emotions and navigate grieving (Sheehan et al., 2016). Suicide raises complex and intense feelings for survivors. They may experience a wide range of emotions, such as guilt, anger, confusion, and profound sadness. Sharing personal information about a loss survivor's story can assist in moderating their loss (Levi-Belz & Hamdan, 2023). Survivors often grapple with unanswerable questions, trying to understand why their loved one took their own life and wondering if they could have done anything to prevent it. Survivors of suicide loss may feel a heightened sense of responsibility for the death of their loved one. They may question their actions, decisions, or missed warning signs, leading to intense guilt and self-blame.

Grief after a suicide loss is stigmatized within the broader society and sometimes even within one's immediate social circles. The lack of understanding and support for suicide survivors can add a layer of complexity to their grief journey. Suicide loss can result in traumatic reactions for survivors. Witnessing or discovering the aftermath of a suicide can have long-lasting psychological impacts.

Additionally, survivors may experience secondary losses, such as strained relationships, changes in social dynamics, or financial challenges, further complicating the grieving process. Due to these unique factors, suicide loss requires specialized support and understanding to help survivors navigate their grief and heal from the profound impact of losing a loved one to suicide.

THEORIES OF LOSS AND GRIEF

Treatment for traumatic grief and loss varies among many theories and processes. Here are three to consider. According to Worden's (2004) task theory, individuals undergo specific tasks as they mourn the loss of a loved one. These tasks are distinct from stages, can overlap, and may be revisited over time. Worden (2004) outlines four areas that individuals should undertake:

- **Accept** the reality of the loss, which involves acknowledging and accepting that the loved one has passed away. It requires facing the reality of the loss and understanding its permanence.

- **Work** through the pain of grieving. This task involves actively experiencing and processing the emotional pain associated with grief. It entails allowing oneself to grieve, expressing emotions, and finding healthy ways to cope with the pain.

- **Adjust** to an environment without the deceased. This task focuses on adapting to a new reality where the presence of the deceased is absent. It involves making necessary adjustments, finding new routines, and establishing a sense of stability in the absence of a loved one.

- **Emotionally relocate** the deceased and move on with life. This task centers on finding a place for the departed loved one in one's memories and emotions, allowing them to live on in a new way. It involves finding a healthy balance between honoring the memory of the deceased and moving forward with one's own life.

Completing these four tasks is essential for individuals to integrate the loss into their lives and continue their personal growth and development (Worden, 2004).

Stroebe and Schut (1999) developed a dual-process model of grief that combines existing grief theories, cognitive stress theories, and coping methods. This model recognizes the importance of considering various stressors following a death. This two-dimensional theory takes a stressor-specific approach to grief, distinguishing between loss – and restoration-oriented stressors. Loss-oriented stressors are directly related to the loss itself, encompassing the challenges and emotions associated with the absence of a loved one. Restoration-oriented stressors, conversely, pertain to the secondary losses that occur after the death, such as changes in family dynamics, financial adjustments, and shifts in responsibilities. The dual process theory emphasizes confronting and avoiding these stressors to adapt to the loss. Avoidance of grief allows individuals to temporarily shield themselves from overwhelming emotions and resume their pre-death roles and responsibilities. However, confronting stressors and expressing sadness and loss is essential for adaptive grieving. Individuals move back and forth between focusing on the loss and rebuilding a new way of life. This dynamic movement enables individuals to grieve the loss while staying connected to the memory of the deceased and simultaneously moving forward with their lives.

Lastly, Neimeyer's (2001) theory of meaning reconstruction encompasses several primary objectives, which include:

a) Assisting those who are grieving in finding or generating meaning not only in the death of their loved one but also in their own life.

b) Exploring the ongoing emotional attachment or connection with the deceased and recognizing how this bond can have positive and healing effects.

c) Addressing both explicit meanings expressed by clients and implicit meanings observed, ensuring that all aspects of meaning are attended to.

d) Encouraging the construction of meaning and integrating it into a newly constructed life narrative.

e) Facilitating the development of meaning at both personal and interpersonal levels.

f) Examining meaning within individual contexts and considering broader cultural contexts.

g) Utilizing a narrative approach to guide individuals in reauthoring their life stories after experiencing loss.

(Neimeyer, 2001)

In summary, Neimeyer's theory focuses on helping bereaved individuals find or create meaning in various aspects of their lives and helping them incorporate this newfound meaning into their life narratives.

INTERVENTIONS FOR TRAUMATIC LOSS AND GRIEF

Seeking therapy for traumatic bereavement is crucial. Brain-based tools that can effectively reduce trauma to the bereaved are Eye Movement Desensitization and Reprocessing (EMDR), a form of psychotherapy initially developed to alleviate distress linked to traumatic memories (Shapiro, 1989). Shapiro's (2001) Adaptive Information Processing model proposes that EMDR therapy facilitates the accessing and processing of traumatic memories and other adverse life experiences, leading to an adaptive resolution. EMDR therapy reduces affective distress, hostile belief reformation, and physiological arousal. During EMDR therapy, the client engages with emotionally disturbing material in brief and sequential doses while simultaneously focusing on an external stimulus. Lateral eye movements, guided by the therapist, are the most commonly employed external stimulus, although various other stimuli like hand-tapping and audio stimulation are also utilized (Shapiro, 1989).

Expressive play therapy interventions are included so play therapists, school counselors, parents, and caregivers can begin to process their losses. According to Neimeyer and Cacciatore's developmental model of grief (2016), some tasks after a traumatic loss can include emotion regulation (downregulation can lead to hypoarousal, and upregulation can lead to hyperarousal) and containment (gaining a sense of boundaries, safety, and security) after the traumatic loss. These tasks combat a loss of connection and work to avoid the potential for isolation after the traumatic loss. Many survivors of suicide loss feel overwhelmed by the stigma and shame, and isolation appears to be the only solution. Traumatic loss can blow apart one's world; as mentioned previously, the goal is to reclaim trust, safety, and a sense of survival to regain self-acceptance after the event. Joining survivors of suicide loss groups can help adults reclaim themselves. Some groups might provide expressive play-based activities (Neimeyer & Cacciatore, 2016).

Loss and grief interventions mirror Neimeyer and Cacciatore's developmental model of grief (2016). The first step is to focus on emotion regulation. *Creative Response Meditation* (Cross & Baker, 2020) assists clinicians in taking time to downregulate through guided imagery. Choose your own 5–10 minute soothing guided imagery. After listening to the 5–10 minute guided imagery of the client's choice, following it by writing, drawing, and creating art from the experience during the imagery, clinicians can deepen their processing of the guided imagery experience. This intervention can be applied to children and adolescents experiencing a need to downregulate. Youth can experience more positive emotions and emotion regulation. Research has shown that positive emotions improve attentional focus, encourage exploration and creative processing, and support the development of practical skills and psychological resources, while negative emotions limit attention and cognition to focus on threats (Fredrickson, 2001). Intense negative affect and trouble with positive affect were linked to higher suicidality (Rojas et al., 2014).

Listen to a Guided Meditation
After, take a pen and paper and draw:

- Images that arose from your meditation.

- Write a response to your mediation.

- Draw or write physical sensations one felt.

- Draw or write down thoughts one had.

- Paint the colors that emerged in one's mind.

- Paint or draw one's emotional state or states that arose during the meditation.

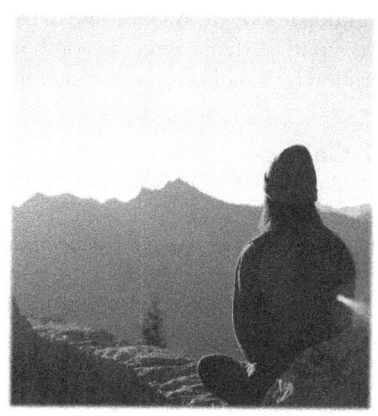

Figure 4.2 Creative Response Meditation

Source: © 2020 Cross, M. R. & Baker, L. *ALL RIGHTS RESERVED.* Cross, M. R. & Baker, L. (2020, October) Creative Response Meditation Intervention. [Conference Presentation]. Healing Traumatic Loss & Grief Through Play Therapy: A Bottom-Up Brain Approach. Expressive Therapies Summit, New York, NY.

Another first stage is the developmental model of grief (2016) by Neimeyer and Cacciatore. *The Unburden Basket* intervention (Cross, 2023) also addresses early grief. Self-acceptance and awareness of how much emotion you are experiencing create a safe containment for release and letting go at this stage if the loss survivor can. Materials needed: small stones approximately two to four inches in size, two baskets, colored permanent markers, and paint pens. This intervention can be done individually or as part of a group experience. One basket is filled with all of the rocks. Numerous rocks should be in the basket so that the weight of all the stones can be felt and provide enough for each participant. Place the empty basket nearby. The filled basket is passed slowly to each participant. Ask the person holding the basket to let themselves feel the basket's weight and see it as the weight of their feelings of loss. They can then choose as many stones as possible out of the basket that match this sense of weightiness. The basket may need to be refilled if this is done in a group. After each person has taken their stones, invite the loss survivor to see how many stones they would like to release by putting them into the empty basket. Their present thoughts and feelings are discussed, and when the participant is ready, they may unburden themselves by giving back the stones. Some participants may hold onto all their rocks, while others may feel ready to release some or all of them. Participants can decorate their rocks using paint pens or permanent markers.

Another first-step intervention from Neimeyer and Cacciatore's developmental model of grief (2016) is *My Grieving House* (Cross & Baker, 2021). Supplies include 11"×17" paper, crayons or markers, stickers, construction paper, scissors, tape, glue, and other appropriate art supplies. The procedure involves folding the paper into an Origami House using 11"×17" paper (smaller paper is possible but more challenging). Discuss what is different in the family now that the person they know has died by suicide. Using the craft and art supplies, have the client decorate the outside of the house to reflect before and the inside to reflect life after their death.

This intervention focuses on using expressive arts to assess the child or adolescent's experience of loss by suicide and the changes that follow. The integration of CCPT in this intervention inserts the relationship between the youth and the play therapist or school counselor as a part of the healing the youth needs. The play therapist creates a safe space for this exploration by building a positive therapeutic alliance on trust.

Leaf Collage

The *Leaf Collage* is adapted from the Remembering Tree (Baker & Cross, 2019a). This middle stage of grief includes developing a continuing bond with the person who died by suicide and creating an opportunity for memorializing and creating a continuing dialogue in a non-physical sense, according to Neimeyer's developmental middle grief (Neimeyer, 2001). Materials include cutting out oak leaves or using precut oak leaves of one's choice, an approximately 4"x6" piece of cardstock, one piece of 8.5"x11" cardstock for the background, one glue stick, black permanent marker, scissors, glue, and collage pictures. Using multiple leaves, write on them to assist the survivor of loss in remembering their loved one. On each leaf, write with black permanent marker memories about the person who died by suicide which the person wishes to reflect on and remember – for example, write the person's name and collage pictures of their hobbies, interests, or favorite photos onto the leaves. Note favorite sayings the person said or a favorite word or joke they used to tell, anything that helps the loss survivor create a memory they want to hold dear. Suppose a loss survivor has many negative memories of their client or loved one; they are welcome to create a grief leaf collage to process their disappointment or select a single positive story or memory to focus on if they wish. It is essential to allow for the loss survivor to be in charge of their collage. They have suffered a traumatic loss; this is an expressive activity, and the loss survivor controls their art.

The uniqueness of suicide loss and finding meaning in the loss is a challenge for many suicide loss survivors. As noted previously, every suicide loss survivor experiences loss differently. From a clinician to a parent, sibling, and caregiver, some people are left with memories they may treasure, and others may feel confused, upset, and angry. Mixed and confusing emotions are common. Seeking in a survivor's mind why, what, how, and where can burden survivors for some time. This subsequent intervention, *Sharing, Tearing, and Finding Meaning* (Baker, 2023), is developed to address some of these issues. Materials include plain and water-colored paper, colored felt pens, and art supplies from crayons, colored pencils, glitter, glue, watercolor pens and brushes, water, and paper towels.

The goal is for the loss survivor to choose a thought or complication they are coping with due to the suicide loss. Some of these issues may be the social stigma of suicide, not feeling able to share the loss due to shame and blame, embarrassment of a loss by suicide, family members' different reactions to the loss, and avoidance of communicating the loss or avoiding the word suicide (Pitman et al., 2018). The loss survivor keeps in mind the stigmatizing issue. Provide five minutes time to write any words that come to mind on a paper. Allow for the free association of any emotions, notice physical tensions or sensations in their body, and once completed, provide the watercolor paper and have the survivor create with color any images or simply colors that come to mind. They are free to draw anything that comes to mind. Once the survivor completes their art, they can share it with the clinician. No interpretation is provided; simply listen, witness, and process as appropriate. As witnessing and sharing occur, open-ended comments toward the client can be helpful, thinking about any meaning they may be coming to regarding the loss of their loved one. Do not push this; just simply be curious. Sometimes, loss survivors wonder if there is any meaning to their loss. Simple open-ended statements may facilitate reflection. "As you create, notice any feelings or body sensations that may be coming up for you" or "What thoughts come to mind as you reflect on your creation?" After the loss survivor has shared, they can keep their art and writing paper if they wish. A clinician may recommend taking a picture of their art for the client's reflection or keeping it in their clinical file for another session. They may also tear up the paper they initially wrote on, letting go of the stigma symbolically. We do not suggest that people tear up or destroy their art; however, like with sand tray, some clients may choose this option. This intervention is a later treatment intervention, as noted in Neimeyer's developmental model, middle grief, in which therapy focuses on validation, understanding, and reconstruction (Neimeyer, 2001).

POSTTRAUMATIC GROWTH

In the mid-1990s, Tedeschi and Calhoun researched responses to trauma and highly distressing life situations to understand better all aspects of trauma response that might aid clinicians in treating their traumatized patients (Tedeschi & Calhoun, 1996). Posttraumatic growth is the positive transformation that can result from overcoming challenging life crises (Maitlis, 2020). Those who have survived trauma or other life crises can begin to see the strength within themselves and are more equipped to manage complex events in the future. Maitlis (2020) also noted other possible changes that may occur from posttraumatic growth, such as how they see others, the ability to have a greater sense of not only intimacy but a sense of belonging, a stronger sense of purpose, and appreciation for life. Posttraumatic growth is a process and an outcome (Tedeschi & Calhoun, 2004). Secondary posttraumatic growth can be seen in healthcare professionals and any profession that works with clients who experience trauma. Secondary posttraumatic growth is connected to how the therapist sees the growth and change in their clients. The more emphatically engaged the therapist is with their clients, the higher the likelihood of experiencing secondary posttraumatic growth (Maitlis, 2020). In other words, witnessing posttraumatic growth in others can have positive transformative effects. The following intervention: *This is Me Now!* (Cross & Baker, 2023) is an intervention to aid the clinician in assessing and understanding the changes that have occurred as the patient has grieved. The play therapist or school counselor can also use this intervention to understand their secondary posttraumatic growth. Four key areas are examined in this intervention: values and beliefs, skills, possibilities, and dreams. The template that follows illustrates the interconnected process and is used to write the answers to the following questions.

> *Values and Beliefs*: What words come to mind when you think of yourself now? What do you want now? What is most important to you now? How do you connect with your inner self or spirit?
>
> *Skills*: What do you enjoy doing? What are you good at? What is your personal style? What do others like about you?
>
> *Possibilities*: Is there anything that holds you back from living fully?
>
> *Dreams*: Where would you go if you could go anywhere? What is it that makes you happy?

Where would you like your life to be in three to five years?

The clinician then creates a collage that uses images illustrating the answers to the questions and supporting the transformation that has occurred. It can also open up awareness for opportunities for further growth and change.

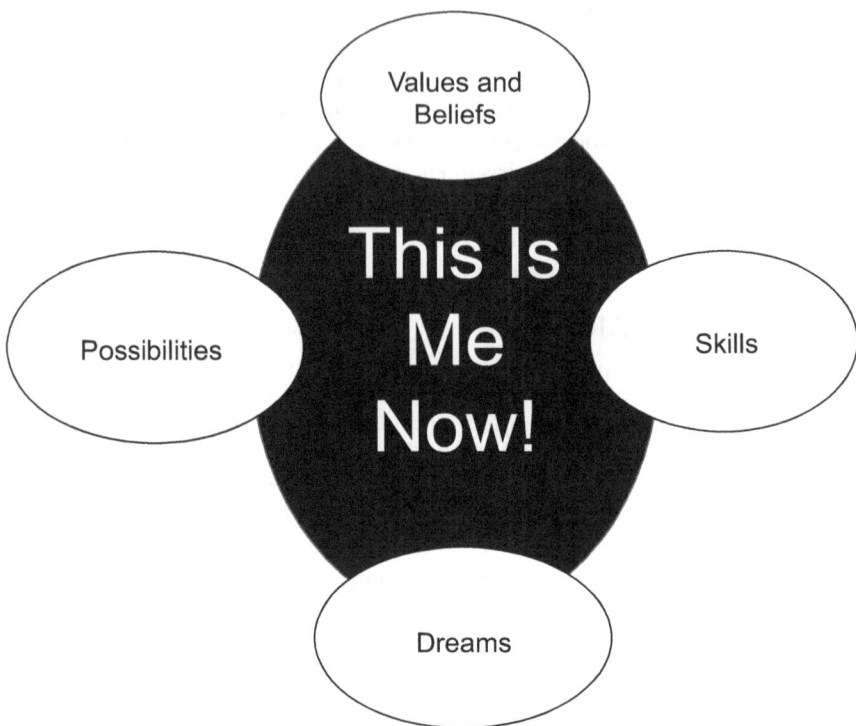

Figure 4.3 This Is Me Now!

Source: Cross, M. R. & Baker, L. (2023, May). This is Me Now! [Conference Presentation]. Making Meaning Through A Journey of Loss: Playful Self-Care To Thrive. Mid-Atlantic Play Therapy and Expressive Arts Conference, Atlantic City, NJ.

CONCLUSION

The dynamic co-creation between play therapists and youth within the therapeutic relationship can involve countertransference and transference, crucial elements in the therapeutic process. Awareness and understanding of countertransference concerns are essential to prevent disruptions that hinder mental health providers from effectively recognizing and addressing suicidality in children and adolescents. On the other hand, transference between the youth and the play therapist can create a healthy alliance, enabling the projection of suicidal thoughts and behaviors to facilitate change.

Self-care for play therapists and school counselors working with suicidal youth needs to be at the forefront of their minds and need for parents and caregivers to address their stress and build resilience when supporting a child or adolescent in coping with suicidal thoughts and behaviors. Suicidality can cause intense feelings of loneliness; treating it requires teamwork. Navigating the complexities of the therapeutic journey means addressing grief and loss for play therapists, educators, parents, and caregivers. Self-care plays a critical role throughout the therapeutic process, particularly in the face of a tragic loss. Play therapists must develop effective coping strategies for themselves and survivors when managing responses to traumatic loss. By recognizing the impact of grief and loss, they can better support themselves and their clients in the healing process. The authors have intended to shed light on the profound significance of the therapeutic relationship, the necessity of self-care, and the understanding of grief and loss for play therapists and others working with suicidal youth. Through continuous exploration and application of these concepts, play therapists and others can enhance their ability to provide compassionate and practical support to those in need.

REFERENCES

Aggarwal, N. K. (2015). Transference in Psychoanalysis: Classical, contemporary, and cultural contexts. In Elsevier eBooks (pp. 545–548). https://doi.org/10.1016/b978-0-08-097086-8.27072-4

American Association of Suicidology. (n.d.). *American Association of Suicidology*. www.suicidology.org/

Baker, L. (2023). *Sharing, tearing, and finding meaning* [Therapy2Thrive Clinical Practice] [Unpublished Intervention].

Baker, L., & Cross, M. R. (2019a, October). *Leaf collage; Adapted from the remembering tree* [Conference Presentation]. Suicide Prevention & Risk Assessment: What Play Therapists Need to Know. Expressive Therapies Summit, New York, NY.

Baker, L., & Cross, M. R. (2019b, October). *What 'Jar' your issues?* [Conference Presentation]. Suicide Prevention & Risk Assessment: What Play Therapists Need to Know. Expressive Therapies Summit, New York, NY.

Compassion fatigue and self-care for crisis counselors. (n.d.). SAMHSA. www.samhsa.gov/dtac/ccp-toolkit/self-care-for-crisis-counselors

Cross, M. R. (2023, May). *The unburden basket intervention* [Retreat Presentation]. *Pathways Through Grief: A Healing Journey*, Danville, CA.

Cross, M. R., & Baker, L. (2020, October). *Creative response meditation intervention* [Conference Presentation]. Healing Traumatic Loss & Grief Through Play Therapy: A Bottom-Up Brain Approach. Expressive Therapies Summit, New York, NY.

Cross, M. R., & Baker, L. (2021, April). *My grieving house* [Conference Presentation]. Healing Traumatic Loss & Grief Through Play Therapy: A Bottom-Up Brain Approach. Expressive Therapies Summit, LA. (Virtual).

Cross, M. R., & Baker, L. (2023, May). *This is me now!* [Conference Presentation]. Making Meaning Through A Journey of Loss: Playful Self-Care To Thrive. Mid-Atlantic Play Therapy and Expressive Arts Conference, Atlantic City, NJ.

Cuartero, M. E., & Campos-Vidal, J. F. C. (2018). Self-care behaviours and their relationship with satisfaction and compassion fatigue levels among social workers. *Social Work in Health Care*, *58*(3), 274–290. https://doi.org/10.1080/00981389.2018.1558164

Ellis, T. J., Schwartz, J. A. J., & Rufino, K. A. (2018). Negative reactions of therapists working with suicidal patients: A CBT/mindfulness perspective on "countertransference." *International Journal of Cognitive Therapy*. https://doi.org/10.1007/s41811-018-0005-1

Fleischhaker, C., Böhme, R., Sixt, B., Brück, C., Schneider, C., & Schulz, E. (2011). Dialectical Behavioral Therapy for Adolescents (DBT-A): a clinical Trial for Patients with suicidal and self-injurious Behavior and Borderline Symptoms with a one-year Follow-up. Child and Adolescent Psychiatry and Mental Health, 5(1). https://doi.org/10.1186/1753-2000-5-3

Fredrickson, B. L. (2001). The role of positive emotions in positive psychology: The broaden-and-build theory of positive emotions. *American Psychologist*, *56*(3), 218–226. https://doi.org/10.1037/0003-066x.56.3.218

Gabbard, G. O. (2020). The role of countertransference in contemporary psychiatric treatment. *World Psychiatry*, *19*(2), 243–244. https://doi.org/10.1002/wps.20746

Gait, S., & Halewood, A. (2019). Developing countertransference awareness as a therapist in training: The role of containing contexts. *Psychodynamic Practice*. https://doi.org/10.1080/14753634.2019.1643961

Hayes, J. J., Gelso, C. J., Goldberg, S. B., & Kivlighan, D. M. (2018). Countertransference management and effective psychotherapy: Meta-analytic findings. *Psychotherapy*, *55*(4), 496–507. https://doi.org/10.1037/pst0000

Jung, C. G. (1966). The psychology of transference: From the collected works of C. G. Jung (Vol. 16) [Print]. Bollingen Princeton Series University Press. https://dokumen.pub/psychology-of-the-transference-from-vol-16-collected-works-9780691218403.html (Original work published 1956)

Legal | NASW-IL. (2023). www.naswil.org/legal

Levi-Belz, Y., & Hamdan, S. (2023). Shame, depression, and complicated grief among suicide loss-survivors: The moderating role of self-disclosure. *European Journal of Psychotraumatology*, *14*(1). https://doi.org/10.1080/20008066.2023.2182820

Maitlis, S. (2020). Posttraumatic growth at work. *Annual Review of Organizational Psychology and Organizational Behavior*, *7*(1), 395–419. https://doi.org/10.1146/annurev-orgpsych-012119-044932

Maltsberger, J. T., & Buie, D. H. (1974). Countertransference hate in the treatment of suicidal patients. *Archives of General Psychiatry*, *30*(5), 625. https://doi.org/10.1001/archpsyc.1974.01760110049005

Miller. (2021). *Child and adolescent and suicidal behavior* (2nd ed.). Guilford.

Neimeyer, R. A. (2001). *Reauthoring life narratives: Grief therapy as meaning reconstruction*. PubMed. https://pubmed.ncbi.nlm.nih.gov/11725416

Neimeyer, R. A., & Cacciatore, J. (2016). Toward a developmental theory of grief. In R. A. Neimeyer (Ed.), *Techniques of grief therapy: Assessment and intervention* (pp. 3–13). Routledge/Taylor & Francis Group.

Pearlman, L. A., Wortman, C. B., Feuer, C. A., Farber, C. H., & Rando, T. A. (2014). *Treating traumatic bereavement: A practitioner's guide*. Guilford Publications.

Pitman, A., Stevenson, F., Osborn, D., & King, M. (2018). The stigma associated with bereavement by suicide and other sudden deaths: A qualitative interview study. *Social Science & Medicine*, *198*, 121–129. https://doi.org/10.1016/j.socscimed.2017.12.035

Prasko, J., Diveky, T., Grambal, A., Kamaradova, D., Mozny, P., Sigmundova, Z., Slepecky, M., & Vyskocilova, J. (2010). Transference and countertransference in cognitive behavioral therapy. *Biomedical Papers of the Faculty of Medicine of Palacký University, Olomouc Czech Republic*, *154*(3), 189–197. https://doi.org/10.5507/bp.2010.029

Prasko, J., Ociskova, M., Vanek, J., Burkauskas, J., Slepecky, M., Bite, I., Krone, I., Sollár, T., & Juskiene, A. (2022). Managing transference and countertransference in cognitive behavioral supervision: Theoretical framework and clinical application. *Psychology Research and Behavior Management*, *15*, 2129–2155. https://doi.org/10.2147/prbm.s369294

Rensko, M. (2017). Countertransference reactions to a suicidal patient. *The American Journal of Psychiatry Residents' Journal*, *12*(1), 18–19. https://doi.org/10.1176/appi.ajp-rj.2017.120106

Rojas, S. M., Leen-Feldner, E. W., Blumenthal, H., Lewis, S., & Feldner, M. T. (2014). Risk for suicide among treatment seeking adolescents: The role of positive and negative affect intensity. *Cognitive Therapy and Research*, *39*(2), 100–109. https://doi.org/10.1007/s10608-014-9650-8

Rosenberger, E. W., & Hayes, J. J. (2002). Origins, consequences, and management of countertransference: A case study. *Journal of Counseling Psychology*, *49*(2), 221–232. https://doi.org/10.1037/0022-0167.49.2.221

Shapiro, F. (1989). Efficacy of the eye movement desensitization procedure in the treatment of traumatic memories. *Journal of Traumatic Stress*, *2*(2), 199–223. https://doi.org/10.1002/jts.2490020207

Shapiro, F. (2001). The challenges of treatment evolution and integration. *American Journal of Clinical Hypnosis*. https://doi.org/10.1080/00029157.2001.10404275

Sheehan, L., Corrigan, P. W., Al-Khouja, M., Lewy, S., Major, D. R., Mead, J., Redmon, M., Rubey, C. T., & Weber, S. (2016). Behind closed doors. *Omega – Journal of Death and Dying*, *77*(4), 330–349. https://doi.org/10.1177/0030222816674215

Stroebe, M., & Schut, H. (1999). The dual process model of coping with bereavement: Rational and description. *Death Studies, 23*(3), 197–224. https://doi.org/10.1080/074811899201046

Taking care of yourself | NAMI: National Alliance on Mental Illness. (n.d.). www.nami.org/Your-Journey/Family-Members-and-Caregivers/Taking-Care-of-Yourself

Tedeschi, R. G., & Calhoun, L. G. (1996). The posttraumatic growth inventory: Measuring the positive legacy of trauma. *Journal of Traumatic Stress, 9*(3), 455–471. https://doi.org/10.1007/bf02103658

Tedeschi, R. G., & Calhoun, L. G. (2004). TARGET ARTICLE: "Posttraumatic growth: Conceptual foundations and empirical evidence." *Psychological Inquiry, 15*(1), 1–18. https://doi.org/10.1207/s15327965pli1501_01

Thompson, I. A., Amatea, E. S., & Thompson, E. (2014). Personal and contextual predictors of mental health counselors' compassion fatigue and burnout. *Journal of Mental Health Counseling, 36*(1), 58–77. https://doi.org/10.17744/mehc.36.1.p61m73373m4617r3

West, J. L., Liang, B., & Spinazzola, J. (2017). Trauma sensitive yoga as a complementary treatment for posttraumatic stress disorder: A qualitative descriptive analysis. *International Journal of Stress Management, 24*(2), 173–195. https://doi.org/10.1037/str0000040

Worden, W. (2004). *Grief counseling and grief therapy: A handbook for the mental health practitioner.* Springer.

Zero suicide (By Education Development Center). (2022). *Zerosuicide.edc.org.* Retrieved August 13, 2023, from https://zerosuicide.edc.org/

PART 2

ASSESSMENT, THEORY, AND TREATMENT OF YOUTH SUICIDE

CHAPTER 5

ASSESSMENT OF SUICIDE FOR YOUTH

Mary Ruth Cross and Leslie W. Baker

SUICIDAL IDEATION

Suicidal ideation refers to thinking about or planning suicide. The thoughts are on a continuum of severity from a wish to die with no method, plan, intent, or behavior to active suicidal ideation with a specific plan and intent (Posner et al., 2011). Suicidal thoughts appear in a "coming and going" fashion, causing the intensity and characteristics of such ideations to vary significantly. Healthcare professionals must understand the diverse nature of suicidal ideation, as it differs in intensity, duration, and form. Given that, no "typical" individual is prone to suicide. Likewise, there are no "typical" suicidal thoughts and ideations. Youth may initially present with suicidal ideation as a warning sign and play therapists and school counselors need to be vigilant in their assessment of suicidal ideation as they embark on the process of assessing youth for suicide.

Screening and Risk Assessment

One of the most challenging aspects of working in mental health with youth is discerning critical factors that impact the entire clinical picture. Screening tools are available to provide a quick look at a youth's level of risk; this can inform a clinician, play therapist, and school-based play therapist of a beginning picture of the situation, suggesting further action. It is crucial to provide an in-depth assessment of suicide beyond a screening tool to see the whole picture. Assessment of suicide takes skill and attention to multiple areas of a youth's life. In ideal circumstances, a play therapist or school counselor is given time to evaluate the child or adolescent before a major crisis. With sufficient time, it allows for a formal assessment to be provided. Assessing suicide risk includes gathering information from multiple sources and examining the client's complete personal history, mental health history, and suicide history.

A developmental history is recommended and can be obtained verbally or through intake. There are many standardized developmental assessments available. Here is a book recommendation for child and adolescent developmental assessments: *The Child Clinician's Handbook* by William G. Kronenberger and Meyer (2001). Clinical associations often provide clinical forms for obtaining a family history, including mental health history, the status of relationships, marriage or non-traditional couplings, births, deaths, and more; clinicians are advised to check with their professional affiliations for possible resources.

Many play therapists have access to electronic record systems (ERH), which may provide assessment forms that can offer intake histories and assessments. In some ERH systems, clinicians can customize these forms to suit specific needs, for example, an intake form tailored for suicide history, including prior attempts if a suicidal history is not provided. Suicide

DOI: 10.4324/9781003358565-7

history includes initial suicide attempts, reaction to attempts, lessons learned from previous attempts, perceived lethality/medical lethality, and probability of rescue.

Suicidal ideation refers to thinking about or planning suicide. The thoughts are assessed on the level of severity from a wish to die with no method, plan, intent, or behavior to active suicidal ideation with a specific plan and intent (Posner et al., 2011). Healthcare professionals must understand the diverse nature of suicidal ideation, as it differs In intensity, duration, and form. Given that there is no "typical" individual who is prone to suicide, likewise, there are no "typical" suicidal thoughts and ideations. Youth may initially present with suicidal ideation as a warning sign, and play therapists and school counselors must be vigilant in assessing suicidal ideation (Harmer et al., 2003).

Assessing a youth's family history can be gained through expressive play-based techniques. Although not designed explicitly for suicide assessment, these interventions effectively assist play therapists and school counselors in viewing family dynamics. They are engaging and creating an opportunity for youth and their families to use the brain's right hemisphere to obtain information that a verbal assessment may not access. The Family Play Genogram, created by Eliana Gil (2016), is an intervention adapted from McGoldrick et al. (1999) genogram wherein the client creates a visual diagram of their family members with an emphasis on understanding the interconnected nature of the family as a system. In Gil's adaptation, play therapists use a large piece of paper to create a genogram, drawing shapes for each family member. Traditionally, circles have represented females, and squares have represented males. Allowing each family member to create their own design for their family members corrects gender stereotyping. Once the shapes are drawn, the play therapist draws lines to connect the shapes, delineating the hierarchy: parents/caregivers, children/siblings, and the state of their relationships.

The Family Play Genogram brings a wealth of information to the family assessment. The play therapist asks each family member to select a figurine to represent themselves. Each figurine is placed within its corresponding shape on the genogram. This technique allows the play therapist to explore metaphors and suggest the character/creature might wish to share information.

This projective technique allows the play therapist to explore the metaphors the miniatures present and to ponder whether their character/creature might have a voice and whether the miniature wishes to share information, such as, "I see your tiger lying on its side. I wonder if 'Tiger' has a voice. What might 'Tiger' want to say?" The critical point is to stay in the metaphor of the character/creature. The play therapist should not interpret the miniature but rather watch, and if words are included, listen. Be curious about who chooses which character/creature, and as a play therapist, gaze upon the diagram and be curious about what the family is telling us.

As play therapists understand family dynamics in assessing suicidal youth, they will progress from gathering developmental history, family history, and suicidal history to assessing risk factors, protective factors, and warning signs.

RISK FACTORS

Risk factors can be identified as elements that weaken or impede the support system and the availability of necessary resources. The American Foundation for Suicide Prevention lists risk factors as characteristics or conditions that increase the likelihood of a person trying to take their life (*Risk Factors, Protective Factors and Warning Signs*, 2022). Risk factors vary depending on developmental as well as chronological age. Recognizing a risk factor as an issue to be taken seriously within the overall clinical picture may be difficult. For example, the death of a relative by suicide denotes a risk factor for a young child. Play therapists must look for patterns of behavior that gauge the risk of suicide or another clinical issue, e.g., patterns of personal behaviors and family history.

PROTECTIVE FACTORS

Once risk factors are examined, the clinician can conduct a further evaluation to enhance resources for young individuals. A protective environment can serve as a barrier to suicide.

The CDC has identified four protective factors for clinicians to examine and implement to prevent suicide (Risk and Protective Factors | Suicide | CDC, n.d.).

Individual Protective Factors

- Effective coping and problem-solving skills.
- Reasons for living (for example, family, friends, pets, etc.).
- Keen sense of cultural identity.

Relationship Protective Factors

- Support from partners, friends, and family.
- Feeling connected to others.

Community Protective Factors

- Feeling connected to school, community, and other social institutions.
- Availability of consistent and high-quality physical and behavioral healthcare.

Societal Protective Factors

- Reduced access to lethal means of suicide among people at risk.
- Cultural, religious, or moral objections to suicide.

WARNING SIGNS

Warning signs that may indicate a suicide attempt include a change in behavior or the presence of entirely new behaviors (Risk Factors, Protective Factors, and Warning Signs, 2022). Most youth who die by suicide show some warning signs; however, not all do, and not all youth who exhibit such behaviors are at risk for suicide. A study in the *Journal of Pediatrics* (Sheftall et al., 2016) showed that impulsivity may be a critical factor in the rate of suicide death among elementary-age children. The research indicated that younger children diagnosed with Attention Deficit Hyperactivity Disorder (ADHD) might be more likely to act on impulsive suicidal thoughts. On the other hand, older youth with mental health problems who died by suicide were more likely to have been diagnosed with depression than with ADHD. Warning signs in younger children can be more subtle and less noticeable than in adolescents. For example, a young child shouting, "I hate you! I do not want to be here any-more," after an argument with a parent, at first glance, may seem to be merely escalating a parent-child conflict. The child could be hinting at a more significant clinical issue requiring an assessment to determine the possibility of imminent suicide. As stated previously, it is essential to note that some children and adolescents who attempt suicide may not show any warning signs. Researchers identified the following factors for clinicians to consider when assessing younger children for suicidality: withdrawal, crying spells, becoming less verbal, and displaying a lack of interest in routine activities (Sheftall et al., 2016). In a 2022 study by Zortea et al., the researchers recommend that psychosocial assessment of suicide risk must explore, with sensitivity, the factors most relevant to the client and their circumstances (see Table 5.1). A psychosocial assessment allows for a deeper understanding of the client's situation and the risk of harm.

After gathering the multiple layers of family history, suicide history, risk factors, pro-tective factors, and warning signs, play therapists and educators can turn to formal clinical assessments to further determine the overall risk of suicide. A risk assessment tool enhances evaluation and can be used safely, provided the clinician knows the family history. Using such a tool without gathering all the previously mentioned information is strongly discour-aged. The following are a few clinical assessments in the literature that have demonstrated

Table 5.1 Suicide Risk Table

Low Suicide Risk	Moderate Suicide Risk	High Suicide Rate
No history of previous atempts. Mild thoughts of self-harm.	Elevated risk due to the presence of suicidal ideation, higher frequency of suicidal thoughts, enduring periods of suicidal ideation.	Elevated risk due to prior history of more than one attempt, presence of triggering event, current suicidal ideation, and social support is limited or absent.
Protective factors are present but there is demonstrated resilience, adequate adjustment, and the presence of hope.	Limited social network, presence of chronic stressors, coping strategies are compromised.	Preparation and planning activities for suicide attempts, history of self-harm behavior, poor stress tolerance, and presence of mental health problems.
No current suicidal ideation, but there may be some lingering chronic or acute factors present.	Presence of capability to attempt suicide, other disorders/problems present, chronic drug or alcohol use.	Sleep disturbance, increased agitation, irritation, isolating, giving away possessions.
Cultural Implications: access to mental health counseling, connection to the community, good problem- solving skills, contact with caregivers and significant others.	Cultural Implications: limited access to mental health counseling, a sense of separateness from the community and significant others, intermittent successful problem solving.	Cultural Implications: litle to no access to mental health care, disconnection from the community, and family, poor problem-solving skills and deepened sense of isolation.

reliability and validity. Further reading, training, and supervision before formal assessment tools are recommended.

SCREENING TOOLS

The Ask Suicide-Screening Questions (ASQ)

The Ask Suicide-Screening Questions (ASQ) is a concise instrument validated by the Joint Commission and suitable for all ages (Horowitz et al., 2012). In order to support the implementation of suicide risk screening, additional resources are available in the ASQ Toolkit. This toolkit, provided at no cost on the website jointcommission.org, is designed for use in medical settings such as emergency departments, inpatient medical/surgical units, and outpatient clinics/primary care. It aids healthcare providers by effectively identifying individuals at risk for suicide. The ASQ Toolkit includes versions tailored for youth and adults. Administering the ASQ involves asking four short screening questions that can be answered within 20 seconds (Horowitz et al., 2012).

Suicidal Behaviors Questionnaire-Revised (SBQ-R)

Osman et al. (2001) report that their empirical analyses of the Suicidal Behaviors Questionnaire-Revised (SBQ-R) offer substantial evidence supporting its efficacy as a reliable measure for assessing suicide risk and distinguishing between individuals at risk for suicide and those who are not. Both clinical and non-clinical settings recommend using the single SBQ-R Item 1 and SBQ-R total scores. The SBQ-R is a self-report questionnaire developed to identify risk factors associated with suicide in adolescents (ages 13–17) and adults. This four-item questionnaire assesses different aspects of suicidal behavior, including lifetime suicidal ideation and attempts, frequency of recent ideation, suicide threats, and the individual's self-assessment of the likelihood of future suicidal behavior (Osman et al., 2001). Each of the four items is rated on Likert scales of varying lengths, and the total scores range from 3 to 18 (Osman et al., 2001).

THE COLUMBIA PROTOCOL

The Columbia Protocol – Columbia Suicide Severity Rating Scale (C-SSRS) is a reputable measure of present suicidality that monitors the regression of symptoms over time. It was developed by Columbia University, the University of Pennsylvania, the University of Pittsburgh, and New York University to evaluate suicide risk. The Columbia Protocol questions have also been incorporated into the SAMHSA SAFE-T model with recommended triage categories (see document SAFE-T Protocol with C-SSRS –Recent). The risk assessment version provides a checklist of risk factors and protective factors for suicide, used along with the C-SSRS (The Columbia Lighthouse Project, 2022a).

Note that the C-SSRS Full version, without the risk assessment, is insufficient to qualify as an evidence-based suicide assessment process. Assessment of the risk and protective factors, in a structured or unstructured way, is required in addition to the suicide inquiry. The Columbia Lighthouse Project provides free online training (The Columbia Lighthouse Project, 2022b).

According to the Columbia Lighthouse website, a play therapist, school counselor, parent/caregiver, and others can use the tool without training. Organizations recommending the C-SSRS Risk Assessment version include the National Institute of Health (NIH), the Substance Abuse and Mental Health Service Administration (SAMHSA), The National Action Alliance for Suicide Prevention (Action Alliance), the Department of Defense, the CDC National Center for Injury Prevention and Control, and the United States Food and Drug Administration (FDA). Research by Posner et al. (2011) stated that the Columbia Lighthouse Project/Center for Suicide Risk Assessment provides evidence in C-SSRS. The supporting evidence was last revised on February 7, 2018. An example applying the C-SSRS to a case will be provided on pages 85 and 93.

Action Planning

As part of the suicide assessment, the therapist must consider the level of risk: high, medium, or low. The level of risk is assessed through clinical judgment and incorporating all other data, including cultural implications, personal circumstances, vulnerabilities, current stressors, history, and especially protective factors and warning signs. For example, having just a few warning signs but many protective factors would suggest a low-risk level. Having many warning signs but few protective factors would indicate an elevated level of risk for a suicide attempt. Play therapists should also note whether the identified risk factors can be reduced or modified. In addition, the therapist should examine what can be done to reduce the harms of the current risk factors, which allows for a clear path toward safety planning. The challenge for the therapist is not only to determine the level of risk but also to take appropriate steps to create safety.

Once the level of risk is assessed, the therapist turns to action (see Table 5.2).

This next step considers safety planning. The safety plan must discern whether hospitalization is recommended to ensure the child or adolescent is safe from self-harm or if sufficient measures can be taken in the home environment to ensure safety.

Safety planning follows a suicide risk assessment. Still, it can be done at any point during the assessment and treatment process. It is important to remember that a safety plan may not be appropriate if hospitalization is warranted, and the child or adolescent is at high risk for suicide or cannot understand and implement a safety plan. A Safety Plan is made for the child or adolescent's needs, including parents, teachers, or special care needs. The Safety Plan is constructed with the therapist and youth sitting side-by-side and with a cooperative, problem-solving approach, which focuses on developing a plan that includes coping strategies, resources, and a commitment to the treatment process and staying alive. In 1973, the original recommendation was that the therapist create a "no harm contract" with the client to ensure a suicide attempt would not be made; however, this was shown to be ineffective for the client and gave the therapist a false sense of security (Norton, 2018). No-harm contracts were used more frequently by the mid-1980s to aid suicide prevention in multiple settings, such as residential treatment, outpatient, and inpatient counseling. One major problem with no-harm contracts is that they are frequently used by individuals not sufficiently trained in mental health and the assessment of suicide.

For safety planning, the Suicide Prevention Resource Center (n.d.) recommends a six-step process. The Stanley-Brown Safety Plan from Two Penguins Studios, LLC is an application designed to aid in the formulation of a suicide safety plan, either independently by the user or collaboratively with a healthcare provider. The app facilitates crafting a

Table 5.2 Suicide Risk and Safety Table

Risk Factors	Protective Factors	Warning Signs	Intervention for Safety
Low Risk Few and modifiable risk factors are present	Strong protective factors are clear and present	Thoughts about death without a plan	Outpatient referral, reduction of symptoms, offer crisis / emergency numbers, connection with trusted caregivers
Medium Risk Multiple risk factors are present	Few protective factors are present	Ideation is current with a plan; however, the intent is not clear	Develop a safety plan with not only precautions but crisis planning included, consider possible hospitalization
High Risk Multiple risk factors are present	Protective factors are not present or are minimal and insufficient at best	Lethal means are available and accessible, and persistent thoughts of suicide with intent is clear	Hospitalization is recommended

succinct emergency plan using the user's language, outlining a network of supports and coping mechanisms to deploy during instances of severe distress or suicidal crises.

1. *Warning Signs*: Using the client's words, list warning signs such as images, thinking processes, moods, and behaviors.

2. *Internal Coping Strategies*: Assess the likelihood of using the safety plan in a collaborative and problem-solving manner so that obstacles and roadblocks can be identified while giving alternative coping strategies to remove the obstacles.

3. *Social Contacts Who May Distract from the Crisis*: List places where the client can safely be around others. List people and other social settings that might work if the first option does not. Continue to assess and plan for obstacles to using this step.

4. *Family Members or Friends Who May Offer Help*: List several people with contact information that the client can reach out to and safely reveal their state of crisis to get appropriate help and care. Role-play or rehearse with the client to improve the likelihood of the client using this step if needed. Continue to assess and plan for obstacles to using this step.

5. *Professionals and Agencies to Contact for Help*: List names and contact information with locations of therapists, urgent care services, Suicide Prevention Hotline number, and other emergency service providers. Role-play and rehearse with the client using this step to improve the likelihood of the client using this step if needed. Continue to assess and plan for obstacles to using this step.

6. *Making the Environment Safe*: Working collaboratively with the client, identify how the client would attempt suicide. Identify ways to limit access to lethal means and secure lethal objects away from the youth.

(Stanley & Brown, 2012)

The safety plan is a guide to managing the client through a crisis. The safety plan needs to be easily accessible so that when there are any thoughts of self-harm, the youth can find opportunities to be safe.

Suicidal ideation and attempts in children and adolescents present differently than they do for the broader population; therefore, therapists must remain aware and vigilant in identifying risk factors and warning signs for youth to implement an effective safety plan (Carbone et al., 2019).

Forster (2016) found disturbing evidence that demonstrated the lack of willingness by medical professionals and others to ask about suicide. If we do not ask, we cannot find out. Difficulties in establishing screening of suicide in medical environments encompass time limitations, handling patients who test positive, unease in discussing suicide-related inquiries, and the associated social stigma. Screening, particularly for youths, can serve as an intervention since it might mark their initial opportunity to openly express distressing thoughts to a trusted figure. Moreover, parents are often unaware of their child's suicidal ideation. (Horowitz et al., 2020). All we must do is simply engage in an honest and sensitive conversation where essential questions are asked. We must engage the at-risk adolescent in honest, sensitive conversation and ask essential questions.

NON-HOSPITALIZATION

When considering hospitalization, a play therapist and a school counselor must determine whether a child or adolescent is in imminent danger to themselves or others. However, the ultimate decision is up to trained law enforcement officers, crisis team members, or contract employees with the final say on placing a 5585 hold on a minor (CA Welf & Inst Code § 5585.50, 2022).

A 5585 refers to the Welfare and Institutions Code under California State Law, which allows the involuntary detainment of a minor experiencing a mental health crisis. Although play therapists and school counselors can provide a suicide risk assessment, most are not authorized to issue a 5585. These contracts are generally set up with law enforcement, crisis teams, or emergency room personnel contracting for services. Again, each state and each county will vary. A play therapist and school counselor must be familiar with the crisis system for children and adolescents where they are practicing. Suppose a play therapist and school counselor have determined by their assessment that a child or adolescent is at high risk. They must not leave the youth alone; they must contact parents or caregivers and call the 988 to reach the National Suicide Lifeline, a 24/7 suicide crisis line, which will, in turn, contact local services. If 922 is unavailable, call 911 for emergency support services. A 24/7 crisis line is available to all, provided the crisis occurs within the local area. If the youth is out of the state, it is best to contact law enforcement in the area where the child or adolescent is in imminent danger. For example, if a play therapist from San Diego is attending a conference in Chicago, Illinois, and their adolescent client calls them stating they are suicidal, the therapist would call San Diego law enforcement and notify them of an imminent suicidal issue and then call the parent and caregivers for immediate response to protect the adolescent. Keep the child or adolescent on the phone. In most cases, the 911 operator cannot transfer a call from one state to another (*911-Frequently Asked Questions*, 2023). Using a landline to call 911 is recommended as the centers often cannot call back on cell phone lines, and calls cannot be routed beyond the local area (*911-Frequently Asked Questions*, 2023) delaying response times.

Once a play therapist or school counselor has called in law enforcement or a crisis team for further assessment, the emergency personnel will privately provide an onsite evaluation with the client, if possible. They may also wish to speak to the school counselor or play therapist separately, leaving another officer or crisis team member with the client to determine the screening tools used to assess the high-risk level. In some cases, a child or adolescent may rescind their threats of suicide and deny they have thoughts or behaviors of suicidality when the crisis team or law enforcement is assessing them. Play therapists, school counselors, and parents/caregivers may be interviewed to gather the complete picture. Sometimes, it is determined not to hospitalize a youth. It is crucial to keep a record in the progress notes of what occurred and why the play therapist or school counselor decided to involve law enforcement or the crisis team. Document the situation in full: record the information received from the client, explain the decisions made, speak to the clinician or officer, take down their opinions and conclusions, report the client's response to the actions taken, make a record of any information that is relevant to the case. If the information is not recorded, in the eyes of the law and ethics, it does not happen. Be sure to include the client's progress notes.

Now what? The professionals and parents/caregivers may feel disrupted, worried, and at a loss for what to do next. Proceeding from this point forward can be difficult for all involved. The first step is to develop a safety plan for the child or adolescent to follow should they again feel at risk of suicide (see case example that follows.) This plan is for youth and should be shared with the parents/caregivers. It is critical to tell the adults caring for the youth to remove any means for self-harm accessible to children and adolescents, including belts, ties, robes, shoelaces, and all sharp objects, and remove and lock up any medicines, including over-the-counter medications. Remove firearms and ammunition from the residence – simply locking guns up is not enough because many youths often have watched closely and not only know where the weapon is but know how to unlock the cases. Also, it is essential to communicate to the parents/caregivers that they must always supervise the youth. In these cases, having the youth sleep in the same room as the adult may be necessary as long as child abuse is not suspected. The parents/caregivers must hide their car keys and find lockboxes for the other unsafe items.

Keep the youth safe; a parent/caregiver may need to take a day or two off work until the suicidal crisis passes. Finding a caregiver is sometimes impossible; finding a relative or caregiver may work. The key here is supervision. Finding a community center that provides daily care for youth may provide some respite for parents/caregivers if the center understands the needs of the youth. It is crucial to set up an appointment for the child or adolescent to see their play therapist as soon as possible; sometimes, increasing play sessions to twice a week may be warranted, and if they are already seeing a psychiatrist, schedule a follow-up appointment. If the child and adolescent have not yet been seen or assessed by a psychiatrist, this crisis may be the time to set up the referral. Chapter 3 addresses why and how to refer to a psychiatrist. The parent/caregivers are asked to contact 988, the local law enforcement/crisis team, or 911 if the crisis returns to an imminent level. How do parents/caregivers know if an imminent crisis is facing them? The Columbia Protocol, also called the Columbia-Suicide Severity Rating Scale (C-SSRS), facilitates the evaluation of suicide risk by utilizing a set of straightforward questions in everyday language anyone can ask (The Columbia Lighthouse Project, 2022a). The responses to these questions aid in determining if an individual is at risk of suicide, evaluating the seriousness and urgency of that risk, and understanding the level of support required. Users of the tool inquire about the following:

- Whether the person has experienced thoughts of suicide and the time frame of those thoughts (suicidal ideation).
- Whether the person took any actions to prepare for suicide and when those actions occurred.
- Whether previous suicide attempts or any ongoing suicide attempts were interrupted by someone else or halted by the person.

The questions used in the Columbia Protocol utilize straightforward and concise language to encourage honest and unambiguous responses. For instance, the questioner may ask:

1. "Have you wished you were dead or wished you could go to sleep and not wake up?"
2. "Have you been thinking about how you might kill yourself?"
3. "Have you taken any steps toward making a suicide attempt or preparing to kill yourself (such as collecting pills, getting a gun, giving valuables away, or writing a suicide note)?"

(The Columbia Lighthouse Project, 2022a)

To optimize the effectiveness and efficiency of the Columbia Protocol, organizations can establish specific criteria or thresholds to determine appropriate actions based on the assessment of each individual. Decisions regarding hospitalization, counseling, referrals, and other necessary measures are guided by the responses of "yes" or "no" to the protocol questions and other factors, such as the recent occurrence of suicidal thoughts and behaviors (The Columbia Lighthouse Project, 2022a). Play therapists, educators, parents/caregivers, and others can find the Columbia Protocol on the website provided in the references. The Columbia Protocol is also available in an application form on Google and iPhone app stores. As noted previously, the clinicians are required to document their progress notes. Be clear and specific. What protocol was followed? How was risk assessed? Why was the crisis team or law enforcement brought in to evaluate a potential 5585? Documentation is essential for treatment, evaluation of the process, and moving forward in the treatment plan.

HOSPITALIZATION

Sometimes, an emergency hospitalization assessment is necessary to ensure client safety. Calling law enforcement or a crisis team may result in faster admittance. The need for hospitalization will be determined based on the child's developmental level, family support, parental resources, and the local hospital's programming for children. Generally speaking, child and adolescent facilities are more likely to offer programs specific to the needs of suicidal youth than large, all-purpose hospitals. Brief suicide interventions, expressive play therapy, CBT, and DBT interventions are generally delivered in a group format, which will be discussed in Chapter 6, Treatment. Parents should provide information on the child's symptoms, behavioral changes, and anything else to assist in the evaluation.

There is always the potential for a traumatizing impact on the child or adolescent due to the complexities of transport and hospitalization. As play therapists, we must keep this in mind. Suppose the indicators show that involuntary hospitalization is needed. In that case, the child or adolescent can be held in the hospital for varying amounts of time as determined by each state. In California, a 5585 can be issued for a 23 to 72-hour psychiatric hold on any minor (under 18 years of age) who displays a credible threat to their safety. If evidence of continued imminent harm to self or others exists, a "5585" can be extended for ten to 14 days without the consent of the parents or guardians. Professionals providing the assessment may request another extended stay, at most 30 days. In certain situations, the individual in charge may be able to recommend a further extension, which would be, at most, 180 days. Parents and caregivers are involved in the process, and if a minor does not have a parent or caregiver, a court will appoint a custodian for the child or adolescent. Although the term "5585" is specific to California, most states have laws concerning involuntary emergency holds for individuals with psychiatric needs. Each state has guidelines regarding the duration of these emergency holds, the authorized individuals who can initiate them, and the patient's rights during the hold. Despite these variations from state to state, there are overarching consistencies regarding these holds. All 50 states and the District of Columbia permit emergency holds to be placed on individuals who pose a danger to themselves or others. While most states specify that the risk must be related to mental illness, others may not have such a requirement. Generally, it is necessary to demonstrate that the threat is imminent, indicating that the individual has the means and the plan to carry it out.

In the hospital, a youth is provided with a general physical exam by a doctor and a psychiatric evaluation by a qualified psychiatrist, which can assess the possible need for medication for mood stabilization and reduction of suicidal ideation. Youth's clothing is reviewed for safety: no shoes, laces, ties from sweatpants, belts, or sharps are allowed. Due to developmental differences and needs, the facilities often have separate wings for children and adolescents.

Confiscated items will be stored at the hospital and returned upon discharge. Youth are provided a bed, meals, and an in-room bathroom with a shower. Programming begins when the doctor assesses the child or adolescent. The young are fed and shown to their bed, often sharing a room with another client, depending on the availability of beds at the facility.

Depending on the facility, programming can include groups that apply expressive play-based therapies, Cognitive Behavioral Therapy (CBT), or Dialectical Behavioral Therapy (DBT). Many facilities have very little funding and may only offer supervision and no inpatient treatment other than physical and psychiatric evaluations. Most facilities do not allow any visitation on the first day of the hold to allow the youth to settle into the new environment and be evaluated. However, professionals providing the assessments may be in direct contact with parents/caregivers to obtain critical information about the child or adolescent, depending on how they were brought into the facility. Youths brought in through emergent means, crisis assessment via crisis teams, and by law enforcement through emergency rooms may have gathered only a minimal amount of information for the inpatient facility. However, in some cases, youth are evaluated onsite at the psychiatric facility by their social workers, and this can allow for a breadth and depth in the information gathering not possible during a crisis. Once onsite assessments are completed and time allows, the facilities offer visitation and connect with parents/caregivers to learn family histories, suicidal histories, and health histories.

AFTERCARE

Once the client has been stabilized and suicide is no longer imminent, the social worker will provide a discharge plan. A family member will likely receive a call to schedule an outpatient appointment with their play therapist upon release from the hospital unless safety concerns lead to more intensive care, such as intensive outpatient programs (IOP) or other clinical environments like a residential treatment program or a treatment center.

Suppose stabilization of the client's mental health is needed, and suicide risk continues to be moderate to high. In that case, residential care may be required for discharge planning. These programs can be expensive; however, some insurance companies may cover this service. If the child is a foster child who has been adopted, funds may be available through the local county to help defray the costs. Residential care is used for profoundly severe cases like those with dual diagnoses (i.e., mental health and substance abuse disorder). Outpatient programs are often three to five days a week and offer coping skills using expressive play-based interventions, CBT, DBT, and some offer family involvement and support. It is common for psychiatric treatment to include psychotropic medications to reduce depression and anxiety and manage suicidal ideation, whether in IOP, residential, or outpatient therapy.

Additional support and aftercare options are found in schools with support groups, academic accommodations, Individual Education Plans (IEPs), or 504 plans. An Individualized Education Program (IEP) is defined within the *Individuals with Disabilities Education Act*, special education legislation. The main objective of an IEP is to assess the strengths and weaknesses of a student with disabilities and to establish a detailed plan outlining the specific educational services the school will provide to support the student's academic progress (U.S. Department of Education, 2019).

Compared to the Individuals with Disabilities Education Act (IDEA), Section 504 has a broader definition of disability. So, even if the child is not eligible for an IEP, a 504 plan may still be able to provide accommodations. Ideally, when the appropriate school, medical, and mental health professionals involved with the child or adolescent work cooperatively as a treatment team, the prospect for safety and suicide prevention increases. The parents and caregivers need to consent to release confidential information so that the treatment team can work together for the common good and safety of the child or adolescent (U.S. Department of Education, 2019).

Jennah had been engaging in play therapy for two years due to her parents' high-conflict divorce and emotional abuse by her father. The therapeutic alliance was well established, and 8-year-old Jennah allowed the healing power of play to help her adjust to her parent's divorce. She could identify her feelings and express herself well enough to meet her needs. She had been able to work through many of the traumatic events she had experienced with her father to increase a sense of safety in her life and have healthier family and peer relationships. Some improvements in her functioning and mental health were accomplished by limiting the time spent with her father. It was hard to imagine then that this child could start to believe that the only way to be safe and free from her intense fear was to kill herself.

There is a documented history that Jennah's father was quick-tempered. When treatment began, Jennah's father was forced by his employer to either go into a substance abuse recovery facility for alcoholism or lose his job. After he returned from the program, he was granted supervised visits. The father was inconsistent in making the supervised visits and staying connected with Jennah, but when the visits occurred, Jennah reported that she enjoyed her time with her dad.

Then, one day, Jennah came into her play therapy session and said she was mad at her dad because he had cheated while playing a game with her. Jennah is a very bright and aware child, so she pointed out the cheating behavior to her dad. Dad's response was to deny it and then make a "scary mad" face that the visitation supervisor did not see. Jennah's play behavior in her sessions became more aggressive, and she expressed frustration. She often voiced bewilderment about how her father was treating her. She asked her therapist why someone would lie "to their kid." Shortly after this, Jennah's dad was granted unsupervised visits, including overnight visits every weekend. Jennah went from seeing her father intermittently and for a limited period in a safe environment to extended stays without protection.

Jennah had a secure attachment to her mother. She trusted her to keep her safe. The father's continued anger at Jennah's mother was evident. To Jennah, there was no place safe enough anymore, and no one could protect her. Jennah spiraled into depression and anxiety. She had difficulty sleeping, refused to sleep in her bed with her mother, called her mother repeatedly while with her father, and cried when her father would not let her see her mother during her soccer games. This behavior made her father incredibly angry, calling Jennah names and saying she was "weak and a baby." Her father emotionally bullied Jennah. Jennah later reported that her father threatened to kill her mother if she said anything about what happened during their visits.

Jennah began refusing to go on the visits, but due to the court orders in place, Jennah had to go. This pushed Jennah further into despair. She said, "Maybe it would be better if I were gone." At school, she engaged in risky plays, like jumping off the highest point of the play structure. Then, one day, when she was supposed to see her father after school, Jennah jabbed a sharp pencil into her leg. She told her teacher she had been playing around, and it slipped. On another day, she rubbed a pair of scissors repeatedly across her arm, leaving visible scratches. Jennah started getting additional support services at school, but her comments about death and dying continued. In her play therapy, she told her therapist that the only thing that would make her feel better was not to see her dad. Jennah's mother worked diligently with her attorney to put protections in place for Jennah but was thwarted in court. The court saw the problem as a custody dispute and neglected Jennah's need for protection.

As things escalated for Jennah, and all attempts to help protect her seemed to fail, her father continued to demand the visits as ordered by the courts. However, there was also a pattern of inconsistent follow-through by the father in ensuring the scheduled visits occurred regularly. Jennah's play behavior showed a child who was shutting down and depressed.

Jennah had many mixed feelings about her relationship with her father. She longed for a kind and playful father but was also very afraid of the father who called her names and always seemed angry at her mother. One day, Jennah told her play therapist that her father was outside the office and that he had called the police to make sure he was able to have the scheduled visit. Jennah escalated into intense fear and said she would try to kill herself if she went with him. The play therapist tried to support Jennah by finding resources to help her. The police officer declined to make any protective steps for Jennah as he indicated this was a custody dispute and not a serious suicide threat.

The therapist reiterated that Jennah had said she would hurt herself if she went with her father. Jennah's fear and anxiety were palpable. The police officer convinced the father to let Jennah go home with her mother and calm down. After this, Jennah's mother returned to court with documentation from school personnel, the school resource officer, the therapist, and medical personnel who evaluated Jennah for possible hospitalization and were able to reverse the previous visitation orders. Jennah's father was allowed phone or video chat conversations with Jennah at prescribed times so they could work on the relationship and Jennah could feel safer. Jennah's father has never called.

One of the difficulties in this case was that so many adults and professionals in Jennah's life did not want to believe that a child this young could honestly be suicidal. The warning signs were there long before Jennah was taken seriously. Thanks to protective measures taken over the month that Jennah was actively suicidal, a tragedy was prevented from happening.

INTERVENTIONS

As Jennah's suicidal ideation became more evident, she engaged with her therapist to create the *Land of Safety* (Cross, 2023), using markers, stickers, and die-cuts of street warning signs, such as a STOP or YIELD sign. These supplies were used to create a game board that identified specific warning signs present for Jennah when thinking about hurting herself. Jennah took on the player role and was represented by a marker whose path was drawn out with separate spaces to step on. In each of the spaces is written a directive, a warning sign, or a protective factor (i.e., "Go ahead one space" or "When I think about going to my dad's house, I get scared" or "I can tell my mom I thought about hurting myself"). The game's goal is to reach "The Land of Safety." Some spaces will have obstacles delaying arrival at the Land of Safety, and some will have a coping strategy for managing the warning sign. The stickers and street sign die-cuts decorate the game board and act as part of the path to the Land of Safety. Once the board game was created and set up, Jennah was asked to choose a sand tray miniature for herself and the therapist to use while playing. Jennah and her therapist took turns rolling the dice and moving along the game board. As the play continued, Jennah was able to participate in assessing her warning signs and begin to focus on positive coping strategies.

One of the dynamics of warning signs is that it can be challenging to ascertain them. Cognitive Behavioral Play Therapy (CBPT) is an excellent theoretical framework for understanding clients' perceptions of suicide. Using the metaphor of how puzzling warning signs can seem, Jennah used the "Puzzling Warnings Intervention" (Figure 5.1, Baker & Cross, 2019) to continue identifying those places and circumstances when she felt unsafe and the thoughts of hurting herself were present. Jennah was given a pre-cut blank puzzle form (a simple handout of a blank puzzle is suggested). Jennah then drew pictures, images, and words from the warning signs she and her therapist had identified onto the blank puzzle pieces. Jennah proudly showed her mother her puzzle at the end of her play therapy session. Jennah was encouraged to take her puzzle apart and put it back together again as often as she liked. Her mother said she could leave it on the coffee table for accessibility.

Due to the high conflict in her family, getting sufficient support from the courts to protect Jennah was exceedingly difficult. Identifying prevention strategies with Jennah was paramount to increasing safety. Jennah created the "BEE SAFE Poster" (Baker, 2019) with the

Talk briefly with your client **to identify and draw out**
warning signs the client can
become more aware of in their puzzle.

Each Participant

1. Using the Puzzle Template

2. Create a picture of warning signs. Choose one
   important warning sign or a few signs to draw on
   the puzzle form. *You can choose more than one.*

3. Decorate the puzzle form.

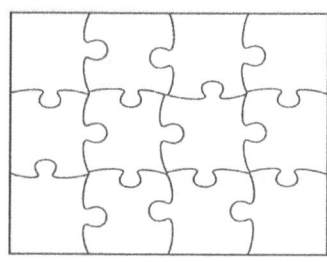

Figure 5.1 Puzzling Warnings

help of her therapist. The BEE SAFE Poster is an expressive art and play-based intervention that helps younger children create a safety plan (see Figure 5.2). The BEE SAFE Poster includes identifying the critical components of safety and suicide prevention. Topics to put on the BEE SAFE Poster, with examples of each, are:

1. My Self-Care Saying – "I want to be safe so I can be me."
2. My Calmers/Get Your Relax On – Read a book, blow bubbles.
3. My Helpers – Mom, Dad, Teacher, Friend, etc.
4. What Do Helpers Do for Me? – Play with me, go for a walk with me, read a book to me.
5. Busy Bee Hands/Busy Bee Brain – Draw, bounce a ball, play a game, make a puppet, and tell a story.
6. My Safe Places to BEE! – At school, with my friends, in my room, on the playground.

Jennah was given a large piece of blank paper. Poster size is ideal, but any large size of paper will do. Then, using die-cuts (or clipart from the internet) of bees, clouds, and stars, each topic is written on the die-cut and placed on the poster. Stars are used for My Self Care Sayings; Bees are used for My Calmers; Busy Hands/Busy Brain and Clouds are used for My Helpers and What Do Helpers Do for Me.

SAFE PLACES TO BEE!

Play engages the child or adolescent in assessing and working through suicidal thoughts and behaviors through the therapeutic power of play. Jennah used a combination of play and expressive arts interventions to rest her overwhelming feelings of fear and anxiety. She is now able to look forward to a life fully lived. Jennah's mother was a key player throughout

BEE Safe Poster – Safety Plan For Younger Children

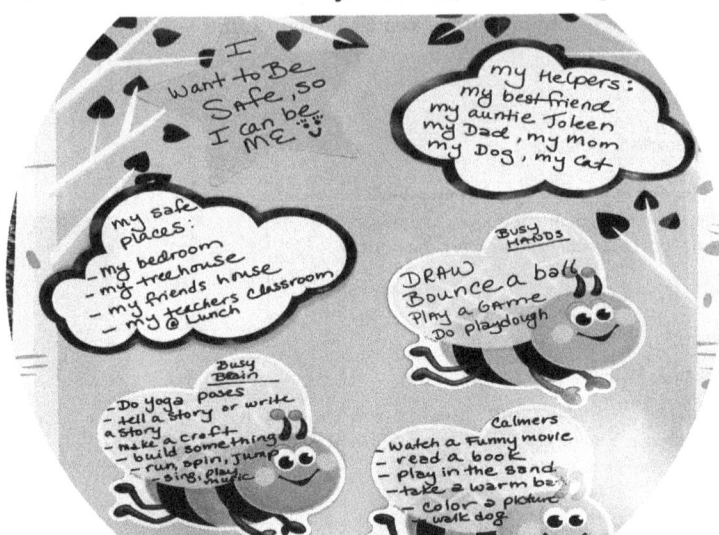

Figure 5.2 Bee Safe Poster

Source: © 2020 Baker, L. *ALL RIGHTS RESERVED.* Baker, L. (2019, October). BEE SAFE Poster Intervention [Conference Session]. Suicide Prevention, Assessment & Treatment of Traumatic Grief for Children & Teens in Play Therapy. International Association of Play Therapy Conference. Dallas, TX.

treatment, helping create a more profound sense of safety and helping the therapist understand the family system and how Jennah responded.

SIX PART STORY MAKING (6PSM)

The following is an example of an assessment strategy that engages play and expressive arts through storytelling to open up a deeper understanding of the child's or adolescent's world. Six Part Story Making (6PSM) was introduced to the play therapy community in 1992 following several years of experimental use, which involved collaboration with Alida Gersie, who first shared the method with Mooli Lahad as early as 1984.

Initially, the purpose of Six Part Story Making was not intended to be an assessment tool. Instead, it was developed within the framework of Dramatherapy as a creative approach to constructing stories and exploring their dramatic and therapeutic potential for individuals and groups.

The 6PSM employs seven levels of analysis to generate a comprehensive understanding of the client's world, encompassing both conscious and unconscious aspects (Lahad & Dent-Brown, 2012; Lahad, 2017). According to Lahad and Dent-Brown, using the 6PSM as an assessment tool involves encouraging the client to construct a fictional story drawing inspiration from fairytales and mythology. This process allows for a deeper understanding of how individuals view their existence and the world around them. The 6PSM enables the therapist to evaluate the picture story the youth drew on seven levels to allow a multi-level understanding of the youth (Lahad et al., 2013).

THE PLAN

Level one – *The coping style*: What are the client's strengths? What are the related languages that have the potential to facilitate change and personal growth? To what degree do coping styles therapeutic sessions? Are there underlying matters of trust or mistrust that need to be addressed?

Level two – *Themes*: How do clients' core beliefs affect their well-being? How would these beliefs influence the therapeutic relationship? Do they lean towards optimism or pessimism? Does their worldview have an age-related theme?

Level three – *Here and Now Questions*: Do they present a challenge for me as a compassionate adult? Am I prepared to tackle them? How can I attentively listen to these questions during their story?

Level four – *Conflicts*: Are the conflicts specific to the client's age group? Have the conflicts in the story emerged during any therapy sessions? Do some of these conflicts serve as the underlying cause of the client's distress? Can the therapist identify any behaviors that may be indicative of these conflicts?

Level five – *Developmental Stage*: What particular stage of development is reflected in the story? What are the anticipated developmental milestones and tasks associated with this psychological phase?

Level six – *The Quest*: How can I interpret the hero's quest within the context of the therapeutic process?

Level seven – *Symbols*: Utilize a symbol interpretation website or book to examine and contrast the meaning ascribed to a particular symbol with its significance within the story, intersecting with conflicts.

(Lahad et al., 2013, pp. 8–10)

To ensure the integrity of the assessment, the therapist must avoid asking leading questions that may guide the client's narrative toward a specific direction or theme. Story-making is presented to the client as a means for them to communicate their thoughts and experiences more effectively. However, they will be asked six questions intended to distance the story from their own life as much as possible and to create a main character who is dissimilar to themselves. This story provides the ideal setting for the projection process and allows children and adolescents the safety needed to share their internal stories more freely.

The play therapist directs the youth or adolescent to fold an 8.5"×11" piece of paper into six boxes or draw six boxes on the sheet to appear like a comic strip or a storyboard. It is recommended to gain a release of information from the youth's parent/caretaker to audio or video record so the story can be transcribed for evaluation.

Using a pencil, colored pencils, pen, or fine-tipped felt pens, have the child or adolescent draw in each square a response to each of these six questions in each section of the paper. Remind the youth that this is an original story that has never been told.

EXAMPLE OF ASSESSMENT OF A SIX PARTS STORY

The original six questions (Lahad, 1997) are:

1. Who is (are) the main character/s (hero/heroine)?

2. What is the task or mission of the main character/s?
3. Who or what can help (if at all)?
4. What is the obstacle in the way, or what prevents the event from happening?
5. How does/do the main character/s cope with the obstacle?
6. What happens next, or how does the story end?

(Lahad, 1997, p. 10)

Once the story has been transcribed, the therapist asks the six questions and reviews the picture story on the seven levels. We recommend Lahad and Dent-Brown's (2012) *Six-Piece Story-Making Revisited* to see a full illustration of this model and how to complete a full assessment using this technique. The goal of the 6PSM is to provide a comprehensive view of the child or adolescent client and their world. The play therapist has the opportunity to evaluate the story of the youth through the seven levels that Lahad et al. (2013) provided. The review can create an exploration into the child's methods of coping with the present, moving forward, and surviving when survival feels tenuous. Expressive play-based interventions assist therapists and school counselors by enabling youth to externalize emotional pain, search the self for coping skills, and nurture resilience in the internal human spirit.

Expressive play therapy interventions allow youth to go beyond words to explore feelings, thoughts, and body sensations, which are part of the processing of suicidality. Unlocking these painful and disturbing STBs can assist the children and adolescents in collaborating with the play therapist and school counselor through trust in the therapeutic bond to find their way back to preferring life over death, connection instead of disconnection. Parents and caregivers can continue to apply expressive interventions at home and continue the bonds, build attachments, and protect and grow a safe and stable environment for them to flourish.

CONCLUSION

A thorough assessment of all areas impacting a child or adolescent's mental health is critical in managing a potential suicide. Assessment includes identifying and understanding the complexities of suicidal risks and warning signs specific to children and adolescents to implement effective coping and preventive strategies. Play-based interventions can be effective when treating at-risk youth. Mental health workers, educators, medical personnel, and law enforcement personnel must not be afraid to ask clear and direct questions (which include the word "suicide" when applicable) to ensure that the right course of action is taken to improve safety. All these professionals can work together as a team to help prevent youth suicide.

REFERENCES

911-Frequently asked questions. (2023, March 23). National 911 Program. Retrieved March 31, 2024, from https://www.911.gov/calling-911/frequently-asked-questions/

Baker, L. (2019, October). *BEE SAFE poster intervention* [Conference Session]. Suicide Prevention, Assessment & Treatment of Traumatic Grief for Children & Teens in Play Therapy. International Association of Play Therapy Conference, Dallas, TX.

Baker, L., & Cross, M. R. (2019, November). *Puzzle warnings intervention* [Conference Session]. Suicide Prevention & Risk Assessment: What Play Therapists Need to Know. Expressive Therapies Summit, New York, NY. CA Welf & Inst Code § 5585.50 (2022).

Carbone, J. T., Holzer, K. J., & Vaughn, M. G. (2019, March). Child and adolescent suicidal ideation and suicide attempts: Evidence from the healthcare cost and utilization project. *The Journal of Pediatrics*, *206*, 225–231. https://doi.org/10.1016/j.jpeds.2018.10.017\

Cross, M. R. (2023). *Land of safety intervention*. [Board Game] [Unpublished Game].

Forster, C. (2016, March). The first step in preventing suicide is to ask. *The Journal of Pediatrics*, *170*, 1–4. https://doi.org/10.1016/j.jpeds.2016.01.009

Gil, E. (2016). *Play in family therapy* (2nd ed.). Guilford Publications.

Harmer, B., Lee, S., Duong, T. V. H., & Saadabadi, A. (2023). Suicidal ideation. In *StatPearls*. StatPearls Publishing.

Horowitz, L. M., Bridge, J. A., Teach, S. J., Ballard, E. D., Klima, J., Rosenstein, D. L., Wharff, E. A., Ginnis, K., Cannon, E., Joshi, P. T., & Pao, M. (2012). Ask Suicide-Screening Questions (ASQ). *Archives of Pediatrics & Adolescent Medicine*, *166*(12), 1170. https://doi.org/10.1001/archpediatrics.2012.1276

Horowitz, L. M., Tipton, M. V., & Pao, M. (2020). Primary and secondary prevention of youth suicide. *Pediatrics*, *145*(Supplement_2), S195–S203. https://doi.org/10.1542/peds.2019-2056h

Kronenberger, W. G., & Meyer, R. G. (2001). *The child clinician's handbook*. Addison-Wesley Longman.

Lahad, M. (1997). The story as a guide to metaphoric processes. In S. Jennings (Ed.), *Dramatherapy theory and practice* (Vol. 3, pp. 31–42). Routledge. *(1) (PDF) Six-Piece Story-Making Revisited*. Retrieved October 1, 2023 from: www.researchgate.net/publication/216774303_Six-Piece_Story-Making_Revisited

Lahad, M. (2017). From victim to victor: The development of the BASIC PH model of coping and resiliency. *Traumatology*, *23*(1), 27–34. https://doi.org/10.1037/trm0000105

Lahad, M., & Dent-Brown, K. (2012). Six-piece story-making revisited. *ResearchGate*. www.researchgate.net/publication/216774303_Six-Piece_Story-Making_Revisited

Lahad, M., Shacham, M., & Ayalon, O. (2013). *The "BASIC Ph" model of coping and resiliency: Theory, research, and cross-cultural application*. Jessica Kingsley Publishers.

McGoldrick, M., Gerson, R., & Shellenberger, S. (1999). *Genograms: Assessment and intervention*. W.W. Norton.

Norton, K. (2018). *No harm contracts.pdf*. The Connection Program. Retrieved September 19, 2022, from: https://theconnectprogram.org/wpcontent/uploads/2018/11/NoHarmContracts.pdf

Osman, A., Bagge, C. L., Gutierrez, P. M., Konick, L. C., Kopper, B. A., & Barrios, F. X. (2001). The Suicidal Behaviors Questionnaire-Revised (SBQ-R): Validation with clinical and nonclinical samples. *Assessment*, *8*(4), 443–454. https://doi.org/10.1177/107319110100800409

Posner, K., Brown, G. M., Stanley, B., Brent, D. A., Yershova, K., Oquendo, M. A., Currier, G. W., Melvin, G. A., Greenhill, L. L., Shen, S., & Mann, J. J. (2011). The Columbia–Suicide Severity Rating Scale: Initial validity and internal consistency findings from three multisite studies with adolescents and adults. *American Journal of Psychiatry*, *168*(12), 1266–1277. https://doi.org/10.1176/appi.ajp.2011.10111704

Risk and Protective Factors | Suicide | CDC. (n.d.). Retrieved September 10, 2022, from www.cdc.gov/suicide/factors/index.html

Sheftall, A. H., Asti, L., Horowitz, L. M., Felts, A., Fontanella, C. A., Campo, J. V., & Bridge, J. (2016). Suicide in elementary school-aged children and early adolescents. *Pediatrics*, *138*(4). https://doi.org/10.1542/peds.2016-0436

Stanley, B., & Brown, G. M. (2012). Safety planning intervention: A brief intervention to mitigate suicide risk. *Cognitive and Behavioral Practice*, *19*(2), 256–264. https://doi.org/10.1016/j.cbpra.2011.01.001

Suicide Prevention Resource Center. (n.d.). https://sprc.org/

The Columbia Lighthouse Project. (2022a, October 13). *About the protocol the Columbia lighthouse project*. The Columbia Lighthouse Project. https://cssrs.columbia.edu/the-columbia-scale-c-ssrs/about-the-scale/

The Columbia Lighthouse Project. (2022b, October 13). *About the protocol the Columbia lighthouse project*. The Columbia Lighthouse Project. https://cssrs.columbia.edu/training/training-options/

U.S. Department of Education. (2019, August 30). *Guide to the individualized education program*. U.S. Department of Education. https://www2.ed.gov/parents/needs/speced/iepguide/index.html

CHAPTER 6

PLAY THERAPY THEORIES
Applications to Suicide in Youth

Mary Ruth Cross and Leslie W. Baker

The theoretical framework a graduate student learns in school can become the foundation for the remainder of a play therapist's career. The theoretical framework, whether humanistic, behavioral, or cognitive, informs case conceptualization and treatment planning. Play therapy offers the child or adolescent a developmentally suitable method of enhancing affect regulation, self-efficacy, problem-solving, and the development of trust within therapeutic relationships (Green & Myrick, 2014). However, Drewes et al. (2011) noted that a more comprehensive treatment approach is needed to address the complex clinical cases that play therapists may encounter in the playroom. This chapter will examine theories most relevant to assessing and treating suicide in children and adolescents.

HISTORY OF PLAY THERAPY

Sigmund Freud's daughter, Anna Freud, introduced play in therapy as a replacement for free association (talk therapy) around 1928 (Freud, 1928). Anna Freud was the first to acknowledge the need for a distinct therapeutic approach for children. Margaret Lowenfeld, a trained medical doctor, eventually turned her attention to the traumatic experiences of children after serving with the British Typhus Unit during the Russo-Polish War. She was impressed with the resiliency she saw in the children. She was also aware of the developmental needs of children and realized that simple "talk therapy" would not be sufficient to facilitate healing in children. She developed the *World Technique* as part of her play therapy practice. Children were invited to create their world in any manner they chose using sand trays and miniature toys. Lowenfeld was a pioneer in the use of play as a therapeutic medium. With Lowenfeld's contributions, Great Britain became a stronghold for child psychotherapy and play therapy (Lowenfeld, 1950). Lowenfeld's work continues to inspire and educate child therapists. The Virtual Sand Tray©® (Stone, 2016) was inducted into the Dr. Margaret Lowenfeld Trust to usher Sand Tray therapy into the 21st century.

In the 1930s, David Levy introduced "Release Therapy," which emphasized using toys in play therapy to help children relive and release negative emotions associated with traumatic events (Levy, 1938). In the 1940s, Carl Rogers established person-centered treatment, which served as the foundation for Child-Centered Play Therapy (CCPT), emphasizing the importance of the therapeutic relationship between the child and the play therapist (Rogers, 1961).

Virginia Axline developed "non-directive play therapy" in the early 1970s and formulated eight principles for therapeutic relationships to guide play therapists in their work with young clients. Sandplay, developed by Frau Dora M. Kalff (1904–1990) from Switzerland,

DOI: 10.4324/9781003358565-8

originated through her integration and refinement of the theoretical work of C. G. Jung, the sand tray World Technique established by Margaret Lowenfeld at her Institute for Child Psychology in the UK, and the principles of engaged witnessing from Tibetan Buddhism applied to the sandplay process. Sandplay is utilized with other therapeutic modalities, such as talk therapy, art therapy, consultation, and traditional play therapy for children. As per an agreement between Kalff and Lowenfeld, only the specific approach aligned with Kalff's methods is called Sandplay (Kalff, 1980).

Clark Moustakas (1950–1980s) focused on the relationship between the play therapist and the play therapy client (Moustakas, 1953), while Garry Landreth (1990–present) became renowned for his book, *Play Therapy: The Art of the Relationship.* Landreth (2012) emphasized the importance of the therapeutic relationship and advocated for the "non-directive play therapy approach." In contrast, Gove Hambridge developed "Directive Play Therapy" or "Structured Play Therapy," promoting rapport-building and the recreation of stressful events in play therapy to facilitate recovery.

In the 1960s, Bernard and Louise Guerney introduced "Filial Play Therapy," which involved training parents or caregivers to use child-centered play therapy at home in conjunction with weekly sessions with a play therapist (Guerney, 1964). This approach aimed to include parents in the therapeutic process.

These play therapists recognized that children and adolescents are not miniature adults and highlighted the importance of specialized training in play therapy for mental health professionals. Colleges and universities increasingly acknowledge the benefits of incorporating play therapy training into their programs.

EXPRESSIVE PLAY-BASED THERAPIES

Expressive Play-based treatment to assist children in navigating emotional issues traces back to Sigmund Freud's daughter Anna, who systematized and expanded play therapy as a valid treatment method. Expressive play therapy aims to aid children in processing emotional distress by providing them with a means of expression through play. Various forms of Expressive Play-based treatment exist, including dramatic and fantasy play, sandtray, and art-focused play. All types of Expressive Play-based therapy have a basis in the belief that play is crucial for the normal development of children and adolescents. Since young people often struggle to articulate and communicate their emotions as adults do, Expressive Play-based therapy offers a natural avenue for youths to reenact and discuss feelings that may impact their daily lives, such as sadness, anger, or worry, with guidance from the child therapist.

Expressive Play-based therapy engages the child and adolescent on many different levels, going beyond the words of traditional "talk therapy" to draw forth subconscious and unconscious material. Landreth noted that play is a child's natural communication medium (Sweeney & Landreth, 2003). The patient becomes the creator, and the therapist monitors the process and witnesses their creations. This method allows the patient to go beyond words, self-expression, and self-discovery. For example, the youth's verbalizations are noted, as are the media they choose, body language, and the youth's emotional state. The play therapist amplifies the metaphor expressively and stays in the play with the child or adolescent as much as possible. For example, while using the sandtray, the play therapist invites the youth to make up a story about what is happening with the images in the sandtray. The story might be, "In a magical land, two kingdoms always liked to fight. One day, the king got furious at the princess, turned her into a small bird, and locked her in a gilded cage." The play therapist could respond with, "I'm wondering what made the King mad." Or "Hmm, that's interesting; what makes the land magical?" The focus is on what is happening in the sandtray rather than directly being focused on the child or adolescent or the interpretation of content.

Building rapport and establishing trust is essential in therapy's initial stages. The child therapist focuses on fostering a therapeutic alliance by allowing the child to explore the therapy space and select play activities suitable for their age. The play therapist may introduce an Expressive Play-based intervention, for example, dollhouse figurines and furniture, that could prompt the child to express feelings or responses about their family life.

Applying Expressive Play-based interventions is common in play therapy and school-based counseling. From pencils and paper, crayons, and coloring to painting or finger painting, understanding how the materials provide containment or more freedom can create more security or, in other cases, too much stimulation for a child or adolescent. The play therapist and school counselor should be familiar with various media and, to avoid overstimulation, allow the child a limited choice of materials. These materials provide opportunities for choice, as children can explore their needs according to the materials' possibilities and limitations.

Additionally, crayons, pens, chalk, etc., allow for abundant expression of emotions. For instance, paints enable fluid movements that evoke a sense of freedom while capturing emotions, although controlling the medium might be challenging for children unfamiliar with painting. On the other hand, fine-tipped markers may be suitable for individuals who seek a greater sense of control and attention to detail, facilitating the necessary expression for regulation. In expressive arts therapy, clients can engage with various artistic modalities and materials, enabling them to select what feels most comfortable and safe based on their sense of security and attachment (Malchiodi, 2013). Making choices in response to specific emotions or situations can be liberating and help foster confidence and a stronger sense of self in the individual. Additionally, the ability of youth to channel their emotional responses through artmaking in play, whether it involves splashing paint or playing drums, exemplifies the decision-making process influenced by their level of comfort and perceived safety.

Through Expressive Play-based therapy, children gradually acquire skills to cope with the challenges they face in their daily lives. This process contributes to developing a sense of competence and enhanced self-esteem, leading to improved adjustment and resolution of any problems they may be coping with.

CHILD-CENTERED PLAY THERAPY THEORY

Child-Centered Play Therapy (CCPT) is a humanistic approach formulated from the original work of Carl Rogers (1961) and later expanded and adapted by Virginia Axline (1969). For many play therapists, this is the theoretical framework they are exposed to when counselors train students. This theoretical framework focuses on the relationship between the therapist and the client. It is through the relationship that healing occurs. The Child-Centered approach is based on the idea that kids can develop and heal in an environment that fosters growth without agendas or restrictions (Schaefer, 2003). The child or adolescent client is the play's director, and the play therapist is the facilitator.

Basic Constructs

Three basic constructs inform this theory: the person, the phenomenological field, and the self. The person is understood to be everything a child or adolescent is, including their self-perceptions of feelings, thoughts, and behaviors. The phenomenological field is the lived experience of all that happens and is experienced in the world by the child or adolescent – the child or adolescent's understanding and perceptions of their behaviors, feelings, and thoughts. The child or adolescent's understanding of reality is what Child-Centered Play Therapy focuses on.

Lastly is the youth's construct of the Self. The Self is developed through interactions to gain a sense of an individuated and differentiated concept of "Me" (Sweeney & Landreth, 2003). In Child-Centered Play Therapy, individuals are accepted and permitted to behave, think, and feel freely without judgment. The corrective experience of unconditional positive regard facilitates the child or adolescent to shift to a more positive self-concept. With these constructs in mind, Child-Centered Play Therapy can be seen as a journey the child or adolescent takes with the therapist to explore and discover themselves.

Goals of CCPT

The focus of CCPT is on the self of the child or adolescent, not on the problem or symptoms. The goals of CCPT, as outlined by Landreth (2012), are designed to help the child or adolescent develop or improve a positive self-concept, become more self-directing, accepting, and reliant, and learn to be more self-trusting and sensitive to how they cope. There is an avoidance of evaluation in CCPT; therefore, children are encouraged rather than praised to position the child/adolescent as leader rather than the adult. Participation in CCPT is always client-directed to ensure that the play therapist is not inserting their agenda into the treatment. The CCPT-informed play therapist will avoid asking questions, offering solutions or suggestions, or becoming the director of the play. Control belongs to the child or adolescent so they can learn to use their strengths and abilities. With CCPT, we give youth a favorable and safe environment to explore and heal themselves. As Axline (1969) reminds us, it is a powerful force within each person to strive for self-actualization. Everyone is entitled to dignity; it is our birthright to gain satisfaction from the impulse to grow.

Therapeutic Limit Setting

Limits emphasize the Child-Centered Play therapist's focus on the process rather than particular behaviors in the play therapy process (Schaefer, 2003). The primary justification for placing restrictions in the playroom includes defining boundaries of the therapeutic relationship, security, and safety for the child, anchoring the session in reality, maintaining a positive and accepting attitude toward the child, creating stability and consistency, promoting catharsis, and enhancing and promoting a sense of self-control and self-responsibility (Schaefer, 2003). Landreth (2012) advocates using the acronym ACT as a therapeutic model for setting limits. First, there must be *A*cknowledgement of the child's thoughts, feelings, and desires; secondly, *C*ommunicate boundaries in a non-punitive and non-authoritative way; and lastly, *T*arget acceptable alternatives. Through limit setting, the child or adolescent can trust the therapist to be authentic in their relationship, and this will be an essential trait when assessing and treating suicidal ideation (Landreth, 2012).

CCPT AND SUICIDE

As noted, the relationship is the healing force in CCPT. Trust and a strong therapeutic alliance can occur through developing the relationship between the client and the therapist. In assessing suicide, research has shown that a direct approach that uses clear and concise language while talking to the youth about suicide and, possibly, interventions directed by the play therapist or school counselor is the most effective way to get an accurate assessment of suicidal thinking and behavior (Miller, 2021). Youth have a basic need for affirmation of the self and self-realization. (Axline, 1969). Maladjustment in the CCPT model is seen as the individual being denied the opportunity to grow freely through their struggles. Suicidal thinking or ideation is often an overlooked research point compared to suicidal behaviors or prevention (Jobes & Joiner, 2019). Suicidal ideation is the thought process of considering all elements of potential suicide.

Suicidal clients often report having thoughts of self-harm and dying far longer than peers or family members are aware of. An adolescent client once disclosed that she wondered what it would be like to drive her car into a tree or what it would be like to drive off a bridge or cliff. She was surprised to learn that this isn't something non-suicidal people think about. Since she got her driver's license, she has been thinking about dying for the last 18 months. With CCPT and the focus being on the relationship between the therapist and the child or adolescent in a non-judgmental and supportive way, it allows for authentic disclosure of suicidal thinking. Because CCPT is a non-directive modality, thematic material emerging from play therapy that suggests suicidal ideation can create a potential clinical problem. Direct questions, as found in the C-SSRS (*The Lighthouse Project, the Columbia Lighthouse Project*, 2022) or other assessment tools, would not be consistent with this theoretical orientation. Although in its purest form, CCPT is non-directive, which could appear as a limitation when working with suicidal youth, it is acceptable to use CCPT in conjunction with directive approaches when it is appropriate to do so, as in assessing for suicidal ideation (Van Fleet et al., 2010). The relational healing power of CCPT provides an essential evidenced-based rationale for working with youth regardless of the level of distress or suicidal ideation (Post et al., 2019). CCPT advocates for parent involvement in their child's therapy.

Effective assessment of suicide within the CCPT model is enabled by candid and trusting conversations between the therapist and the client. When the therapist establishes this therapeutic relationship from the beginning, the inherent methods of CCPT are easily applied. The clinical skills needed in risk management begin by listening with an intent to learn. The therapist expresses genuine empathy through paraphrasing and validating feelings. The therapist utilizes unconditional positive regard and authentic responses to normalize the youth's expressions. CCPT creates a safe and sacred space for the client to trust the therapist sufficiently to be truthful about suicidal thinking and behavior.

Case Example

A 6-year-old, Kevin, is referred to play therapy due to aggressive behavior at school. Kevin comes into the playroom and immediately goes to the sandtray. Kevin creates a forested graveyard scene with coffins and tombstones. He puts a circle of crocodiles around the outer edge of the sandtray. As Kevin makes the scene, the play therapist says, "Oh, I see you are looking at the toys and putting them in the sandtray." Kevin just nods and works quietly, adding images and mumbling under his breath. The play therapist responds calmly, "I hear you talking under your breath as you *move the toys in or put toys into* the sandtray."

Kevin:	"Yeah, sometimes people die."
Therapist:	"You sometimes think that people die."
Kevin:	*"Yeah, sometimes kids die too."*
Therapist:	"Um, hmm, yes, sometimes kids die too."

The CCPT play therapist focuses on being fully present to the child or adolescent and does not interpret nor direct the play. The child is seen, heard, and valued through witnessing by the play therapist. It is the relationship with the child and deep respect from the play therapist who assumes that the child or adolescent has the inherent ability to heal and work through their issues.

Interventions

In a recent study by Burgin and Ray (2022), CCPT was effective in reducing depressive symptoms in children and improving overall behavior problems. Young children from economically disadvantaged backgrounds identified as at-risk showed improvement by CCPT treatment. The perspective of CCPT is to view the child or adolescent as always moving towards self-actualization and greater functionality. Through the relationship between the therapist and the child or adolescent, founded on unconditional positive regard, the innate internal processes of empathy can be opened up to decrease aggression, whether directed at the self (creating self-harm) or others. The sense of belonging humans need to feel increases in direct proportion to the level of suicidal ideation they experience. The therapeutic relationship in CCPT directly combats this problem. The permissiveness in CCPT must also be balanced with an appropriate behavioral limit setting so that inappropriate or harmful behaviors are addressed in a way that aids the child or adolescent in feeling safe and then learning behaviors that will allow self-expression in more appropriate ways. The CCPT way of limit setting maintains acceptance of the child or adolescent while communicating understanding and trust and that the behavior is unacceptable (Ray, 2011). Limits are set when harm is imminent. Ray (2011) points out that the play therapist learns to trust the child, not suspect the child. CCPT play sessions begin with an introductory statement about limits, "This is our special play time together. You can do just about anything here. If there is something you can't do, I'll let you know." A CCPT play therapist might use language to set a limit: "You are not for hurting" or "I am not for hitting." Positive boundaries will contribute to confidentiality and trust.

The intervention is the relationship between the child or adolescent and the play therapist, a vital focus of CCPT. The CCPT play therapist provides facilitative responses that promote the "good growing ground" of therapy (Homeyer & DeFrance, 2013, p. 145). Techniques and interventions rely on facilitative responses like reflecting on the content and feelings and communicating to the child or adolescent that the therapist is focusing on them, not a preconceived agenda. In addition, the play therapist is fully and completely involved in the play as the child directs and uses questions to clarify the youth's reality but not to prove some theory or hypothesis. CCPT also uses structuring to convey the logistics of therapy. Structuring is offered through the lens of the youth's questions and always returns responsibility to the child. For example, "In here, it's you that decides" (Homeyer & DeFrance, 2013, p. 146).

COGNITIVE BEHAVIORAL PLAY THERAPY THEORY

Aaron Beck first conceptualized cognitive therapy (1989) as a model incorporating cognition, physiology, and behaviors to understand emotional disorders fully. This model contends that verbal processes mediate behavior. Knell (1998) realized that this model could be modified to work with children and adolescents to incorporate play therapy. In the Cognitive Behavioral Play Therapy (CBPT) model, Knell reiterated the fundamental principles from Beck's model and applied them to play therapy (Knell, 1998). Structural and directive, CBPT is a brief, time-limited, problem-oriented, and educational therapy.

Goals

Goal setting is an integral part of the CBPT model. Although this is antithetical to the CCPT model of letting the client be the play's director, the therapist's direction throughout treatment is based on the child or adolescent's lead or the assessment of needs the therapist has made. Information gathered from parents, caregivers, teachers, and others is all used to choose the direction for treatment. The toys become the vehicle for the child to verbalize problems and work on coping strategies. The therapist's use of modeling is an efficient and critical component of CBPT as it encourages learning about acquiring, strengthening, or weakening behaviors (Schaefer, 2011).

Interventions

The CBPT model can incorporate critical behavioral interventions such as systematic desensitization, contingency management, positive reinforcement, shaping, stimulus fading, extinction of other behaviors, self-monitoring, and activity schedule. Cognitive interventions include recording dysfunctional thoughts, countering irrational beliefs through cognitive change strategies, and using positive self-statements or affirmations to improve coping (Schaefer, 2011). Bibliotherapy, a therapeutic intervention that employs books and other forms of literature as an adjunct to playing therapy and other modalities to meet treatment goals and create change, can be easily used to reinforce learning and integrate coping strategies.

CBPT AND SUICIDAL THOUGHTS AND BEHAVIORS

It is recommended in suicide assessment research that being direct and using clear yet supportive language is necessary to get an accurate and honest response to queries about suicide (Miller, 2021). In a commentary about suicide, noted suicidologists Jobes and Joiner have found that suicidal ideation must become an essential intervention target in and of itself because, in the singular pursuit to prevent suicide deaths, better identification and more effective treatment of suicidal ideation upstream will invariably lead to many fewer suicide attempts and many fewer suicide deaths downstream (Jobes & Joiner, 2019). In essence, if we pay attention to what children and adolescents think about suicide, even in the minutest of ways, it will lead to fewer deaths by suicide. The CBPT model focuses on what a child or adolescent thinks, feels, behaves, and believes about suicide. CBPT can assist the play therapist in helping youth cope with and alter their STB.

Case Example

Claret, an 11-year-old pre-adolescent, comes into the school counseling office complaining, "It would be better if I never woke up, and then I would never have to come to school." The school counselor knows that Claret has a history of being a parent with substance use issues. She is now living alone with her mother in Section 8 housing. The school is providing her with lunch. She has risk factors for suicide and is now presenting with a warning sign. The school counselor has a positive rapport with Claret, considers her risk factors, warning signs, and protective factors, and utilizes the C-SSRS to assess her immediate level of suicide. The school counselor determined that Claret only considered "not waking up" to avoid a school bully. Claret denies any plan or desire to harm herself beyond her wish to avoid the bully.

The school counselor intervenes with Claret's mother and tells the mother that Claret is coping with suicidal thoughts regarding a bully at school. The purpose of the disclosure to Claret's mother is to assist Claret at home as well as at school. The school counselor protects Claret from bullying behavior, and a child with bullying behavior is given a referral for assistance.

The school counselor meets with Claret and works with her on negative suicidal thoughts with a thought-stopping activity called the *Thought-Stopper Band Intervention*. First proposed in 1928 (Bain, 1928), this method involves identifying a detrimental, anxious, or counterproductive thought. Whenever clients become aware of such a thought, they intervene by saying "stop" or employing a physical gesture, like softly snapping a rubber band on their wrist. Incorporating affirmative self-statements helps foster encouragement and motivation (Prasertsri, et al., 2011).

Thought Stopping Band Intervention (Baker, 2023a) materials include a wide rubber band of approximately 6"x.75", sized to the child or adolescent one is working with. The rubber band needs to be loose enough not to cause a mark and wide enough to write a positive prompt. The goal is for the youth to think of a positive thought that is true and helpful to negate a negative, suicidal thought. For example, if the negative thought is "I should not wake up, so my problems will go away." The youth could write on the band, "*I CAN ASK FOR HELP! I AM GREAT AT GETTING HELP!*" If the child or adolescent has a negative thought, they can "lightly snap" the band on their wrist (a behavioral cue) and then read the band and say the statement aloud or in their mind. Reinforce positive affirmation by following through and sharing their progress with their school counselor.

Collage Affirmation Cards (Baker & Cross, 2022) are another helpful intervention in CBPT. The materials include one permanent marker and one to two sheets of colored cardstock, a collection of three sheets of tissue paper – two plain and one printed – torn into pieces, decoupage glue, and one paintbrush. The youth places the tissue paper pieces onto one side of the cardboard and decoupage glues the tissue down. Let dry. Once dry, the youth cuts any cardboard shape large enough to have an affirmation written about 2"x3" long as a rectangle. Take the permanent marker, and depending on the age of the youth, have them write an affirmation on the back of the card. The cards can be in a tissue box, covered with more tissue paper decoupage, or any container a child or adolescent desires. Some youth with cell phones prefer to take photos and create an album of their photos, and they like to look at the photo affirmations when needed.

The intervention known as "self-affirmation" is founded on the theory that people can reinforce their sense of self-worth, a comprehensive notion of ethical and adaptive adequacy, during times of psychological distress.

Affirmations ease stress and counteract defensive behaviors. The beneficial effects of self-affirmations have been demonstrated in numerous areas where continuous threats to self-worth can hinder adaptive defenses. By widening the recognized foundations of self-worth, affirmations make these threats less severe. While affirmation interventions have proven potent, their effects are context-dependent (Walton & Crum, 2022). Research based on the self-affirmation theory indicates that MRI studies have found evidence of enhanced neural pathways when individuals engage in self-affirmation activities, like the daily repetition of positive affirmations (Cascio et al., 2015). When aiding clients in creating their positive self-statements, they must view these statements as believable and beneficial. If a client struggles to formulate an affirmation statement, guide them with insightful starter questions:

What values do you take the most pride in?
What values help you when you are under stress?
Can you remember an instance where you were proud of managing a stressful situation?
What do people typically commend or compliment you for?

Research also indicates that value-centric affirmations utilized by middle school children can protect and inoculate against stress. Self-affirmation interventions are interesting, insightful, and scientifically supported (Walton & Cohen, 2011). Self-affirmation theory has been extensively researched and suggests that individuals are driven to protect the integrity of the self, which can be achieved by affirming personal values or qualities (Critcher & Dunning, 2014).

When people face a threat, they may engage in self-affirmation, reminding themselves of their values, strengths, and past achievements. By self-affirmation, youth can cope better with the threat, maintain self-integrity, and continue to see themselves as good, virtuous, and capable (Critcher & Dunning, 2014). Self-affirmations work through a variety of psychological mechanisms. First, they evoke a more expansive self-conception. Focusing on different areas of life that are important to us, such as our faith or relationships, we realize

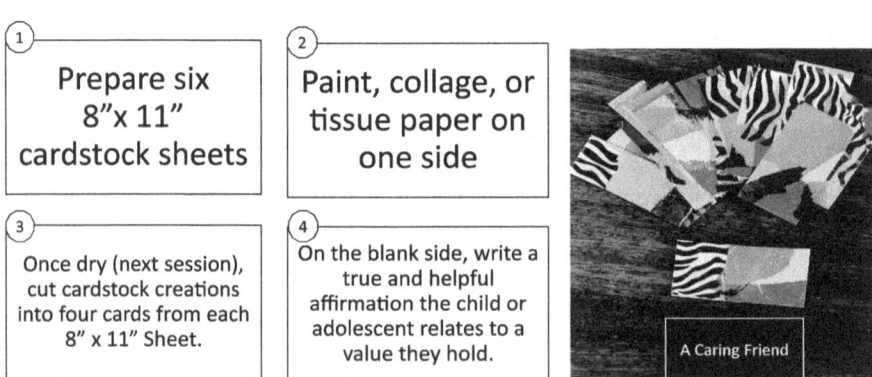

Figure 6.1 Affirmation Collage Cards

that our sense of self-worth and self-regard are multi-faceted and not solely dependent on the threatened area. Second, self-affirmations facilitate positive feedback loops between the individual and the social system (Cohen & Sherman, 2014). When individuals affirm their values and attributes, they receive positive feedback from the social environment, boosting their self-esteem and confidence (Cohen & Sherman, 2014). Lastly, self-affirmation can increase our self-efficacy or belief in handling difficult situations. When we remind ourselves of our past successes and inherent strengths, we increase our confidence in our ability to address future challenges. This increased self-efficacy can help us to persist in the face of adversity and resist temptations to give up or resort to unhealthy coping mechanisms. In summary, self-affirmations can have long-lasting and far-reaching effects by enhancing our self-concept, creating positive feedback loops with our social environment, and increasing our self-efficacy (Cohen & Sherman, 2014).

DIALECTICAL BEHAVIOR THERAPY THEORY

Dialectical Behavior Therapy (DBT) was initially developed for chronically suicidal patients. The intention was to address the intractable problems by confronting the behaviors with Eastern mindfulness practices. A synthesis of opposites is the focus of DBT in that dialectical thinking patterns replace rigid dichotomous ones (Dimeff & Linehan, 2001). This theoretical framework's fundamental concept is that the combination of validation and acceptance is accomplished while helping the youth change. DBT mindfulness is the attention one gives to being present. The therapist or others involved with the youth assume a non-judgmental stance that focuses on effectiveness. Robins and Rosenthal (2012) put it this way: "Dialectical tension and synthesis most central to DBT are that between acceptance and change" (p. 164). It is through mindfulness that greater acceptance of reality happens. In a randomized controlled trial, the results supported using DBT in a six-month format to treat non-suicidal self-harm, suicidal behavior, and ideation (Stanley et al., 2007). Further, DeCou et al. (2019) found evidence that DBT can impact suicidal ideation. On the other hand, Jobes and Joiner (2019) warn that other clinical interventions and treatment strategies for suicide attempts have limited to no impact on suicidal ideation.

The four stages of DBT include pre-treatment, which focuses on connecting the child or adolescent to the treatment process and the therapist. Stage one is the most intensive (Dimeff & Linehan, 2001; Dimeff et al., 2020). The elements of stage one include stabilizing the client to improve behavioral control and identify targets for treatment. Suicide targets would be focused on decreasing suicidal and life-threatening behaviors, decreasing acts and behaviors that interfere with therapy, and decreasing behaviors that interfere with the quality of life. In stage two, the focus is on achieving happiness, reducing ongoing disorders, and reducing problems with living. Stage three is focused on resolving a sense of incompleteness to achieve joy. Stage four synthesizes the previous stages to replace out-of-control behaviors and feelings of inadequacy with enhanced control, resolution of everyday problems, and increased well-being (Dimeff et al., 2020).

Once targets have been identified, priorities are assigned based on a target hierarchy. The target hierarchy is as follows: a) suicidal/homicidal or other life-threatening behaviors, b) therapy-interfering behaviors, c) behaviors that severely interfere with the quality of life, and d) behavioral deficits that prevent change. The therapist helps the youth with increasing emotion regulation, distress tolerance, and skillful responses to interpersonal problems.

Progress in DBT is not linear. Treatment can flow from stage one to stage two and back again. The therapist understands that each statement of a position the client makes contains its antithesis or opposite position within it. For example, "I wish to die" suggests an action that could be accomplished secretly. Still, the action actually taken – the statement itself – is an interpersonal expression of the speaker's feelings. Dialectical change comes when the two opposing points are resolved into synthesis (Dimeff et al., 2020).

The application of mindfulness varies based on the therapeutic approach and the anticipated advantages of incorporating mindfulness into the treatment. The utilization of mindfulness in Dialectical Behavior Therapy (DBT) is fascinating, especially regarding the role of acceptance without judgment and non-reactivity in effecting change. Mindfulness in DBT emphasizes recognizing and accepting emotional conditions (Stanton & Dunkley, 2019). The findings from the analyzed studies suggest that mindfulness contributes to the overall efficacy of DBT. However, the precise processes of change and the overall magnitude of the effect have yet to be determined due to the small participant numbers and the absence of controls in some of the studies (Eeles & Walker, 2022).

DBT AND SUICIDE

Case Example

Keisha, a 12-year-old girl, presents with child sexual abuse from a daycare staff at her after-school program. All the reports are made, and the investigation is completed. The pre-adolescent is referred to the community play therapist regarding her trauma and her threats of suicide. She is also cutting on her thighs and wrists and starving herself, stating, "My tummy hurts; I am so afraid I am going to have his child." Despite receiving a negative pregnancy test, she fears becoming pregnant. The parents are coping with mood swings and rage. She is refusing academics, food, and rules. She leaves the home and reports having unsafe sex with anyone she meets online. She states, "I am a whore; it doesn't matter if I live, die, or cut. He ruined me. I am a whore; I hate myself."

The play therapist utilizes assessment and crisis intervention. Keisha is dismissed from residential care, and the parents request twice-per-week outpatient therapy with the understanding that hospitalization is a real possibility. A safety plan is created, and the family is sent to family DBT to work on the DBT skills as a group. The play therapist uses DBT-PT to address Keisha's dysregulation by recognizing and accepting her emotional conditions without judgment.

Intervention The *Relax Mat – Yoga & Mediation Intervention* (Baker, 2023b). Supplies needed for this intervention include a light-colored yoga mat and other colored permanent marker pens. The youth will complete four areas on the four sides of the yoga mat:

1. Calming Phrase or Mantra.
2. Draw or write out two to four yoga poses.
3. Write or draw song lyrics, poems, or quotes.
4. Write or draw a few calming activities to do.

This mat becomes a safe place. A place to be mindful, meditate, calm, breathe, and find peace in words, actions, and support.

Relax Mat Supply List

- Yoga Mat, plain neutral color
- Colored and dark Sharpies
- Write on four sides
  - Calming Phrase or Mantra
  - Yoga Poses (2-4 poses)
  - Songs, poem, or quote
  - Calming Activities to do

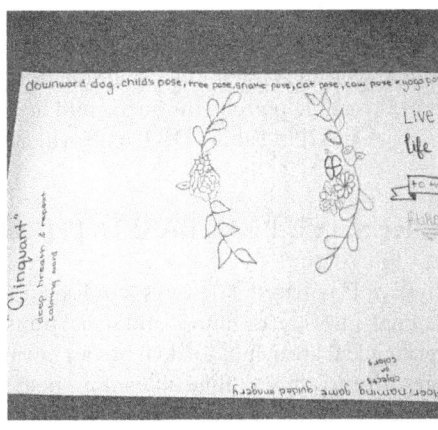

Figure 6.2 Relax Mat – Yoga & Mediation Intervention

Source: Cross, M. R. & Baker L. (2021, October) Play Therapy Continuum [Conference Presentation] Healing Traumatic Grief & Loss Through Play Therapy: A Bottom-Up Approach. Association for Play Therapy International Conference, Little Rock, AK.

Mindfulness and DBT

Over the past decade, Mindfulness-based Interventions (MBIs) have attracted substantial attention due to their effective outcomes. A systematic review explored evidence-based research on the efficacy of MBIs as a therapeutic intervention for suicide and to provide recommendations that could guide future research. The review identified 13 studies, six randomized controlled trials, two controlled studies, and five pre/post-observational studies. The results primarily favored MBIs as an effective strategy for managing suicidal behavior. The interventions demonstrated encouraging outcomes in tackling suicidal behavior. Nonetheless, to understand how MBIs contribute to reducing suicidal behavior, there is a need for larger-scale, high-quality trials with active control and long-term intervention efficacy studies (Raj et al., 2020).

Another DBT technique the play therapist worked on was Keisha's *Chain Analysis* (Linehan, 2014). The goal of the play therapist was to assist the sexual abuse survivor in understanding what triggers Keisha's behavior to go out and seek more abusive sexual encounters. Using single-chain analysis, the therapist obtained a detailed account of the events that led from a single instance of a particular behavior to its resulting consequences. Chain analysis offers a structured approach to assessment that assists both the play therapist and adolescent in gathering pertinent information to comprehend the triggers and sustainers of a target behavior. The chain analysis includes vulnerability factors, the triggering event, links (thoughts, emotions, actions, and other occurrences relating to the self and others), the target behavior, and short- and long-term outcomes (Rizvi, 2019).

Remember that the primary role of chain analysis is to scrutinize a single occurrence of a specific behavior to generate solutions that will effectively impact its future events. Identify the critical controlling factors and avoid rote assumptions. Assess all the information to understand the progression from one link to another (Rizvi, 2019).

After working with the adolescent survivors, Keisha began to problem-solve the triggers: a demanding parent, abusive scolding for skipping school and bad grades, and seeking online attention, which led to unsafe sexual situations and reenactments of sexual assault. The play therapist worked on problem-solving and how to cope with homework. Keisha and her parent were referred to Family DBT to provide skills for the family to manage their emotions.

EXPRESSIVE PLAY-BASED THEORY

Expressive Play-based Theory is a holistic approach that considers and addresses a client's emotional, physical, cognitive, and social traits (*Expressive Arts Therapy*, 2023). It is founded on the principle that each individual has an intrinsic reservoir of understanding and carries the innate drive to achieve their maximum potential (*IEATA International Expressive Arts Therapy Association* ®, 2017). Humanistic psychologists occasionally use the term phenomenological. The humanistic approach examines personality by focusing on individual experiences (*Expressive Arts Therapy*, 2023). Expressive Play-based Theory allows this lived experience to move from the internal to the external through play and artful modalities, such as dance therapy, music therapy, drama therapy, art therapy, and poetry therapy (*IEATA International Expressive Arts Therapy Association* ®, 2017).

Basic Tenets

One can promote profound personal development and strengthen children and adolescents coping with STB by using visual arts, motion, drama, music, writing, and various creative endeavors. Note that merely engaging in creative activities like having a client move or draw is not commensurate with practicing Expressive Play-based Therapy (*Expressive Arts Therapy*, 2023). The Expressive Play-based Theory encompasses a dynamic, multi-faceted approach to psychology, organizational progress, community arts, and education (*Expressive Arts Therapy*, 2023). By merging artistic methods and seamlessly transitioning from one to another, we tap into our innate abilities for healing, understanding, enlightenment, and innovation.

Expressive Play-based Theory incorporates and values multiple modalities, often combining various art forms in a single session (*Expressive Arts Therapy*, 2023). The focus is on the therapeutic potential of the artistic journey, highlighting the youth's ability to manifest thoughts, feelings, and life experiences through creative expression (*IEATA International Expressive Arts Therapy Association* ®, 2017). This model of play therapy focuses on diversity, equity, and inclusiveness.

Case example: Kalani, an 8-year-old Sri Lankan boy, is referred to a school-based play therapist for suicidal thoughts and behaviors (STB). He was overheard by a student on the playground saying to himself, "I just wanna die, I don't wanna be here no more, this is a bore, I just don't wanna be here no more." The student reports her concern to the school counselor, and he brings Kalani into his office and provides **Suicide Safe Mobile App** by SAMHSA (Substance Abuse and Mental Health Services Administration, n.d.), which includes a five-level assessment including his risk factors, warning signs, and protective factors, and utilizes the C-SSRS to assess his immediate level of suicide. It is determined Kalani is at a moderate level of suicide but does not warrant hospitalization. Parents are notified, and a plan for in-school treatment twice a week is set up. Kalani is sent to his pediatrician for further assessment, and the pediatrician will follow up with a medication referral to a psychiatrist should this be warranted.

The school counselor, Eric, begins working with Kalani in his school-based program. The school provides one private session and one group session per week. Kalani starts the group sessions and is interested in meeting other children his age who are struggling with STB. Eric leads the Expressive Play-based Therapy group and then has the youth do the *Magic Rainbow Wand Intervention.*

The Magic Rainbow Wand (Cross & Baker, 2020b) supplies:

- Small wooden dowel – approximately 1 ft.
- Acrylic paint and brushes
- Hot glue tool and glue sticks
- Ribbon – various colors
- Blank medium-size stickers (spice bottle stickers)
- Paper – approximate size of the stickers for art creation
- Colored permanent markers

Procedure: This intervention is done with several steps to allow the child or adolescent time to reflect on expressing their emotions when they experience STB.

1. Using the paint, decorate the wooden dowel with color combinations appealing to the client and set it aside to dry before moving to the next step.
2. Invite the child or adolescent to talk about the suicidal thoughts or behaviors they have experienced, and the feelings connected to them. Paint or create these emotions and then explore the client's feelings. Create a second set of art (painting, poetry, or drawings) of what the client could do to manage the emotions. (Listen to music, dance, create a poem, create a play.)
3. The client then chooses a ribbon of any color and cuts it to the length that matches the intensity of the feeling, e.g., if it is a mild reaction, the ribbon would be short; if it is more intense, the ribbon might be longer. Tape each ribbon to the decorated dowel.
4. Using the blank stickers, adhere, with a glue gun, the art piece to the sticker that recalls the suicidal thought or feeling, then glue the corresponding coping strategy art piece on another sticker. Attach the two stickers back-to-back at the end of one of the ribbons. Repeat until all the ribbons have stickers on the end.
5. Have the child or adolescent create a dance, a song, or any creative expression they choose to integrate the wand into the play.

(Cross & Baker, 2020b)

This intervention examines the feelings attached to current or recent STB to improve overall coping. Expressive Play-based Theory constructs support the theoretical underpinnings of this intervention. In short, becoming aware of what one feels and expressing these feelings creatively and interactively, such as waving the wand, casting a spell, making a wish, or dancing with the rod, creates a coping strategy for the youth (Cross & Baker, 2020). The group Kalani attended was divided into pairs to create a dance or play with their Magic Rainbow Wands. They shared their dances and plays with their group, and the children provided feedback such as "Wow! I do have big feelings!" Some children do not want to take it home because of parental responses. Others want to keep it in the playroom to be used repeatedly with new dances and new stories.

PRESCRIPTIVE PLAY THERAPY THEORY

The Association for Play Therapy lists seminal and historically significant theories that drive play therapy, such as Adlerian, Child-Centered, or Jungian Play Therapy, to list a few. Although not considered a seminal theory, Prescriptive Psychotherapy has gained in popularity since the 1970s when it was first described (Beutler & Harwood, 2015/2000) and has evolved into what is known in play therapy as Prescriptive Play Therapy. At first, this theoretical orientation would appear eclectic and unfocused; however, just like any psycho-therapeutic theory, there are basic tenets and core practices that, once understood, reveal the more profound value of this model, mainly as it is applied to the assessment and treatment of suicide in children and adolescents.

Basic Tenets

There are six core principles or tenets of Prescriptive Play Therapy: individualized treatment, differential therapeutics, transtheoretical approach, integrative psychotherapy, prescriptive matching, and lastly, comprehensive assessment (O'Connor, 2016). First, as an individualized treatment model, Prescriptive Play Therapy sees each client as having unique needs. It, therefore, needs individual interventions that are tailor-made to the client, which is a driving force in this theory. Each client is assessed and understood through their unique presenting problem and needs. In Prescriptive Play Therapy, we treat the individual, not the problem. The therapist must clarify that what will work with one client will not necessarily work with another.

The second foundational belief is "differential diagnosis." Differential diagnosis refers to the idea that one-size therapy does not fit all. Prescriptive Play Therapy debunks the "Dodo Bird Verdict," which says psychotherapy approaches will be equally effective for all disorders. In the Prescriptive Play Therapy model, the solutions to the client's problems and challenges vary so that the proper play intervention will fit that client.

Prescriptive Play Theory is called a transtheoretical approach. This structure draws on three fundamental constructs: clinical experience, empirical evidence, and what the client wants to focus on (O'Connor, 2016). The play therapist then chooses from different theories the techniques that best fit the therapeutic needs of the clients. Schaefer and Drewes (2013) noted that the most effective core change agents best suit the client and do not adhere to one theoretical perspective. The more play interventions the therapist can offer to remedy the client's problem, the more influential the treatment can be (Stein & Goldstein, 2013).

The fourth core principle of Prescriptive Play Therapy is integrating interventions from various theoretical perspectives to meet the client's needs is best described as a multimodal approach. The therapist considers the presenting problem and the client's strengths and challenges and then mindfully applies two or more theories that match the client through appropriate interventions and techniques. Many play therapists have a firm grasp of one theoretical orientation, such as Child-Centered Play Therapy. As they learn and grow as clinicians, they assimilate other ideas and schools of thought to apply multiple interventions (O'Connor, 2016).

The fifth core principle of Prescriptive Play Therapy Theory involves prescriptive matching refers to the therapist matching the interventions to the diagnosed disorder. The matching is made by choosing the agents of change that treat the disorder's underlying cause, not just the symptoms. For example, when working with youth who have suicidal ideation, the change agent of direct teaching is a good match since it is essential to help the client understand their thinking and the underlying cause. A non-directive approach would not be a good match as children and adolescents may avoid the difficulty of talking about self-harm and suicidal thinking or behavior.

The sixth core component of Prescriptive Play Therapy Theory is a comprehensive assessment which is necessary to facilitate the overall treatment plan. A thorough evaluation includes the following: a complete understanding of the presenting problem and the history of the problem, family history, past attempts to work on the problem, developmental history, trauma history, medical history, family system, and family support. This information can be gained through intake interviews with parents/caregivers, behavioral checklists, sensory checklists, initial play therapy sessions with the child, dyad play therapy sessions with each parent, and standardized instruments. The assessment process is ongoing throughout treatment to ensure that treatment goals are achieved and revised as necessary.

Prescriptive Play Therapy and Suicide

Applying the Prescriptive Play Therapy model to assessing and treating suicide in children and adolescents allows the therapist to incorporate interventions and techniques from evidence-based protocols such as Cognitive Behavioral Play Therapy and Dialectical Behavior Therapy that integrates Expressive Play-based Therapy (Drewes, 2009). Cognitive Behavioral Play Therapy is based on theories of emotional development, which are developmentally sensitive and incorporate various interventions that address thoughts, feelings, and behavior with the play-based paradigm. Dialectical Behavioral Play Therapy is a flexible psychotherapy that comprises elements of behavior therapy, cognitive behavior therapy, and mindfulness. It incorporates interventions within the play-based paradigm. Expressive Play-based Therapy offers a comprehensive and interconnected method that caters to an individual's emotional, physical, cognitive, and social dimensions. It operates on the belief that every person possesses a natural core of insight and has the inherent ability and motivation to realize their fullest potential. Play therapy, Cognitive Behavioral Therapy (CBT), and Dialectical Behavioral Therapy (DBT) afford research-based theory and interventions. Expressive Play-based Therapy integrates play that examines and encourages healthy sensory-motor functioning, emotion identification and regulation, behavioral regulation, and attachment play. Cognitive Behavioral Therapy Play Therapy (CBT-PT) focuses treatment interventions on thought-stopping and restructuring, thoughts, and affirmations, refocusing beliefs, and changing behaviors. Dialectical Behavior Therapy Play Therapy (DBT-PT) focuses treatment interventions on mindfulness and meditation, behavioral chain analysis, and coping skills.

In Expressive Play-based Therapy, when treating a child or adolescent with suicidal ideation, the play therapist must use all of their resources to create an individualized treatment plan that assesses for risk factors, protective factors, and warning signs, matching client needs with interventions that heal and protect.

Case Example

A 13-year-old female, Mona, presents to the play therapist as a transgender youth wishing to have his parents honor his male pronouns (he/him) and be called by his traditional Hawaiian name, Kekoa. He is suicidal, struggling with self-harm, and is hospitalized once after asking his parents to accept him and take him to the pediatrician. The hospital discharges him to outpatient play therapy. At the initial meeting, the parents tell the play therapist they oppose their daughter's wishes. Although they understand his struggle, they only bring him to therapy to stop his suicidal behavior. The play therapist builds rapport and trust using play interventions, including Non-Directive CCPT, by allowing him to explore the playroom, express his feelings and his story with the play therapist witnessing, and build rapport with supportive reflection. He picks up the watercolor pen set, and the play therapist encourages him to paint and draw anything he likes.

The play therapist's goal is to witness, support, listen carefully, and provide thoughtful comments as needed. Prescriptive Play Therapy allows for the therapeutic matching of theory and interventions. This case, due to suicidal thoughts and behaviors, also required directive interventions to provide a comprehensive suicide assessment, including family history, suicide history, and medication history, using the Columbia Protocol – Columbia Suicide Severity Rating Scale (C-SSRS) (*The Lighthouse Project, the Columbia Lighthouse Project*, 2022) incorporated within the **Suicide Safe Mobile App** by SAMHSA (Substance Abuse and Mental Health Services Administration, n.d.).

This assessment tool allows for both past and current assessments. A skilled play therapist can be direct, compassionate, and caring while weaving directive interventions into a child-centered approach. Once assessed, the play therapist uses the *Safety Planning Application* intervention (Inquiry Health LLC, n.d.). The Safety Plan Application encourages the individual to create a customized list of warning signs that a crisis may develop, coping strategies for dealing with suicidal urges, places for distraction, friends and family members to reach out to, and professionals to call on.

The benefit of this type of safety plan is that it resides on the youth's phone, and generally, Kekoa takes it wherever he goes. Should he experience a crisis of STB, he can open the safety planning app and explore his warning signs, coping skills, distractions, reasons to live, and people to contact (Inquiry Health LLC, n.d.). Contacts listed on his app include his mother, Kalea, his therapist, and 988, the international suicide lifeline. In real time, he can message or speak directly to the Crisis Text Line by texting *HOME–741-741* and get help immediately (*Crisis Text Line | Text HOME to 741741 Free, 24/7 Crisis Counseling*, 2022). The feature also includes instructions to go to the emergency room or urgent care should he feel he needs more direct care. The play therapist demonstrated the safety plan application from his phone and assisted Kekoa in downloading it to his phone. The therapist did their ethical due diligence and, in their consent, outlined that phone-based application technology is used in play or a crisis. The play therapist must also read the privacy rules on this application to determine that there is no tracking for personal information. The key is to maintain client privacy. Many applications collect some non-identifying data, keeping the client's personal information private. If tracking of personal information is allowed, find out what information is collected.

In most cases, due to the limits of confidentiality, this would not be an application used in therapy. After the session, Kekoa was willing to share the Safety Plan app with his mother, who was pleased to see that she was on his crisis list. The therapist explained to the parents how to use the Columbia Protocol application, which allows anyone to do a simple Columbia Suicide Severity Rating Scale (C-SSRS) Assessment with their loved one (*The Lighthouse Project, the Columbia Lighthouse Project*, 2022). They simply download the app and ask the questions on the screen. The app will calculate their loved one's answers and recommend the next steps. The C-SSRS, the most evidence-supported tool of its kind, is a simple series of questions that anyone can use anywhere in the world to help prevent suicide (*The Lighthouse Project, the Columbia Lighthouse Project*, 2022).

For Kekoa, improving his sense of self-worth and positive self-identification is essential to help combat some STB. The play therapist uses the *Greatness Tags Intervention* (Tyler, 2019), which uses positive self-affirmations and a visual aid to help Kekoa integrate a solid positive self-esteem with a sense of belonging to his family and community. The needed supplies include large blank gift tags, watercolor paints/markers, small stickers/bling, ribbon (several colors about .5" to 1" thick), fine point marker, printed-out phrases or words, or collage words (optional). Kekoa and his play therapist started using watercolor paints to create a background of their liking on a blank gift tag. The painted tag is set aside to dry (it usually dries quickly). Then Kekoa and his play therapist discuss what he sees as strengths or positive qualities about himself and how he behaves. The play therapist helps find words representing his greatness through printed resources, collage materials, or writing it out freehand. Once the painted gift tag is dry, it is decorated with the rest of the art supplies, including words, phrases, stickers, etc., to affirm his greatness further. Kekoa inserts a blue and green ribbon into the top of the gift tag, bookmark-style, to complete his Greatness Tag. This intervention (Tyler, 2019) focuses on building self-esteem and having positive self-constructs and also supports the healing process from suicide loss. CBPT and DBT are the theoretical bases for this intervention. They demonstrate a mindfulness approach that empowers the child or adolescent to retreat from any possible self-blame or sense of responsibility for the loss and shift from maladaptive thinking to positive coping strategies through affirmations (Kennedy & Pearson, 2020).

'Ohana was a concept important to Kekoa. The idea of 'ohana extends beyond forming loving bonds solely with biological family (Kanuha, 2005). Adopting the 'ohana mindset means cultivating a feeling of family loyalty and affection towards everyone in the broader human community. 'Ohana is an important cultural concept in Kekoa's family, and the play therapist wanted to address Kekoa's feelings of perceived burdensomeness and thwarted belongingness as he felt he did not belong to the 'ohana. His play therapist invited him to do the *Heart Prints* (Cross & Baker, 2020a) intervention. This intervention connects to those who have left an important "print" on one's heart. The needed supplies include 8"×11" felt rectangles of various colors, scissors, and glue.

Kekoa is encouraged to review and list the important people in his life. He and his play therapist then discuss what qualities make them important to him. Once the essential people are identified, Kekoa uses a green felt square to cut out a large heart shape. Then, using the other colors of felt squares, he creates smaller hearts, each of a different color, for each person listed as essential to him.

Once all the hearts are cut out, Kekoa uses the glue to affix the smaller hearts to the large heart. Kekoa is asked to hold the finished Heart Print close to him and allow the way these crucial people feel about him to enter into his feelings. Kekoa is then asked to show where he is experiencing the feeling in his body and then to allow his body to act out the movement that corresponds with the feeling. He says he feels a little awkward at first and then begins to circle his arms slowly in front of his chest, and then opens his arms wide and throws his arms around himself, holding the hug and letting himself feel the love and support he says these important people give him. Kekoa is encouraged to find a place at home to put the assembled heart as a reminder of these meaningful relationships. A strong sense of belongingness is a powerful deterrent to STB.

Another adaptation for this intervention is to create the large heart as a puppet, and as each new heart is added, the hearts can talk to each other using imaginative play. Some older youths may feel awkward performing this activity, so alter it as needed.

This intervention integrates expressive art with mindfulness and somatic experiencing found in the DBT model. Kekoa was able to gain visual awareness of those people in his life who could be a resource for him, especially when having STB.

CONCLUSION

The case example of Kekoa demonstrates how being well grounded in one's theoretical orientation not only informs treatment planning but aids in conceptualizing all of the unique dynamics of the case clearly and consistently. Prescriptive Play Therapy allows the play therapist and school counselor to formulate a treatment plan tailor-made to the client based on sound evidence-based theory. This chapter comprehensively looked at Child-Centered Play Therapy, Cognitive Play Therapy, Dialectical Therapy, and Expressive Play-based Therapy. Prescriptive Play Therapy theory can integrate any of these theories, among others, to better develop a personalized prescriptive matching for the child or adolescent depending on their particular needs. Prescriptive Play Therapy theory allows the clinician to understand the connection between the theory, the intervention, and the individualized needs of a suicidal youth. The interventions presented enable clinicians to facilitate safety planning and suicide prevention efforts while engendering hope when there is despair. Over time, these models aid children and adolescents to become more regulated with the goal of decreasing the likelihood of suicidal ideation or suicidal behaviors.

REFERENCES

Axline, V. M. (1969). *Play therapy: The groundbreaking book that has become a vital tool in the growth and development of children*. Ballantine Books.

Bain, J. A. (1928). *Thought control in everyday life*. Funk & Wagnalls.

Baker, L. (2023a, June). *Thought stopping band intervention* [Conference Session]. A Play Therapy Approach to the Assessment & Treatment of Pre-Adolescent & Adolescent Anxiety. Mid-Atlantic Play Therapy Training Institute, Atlantic City, NJ.

Baker, L. (2023b, June). *Relax mat – yoga and meditation intervention* [Conference Session]. A Play Therapy Approach to the Assessment & Treatment of Pre-Adolescent & Adolescent Anxiety. Mid-Atlantic Play Therapy Training Institute, Atlantic City, NJ.

Baker, L., & Cross, M. R. (2022, August). *Collage affirmation cards* [Conference Presentation]. Restoring Hope to Youth: Assessment, Treatment, and Prevention of Suicide. Illinois Association for Play Therapy Conference, Chicago, IL.

Beutler, L. E., & Harwood, T. M. (2000). Introduction to prescriptive therapy. In *Prescriptive psychotherapy: A practical guide to systematic treatment selection* (Online ed., October 1, 2015). Oxford Academic. https://doi.org/10.1093/med:psych/9780195136692.003.0001

Burgin, E. E., & Ray, D. C. (2022). Child-centered play therapy and childhood depression: An effectiveness study in schools. *Journal of Child and Family Studies, 31*(1), 293–307. https://doi.org/10.1007/s10826-021-02198-6

Cascio, C. N., O'Donnell, M., Tinney, F. J., Lieberman, M. D., Taylor, S. E., Strecher, V. J., & Falk, E. B. (2015). Self-affirmation activates brain systems associated with self-related processing and reward and is reinforced by future orientation. *Social Cognitive and Affective Neuroscience, 11*(4), 621–629. https://doi.org/10.1093/scan/nsv136

Crisis Text Line | Text HOME to 741741 free, 24/7 crisis counseling. (2022, December 1). Crisis text line. www.crisistextline.org/

Critcher, C. R., & Dunning, D. (2014). Self-affirmations provide a broader perspective on self-threat. *Personality and Social Psychology Bulletin, 41*(1), 3–18. https://doi.org/10.1177/0146167214554956

Cross, M. R., & Baker, L. (2020a). *Heart prints* [Conference Session]. Treatment of Traumatic Grief & Loss for Youth in Play Therapy Expressive Therapies Summit, Los Angeles, CA.

Cross, M. R., & Baker, L. (2020b). *The magic rainbow wand* [Conference Session]. Treatment of Traumatic Grief & Loss for Youth in Play Therapy Expressive Therapies Summit, Los Angeles, CA adapted from Gomez, A. M. (2012). *EMDR therapy and adjunct approaches with children: Complex trauma, attachment, and dissociation.* Springer Publishing Company.

DeCou, C. R., Comtois, K. A., & Landes, S. J. (2019). Dialectical behavior therapy is effective for the treatment of suicidal behavior: A meta-analysis. *Behavior Therapy, 50*(1), 60–72. https://doi.org/10.1016/j.beth.2018.03.009

Dimeff, L. A., & Linehan, M. M. (2001). Dialectical behavior therapy in a nutshell. *The California Psychologist, 34,* 10–13. www.ebrightcollaborative.com/uploads/2/3/3/9/23399186/dbtinanutshell.pdf

Dimeff, L. A., Rizvi, S. L., & Koerner, K. (2020). *Dialectical behavior therapy in clinical practice, second edition: Applications across disorders and settings.* Guilford Publications.

Drewes, A. A. (2009). *Blending play therapy with cognitive behavioral therapy: Evidence-based and other effective treatments and techniques* (eBooks). John Wiley & Sons. http://ci.nii.ac.jp/ncid/BA8992539X

Drewes, A. A., Bratton, S. C., & Schaefer, C. E. (2011). *Integrative play therapy.* John Wiley & Sons.

Eeles, J., & Walker, D. (2022). Mindfulness as taught in dialectical behaviour therapy: A scoping review. *Clinical Psychology & Psychotherapy, 29*(6), 1843–1853. https://doi.org/10.1002/cpp.2764

Expressive Arts Therapy (By Appalachian State University). (2023). *Expressive Arts Therapy.* Retrieved August 18, 2023, from https://expressivearts.appstate.edu/

Freud, A. (1928). *Techniques of child analysis.* Nervous and Mental Disease Pub. Co.

Green, E. D., & Myrick, A. C. (2014). Treating complex trauma in adolescents: A phase-based, integrative approach for play therapists. *International Journal of Play Therapy, 23*(3), 131–145. https://doi.org/10.1037/a0036679

Guerney, B. G. (1964). Filial therapy: Description and rationale. *Journal of Consulting Psychology, 28*(4), 304–310. https://doi.org/10.1037/h0041340

Homeyer, L. E., & DeFrance, E. (2013). Play Therapy. In C. A. Malchiodi (Ed.), *Expressive therapies* (pp. 141–161). Guilford Publications.

IEATA International Expressive Arts Therapy Association ®. (2017). Retrieved August 18, 2023, from www.ieata.org/

Inquiry Health LLC. (n.d.). GitHub – suicide safety plan/safety plan: Suicide safety plan is a free mobile application for suicide prevention. *Github.* Retrieved August 13, 2023, from https://suicidesafetyplan.app/

Jobes, D. A., & Joiner, T. E. (2019). Reflections on suicidal ideation. *Crisis-the Journal of Crisis Intervention and Suicide Prevention, 40*(4), 227–230. https://doi.org/10.1027/0227-5910/a000615

Kalff, D. M. (1980). *Sandplay: A psychotherapeutic approach to the psyche.* Temenos Press.

Kanuha, V. K. (2005). *Nā 'Ohana*: Native Hawaiian families. In M. McGoldrick, J. Giordano, & N. Garcia-Preto (Eds.), *Ethnicity and family therapy* (pp. 64–74). The Guilford Press.

Kennedy, F. C., & Pearson, D. (2020). *Integrating CBT and third wave therapies: Distinctive features.* CBT Distinctive Features.

Knell, S. M. (1998). Cognitive-behavioral play therapy. *Journal of Clinical Child Psychology, 27*(1), 28–33. https://doi.org/10.1207/s15374424jccp2701_3

Landreth, G. L. (2012). *Play therapy: The art of the relationship.* Routledge.

Levy, D. M. (1938). "Release therapy" in young children. *Psychiatry MMC, 1*(3), 387–390. https://doi.org/10.1080/00332747.1938.11022205

Linehan, M. (2014). *DBT? Skills training manual* (2nd ed.). Guilford Publications.

Lowenfeld, M. (1950). The nature and use of the Lowenfeld world technique in work with children and adults. *The Journal of Psychology, 30*(2), 325–331. https://doi.org/10.1080/00223980.1950.9916070

Malchiodi, C. A. (2013). *Expressive therapies*. Guilford Publications.

Miller, D. N. (2021). *Child and adolescent suicidal behavior: School-based prevention, assessment, and intervention*. Guilford Publications.

Moustakas, C. E. (1953). *Children in play therapy: A key to understanding normal and disturbed emotions*. McGraw-Hill.

O'Connor, K. (2016). *Handbook of play therapy* (2nd ed.). Wiley.

Prasertsri, N., Holden, J. E., Keefe, F. J., & Wilkie, D. J. (2011). Repressive coping style: Relationships with depression, pain, and coping strategies in lung cancer outpatients. *Lung Cancer, 71*(2), 235–240. https://doi.org/10.1016/j.lungcan.2010.05.009

Post, P., Phipps, C. B., Camp, A., & Grybush, A. L. (2019). Effectiveness of child-centered play therapy among marginalized children. *International Journal of Play Therapy, 28*(2), 88–97. https://doi.org/10.1037/pla0000096

Raj, S., Ghosh, D., Verma, S., & Singh, T. (2020). The mindfulness trajectories of addressing suicidal behavior: A systematic review. *International Journal of Social Psychiatry, 67*(5), 507–519. https://doi.org/10.1177/0020764020960776

Ray, D. C. (2011). *Advanced play therapy essential conditions, knowledge, and skills for child practice*. Routledge.

Rizvi, S. L. (2019). *Chain analysis in dialectical behavior therapy*. Guilford Publications.

Robins, C. J., & Rosenthal, M. Z. (2012). *Dialectical behavior therapy* (eBooks, pp. 164–192). John Wiley & Sons, Inc. https://doi.org/10.1002/9781118001851.ch7

Rogers, C. R. (1961). *On becoming a person: A psychotherapists view of psychotherapy*. Houghton Mifflin.

Schaefer, C. E. (2003). *Foundations of play therapy*. John Wiley & Sons.

Schaefer, C. E. (2011). *Foundations of play therapy* (2nd ed.). John Wiley & Sons.

Schaefer, C. E., & Drewes, A. A. (2013). *The therapeutic powers of play: 20 core agents of change*. Wiley.

Stanley, B., Brodsky, B. S., Nelson, J. D., & Dulit, R. A. (2007). Brief Dialectical Behavior Therapy (DBT-B) for suicidal behavior and non-suicidal self-injury. *Archives of Suicide Research, 11*(4), 337–341. https://doi.org/10.1080/13811110701542069

Stanton, M., & Dunkley, C. (2019). Teaching mindfulness skills in DBT. In M. A. Swales (Ed.), *The Oxford handbook of dialectical behaviour therapy*. Oxford University Press.

Stein, N., Goldstein, A. P., & Krasner, L. (2013). *Prescriptive psychotherapies: Pergamon general psychology series*. Elsevier Gezondheidszorg.

Stone, J. (2020, September 19). Virtual Sandtray App®© https://jessicastonephd.com/virtual-sandtray/

Substance Abuse and Mental Health Services Administration. (n.d.). *Publications and digital products: Suicide safe mobile app*. https://store.samhsa.gov/product/suicide-safe

Sweeney, D., & Landreth, G. (2003). Chapter 4: Child centered play therapy. In C. E. Schaefer (Ed.), *Foundations of play therapy* (pp. 76–98). John Wiley & Sons.

The Lighthouse Project The Columbia Lighthouse Project. (2022, August 23). The Columbia Lighthouse Project. https://cssrs.columbia.edu/

Tyler, L. (2019, May). *Using the nurtured heart approach and play therapy to discover greatness in your clients and you!* [Conference Session]. Spark It Up Play Therapy Retreat, Danville, CA.

VanFleet, R., Sywulak, A. E., & Sniscak, C. C. (2010). *Child-centered play therapy*. Guilford Press.

Walton, G. M., & Cohen, G. L. (2011). A brief social-belonging intervention improves academic and health outcomes of minority students. *Science, 331*(6023), 1447–1451. https://doi.org/10.1126/science.1198364

Walton, G. M., & Crum, A. J. (2022). *Handbook of wise interventions: How social psychology can help people change*. Guilford Press.

CHAPTER 7

TREATMENT OF SUICIDAL THINKING AND BEHAVIORS IN CHILDREN AND ADOLESCENTS USING PLAY THERAPY

Leslie W. Baker, Mary Ruth Cross, and Kim Vander Dussen

WHAT WE NEED TO KNOW

Training in understanding the dynamics of suicidology is a mandatory requirement in graduate school programs and licensing boards; however, the application and integration of what has been learned by the play therapist or school counselor need to be explored further for more efficacious play therapy treatment. Most importantly, child therapists and school counselors must understand that suicidal ideation is not only found in adults. Statistics underscore the importance of all play therapists and school counselors working with children and adolescents to fully grasp the clinical issues that may be present through a developmental lens.

Developmentally, suicidal thoughts and behaviors (STB) manifest differently in younger children than adolescents (Maughan et al., 2013). This chapter will examine the main overriding principles theoretically relevant to the treatment of suicidal thoughts and behaviors in children and adolescents. The application of theories in the treatment planning and implementation of the goals and interventions that play therapists and educators utilize with children and adolescents will reduce STB. Another essential component in the treatment is wrapping in the parents and caregivers as children and their carers are fundamental to youths' success in development.

Play therapy treatment models that have evidence to support their effects on children include Child-Centered PT, Cognitive-Behavioral PT, Sandtray PT, Theraplay©, and more (Bratton & Lin, 2015).

According to Bratton and Lin (2015), play therapy demonstrates beneficial outcomes in:

- Social skills and social adjustment
- Self-image
- Language and academic achievement
- Trauma symptoms
- Internalized problems, including anxiety
- Functional impairment
- Caregiver/child relationships
- Externalized behavior problems, including ADHD symptoms, aggression, conduct problems, and disruptive behaviors

Four meta-analyses of controlled outcome studies have been conducted in recent years, encompassing more than 130 individual studies and nearly 4,000 participants. These meta-analyses provide substantial evidence confirming the effectiveness of play therapy in

DOI: 10.4324/9781003358565-9

addressing a wide range of presenting issues among diverse populations in real-world settings. These studies have limitations from small sample sizes, lack of replication, lack of research on specific outcomes, and more. More research needs to be replicated and the results disseminated to increasingly inform clinicians and educators about the efficacy limitations of play therapy (Bratton & Lin, 2015).

Play therapy is formulated around the *Therapeutic Powers of Play* (TPoP), as Schaefer and Drewes (2014) outlined. The 2005 meta-analysis by Bratton et al. is the most potent research supporting the efficacy of play as being therapeutic. Charles Schaefer first started researching and identifying a list of TPoP in 1993 (Schaefer & Drewes, 2014).

Play is how children communicate what is happening and learn strategies that help them grow and develop. The TPoP facilitates communication, fosters emotional wellness, enhances social relationships, and increases personal strength. As treatment begins and areas of the youth's life are reviewed in a developmental assessment, the play therapist or school counselors create a conception of the case applied to the TPoP. A child experiencing bullying at school may need interventions focusing on empowerment and increasing personal strength. To further illustrate this point, we look at the case of a 9-year-old Caucasian male, Marcus, presenting with suicidal thoughts and behaviors. In the initial therapy session, his parents stated that suicidal ideation was due to a history of sexual abuse by a babysitter. The parents noted that Marcus came to treatment after the family had reported to the local police, and the child had been processed through the legal system, having been interviewed by a child-friendly interview center and Sexual Assault Response Team (SART), which examined the boy at a local hospital. The law enforcement determined that the case was unsubstantiated due to a lack of physical evidence from the SART examination and the child's inability to testify in a court of law. The parents noticed the child was struggling with sleep anxiety, fear of going to the bathroom alone, and worries about leaving his parents for school or social events. The parents sought help for their child from a credentialed play therapist.

To have an informed and effective treatment plan for any clinical issue, the play therapist looks to the healing power of play. We can apply this directly to treating suicide in children and adolescents. It is important to note that play does more than just use change agents; it also does more than moderate the intensity or course of therapeutic change. Play therapy contributes to the production of change (Drewes & Schaefer, 2015). In other words, play transforms and heals the child or adolescent's distress or problems; for youths struggling with STB, play can save a life.

The four *Therapeutic Powers of Play* are, first, *facilitating communication,* and its agents of change are self-expression, access to the unconscious, direct teaching, and indirect teaching. Second is *fostering emotional wellness,* and the core agents of change are catharsis, abreaction, positive emotions, counterconditioning of fear, stress inoculation, and stress management. Third, *enhancing social relationships* includes these agents of change: therapeutic relationship, attachment, social competence, and empathy. Fourth, *increasing personal strength* consists of these core agents of change: creative problem-solving, resiliency, moral development, accelerated psychological development, self-regulation, and self-esteem (Schaefer & Drewes, 2014).

In conceptualizing the previous case through the lens of TPoP, the play therapist must consider the treatment issues and what type of play would be most beneficial for the client. In the case of Marcus with his trauma history, the play therapist would understand the impact that trauma has on children and then would focus on fostering emotional wellness, increasing personal strength, and enhancing social relationships as a way to resolve and heal the trauma so that Marcus could return to his typical developmental trajectory.

Interventions the play therapist would choose to highlight the 20 core agents of change noted previously, but one would only focus on change agents appropriate for this case. For Marcus, the play therapist chose catharsis, positive emotions, and the counterconditioning of fears to address Marcus's trauma issues.

An intervention this play therapist implemented for catharsis for Marcus is the *Squish & Smash Intervention* (Baker, 2023b), which utilizes white molding clay (air dry), a wooden mallet, and washable felt pens. The goal is for the child to create a character of their choice, coloring the white clay with washable felt pens (swipe the color onto the white clay and work the color into the clay). Once the figure is created, the child can squish and smash their character to their heart's content. This intervention can provide catharsis for emotions of anger, fear, and sadness to assist Marcus in processing his experience with the police and or SART exam. The process of catharsis allows a child space for positive emotions. It can be challenging for traumatized youth to experience "positivity" immediately.

In the middle stage of treatment, the play therapist also focused on using the change agent of positive emotions to improve self-awareness and integrate a trusting relationship with the play therapist. Kottman (2014) recommends the following guidelines to implement and facilitate positive emotions throughout treatment naturally: create a safe space, be fun and have fun, with the therapist not only experiencing positive emotions but expressing them, give permission, and engage with parents and caregivers to help them encourage positive emotions outside of the play therapy room. The play therapist created an alliance with Marcus by allowing him to play any way he liked. It is common for abused children like Marcus to have fears and anxiety. Marcus felt his boundaries had been crossed, and his world had become unsafe. Using the change agent of counterconditioning fears, the play therapist used gameplay and imaginative play to work through fear.

The following is an example of a counterconditioning intervention utilized with Marcus. In The *Superhero Gadget* by Rubin (2006), the child makes a gadget using Play-Doh, clay, or Legos™ that have different powers – for example, with a gadget like a "Cool Ruler," the child identifies the power of the gadget, how to use it, the name of the gadget and who can use it – then the child and therapist play out using the gadget to help identify and resolve fears. Marcus enjoyed creating his Superhero and giving his Superhero powers, like protection, invisibility, and zapping powers!

According to parental reports, participation in CCPT (Child-Centered Play Therapy) resulted in notable and meaningful reductions in aggression, self-regulation improvements, and empathy (Wilson & Ray, 2018), all symptoms one may see in a suicidal youth. Child-Parent Relationship Therapy (CPRT) is a program for young children with behavioral, emotional, social, and attachment difficulties. It is rooted in the principles of CCPT theory, attachment theory, and interpersonal neurobiology. CPRT believes establishing a secure parent-child relationship is vital for a child's well-being. Parents are equipped with skills to respond effectively to their children's emotional and behavioral needs within a supportive group setting. Simultaneously, children understand that their parents can be relied upon to provide love, acceptance, safety, and consistent security. Results of a study by Opiola and Bratton (2018) showed statistically significant findings and substantial treatment effects across all measures, affirming the effectiveness of CPRT compared to Treatment as Usual (TAU). Specifically,

CPRT successfully reduced global behavior problems in adopted children, alleviated stress in the parent-child relationship, and increased parents' display of empathic behaviors. These outcomes were evaluated by unbiased observers unaware of the study's details. This research indicates that for children and adolescents with attachment issues, CCPT and CPRT may start repairing expressed or unexpressed feelings of thwarted belongingness or perceived burdensomeness. Is it possible to mitigate the emotional pain of STB and allow alternative thoughts and behaviors through play? The answer is a resounding "Yes!"

The treatment plan for Marcus focused on fostering communication, encouraging self-expression, and sharing his suicidal ideation with direct, straightforward language. The play therapist developed interventions for expressing anger, including a sandtray where he used miniature figures to work through the power struggle scenarios in which he could "win" the day. The play therapist also utilized art interventions to encourage catharsis. Board games assisted him in impulse control, allowing him to slow down his reactions and express his emotions safely. The play therapist helped the child role-play, telling someone in charge when he was experiencing inappropriate touching by the babysitter (or someone older or bigger than him), who then told him to keep the touching a secret. He could time himself out by seeking refuge in the school office. This intervention aimed to eliminate loud resistance to being dropped off at school.

Dr. Margaret Lowenfeld created *The World Technique* in 1979 (reprinted as *Understanding Children's Sandplay: Lowenfeld's World Technique*, 1993), adapted by Baker (2018) as the *Minirock Box* intervention to aid in reducing separation anxiety for youth in a school-based program. The play therapist utilized a small wooden blue bottom box with a lid filled with small, smooth river rocks. The parents purchased 20 miniature figures. The miniatures comprised multiple figures similar to those often found in a therapist's sandtray. These sandtray images represent symbols of earth, trees, wind, fire, water, animals, people, miniatures culturally suitable to the child and their family and ancestors, houses, and fantasy items. The sandtray images were given to the teacher, and each time the child successfully walked to the class-room, the child was given ten minutes to play in the *Minirock Box*. The child was initially given six original miniatures, and over time, the child earned the other miniatures at each triumphant classroom arrival. This intervention promoted an orderly arrival to school as parents walked the child safely to the classroom. The child demonstrated an ability to ask for assistance from the school counselor to manage anxiety. The child was able to draw pictures of their feelings of fear and give them to the school counselor, and over time, the images of worry became less menacing. These are dramatic changes from the initial presenting issue of frequent suicidal thoughts and behaviors.

BRAIN AND SUICIDE

The impact of developmental trauma and adverse experiences has been well documented (Dye, 2018; Cronholm et al., 2015; Gur et al., 2019). The relationship between these experiences, brain development, and present functioning is a critical component of the Neurosequential Model developed by Dr. Bruce Perry and the Neurosequential Network. Note that the Neurosequential Model is not theoretical or clinical but is a clinical problem-solving tool that deepens case formulation and guides intervention. Understanding how the brain develops and the impact of developmental experience on a child's brain is one of the model's core components. In designing interventions for children impacted by suicide, it is necessary to contextualize chronic stress and trauma and its impact on development. The brain organizes itself in a sequential and predictable pattern. Its structure and functioning reflect developmental experience. While different brain regions are responsible for many functions, what will be discussed in what follows are those most frequently referenced in the Neurosequential Model (Perry, 2020).

Sequentially, the brain stem develops first and is primarily responsible for some basic regulatory functions; blood pressure, heart rate, and body temperature are all managed here. The core relational and regulatory networks originating in this area are most sensitive to developmental trauma in the first months and years of life. The midbrain or diencephalon is responsible for motor regulation, arousal levels, and appetite. Between the ages of 2 and 6, it is especially vulnerable to the impacts of developmental trauma. Perhaps one of the most well-understood regions outside the cortex is the limbic system, the location of our emotional networks, particularly anger, fear, and feelings of attachment. The cortex houses the core executive functions, abstract and concrete thought, the ability to reason, and our feelings of affiliation and belonging. During late childhood and adolescence, the cortex is sensitive to the impacts of experience. It should be noted that all of these regions may be impacted by the loss of a loved one to suicide or other developmental trauma (Hambrick et al., 2019).

Regarding the impact of developmental trauma, another key concept to understand is state-dependent functioning. In brief, the brain has a collection of afferent networks that function to moderate primary regulatory networks. One function they serve is to work in conjunction with the stress response system, which originates in the most primitive parts of the brain to maintain homeostatic states. These networks are consistently responding to stimuli from the external and internal world. That information will then be processed at different levels of the brain by means of one series of networks that continually monitor internal and external experiences and a second set of networks that interpret those experiences and organize responses. When interpreting these experiences as non-threatening, familiar, etc., the brain remains calm and reflective. The calm brain allows an individual to experience higher order thinking and creativity. However, as stress increases and the threat increases, the state of cognition and behavior becomes more reflexive. Over time, with ongoing stress, trauma, and chronic unpredictability, these reflexive states of responding become more fixed and entrenched in individuals (Perry et al., 1995).

Given the impact of stress and trauma on the developing brain and the importance of state-dependent functioning, some considerations can be made in treatment planning and intervention. For a young child struggling with suicide, it can be inferred that their state-dependent functioning is entirely compromised, and the child is reacting to internal and external cues with reflexive thoughts and behaviors. These reflexive thoughts and behaviors suggest that more primitive areas of the brain, those not responsible for cognition but rather regulatory and relational networks, need additional support. Here is where somatosensory experiences and play therapy, heavily based on the context of strong relational bonds, can provide critical intervention and support. Talking and reasoning with suicidal ideation and intent can feel fruitless when the ability to reflect cognitively is compromised. Therefore, interventions should target the most disorganized level of the brain with consideration for the current state and history of developmental risk, trauma, and adversity (Gaskill & Perry, 2014, 2017).

UNDERSTANDING THEORY AND TREATMENT FOR SUICIDE

The theory to which the play therapist ascribes creates the framework to conceptualize and fully understand each client's dynamics. In treating suicidal children and adolescents, treatment must include a good understanding of not only child development but evidenced-based approaches for treating suicide, as well as neurobiology and how the brain works in times of stress and trauma. Most specifically, the authors will give examples of bottom-up approaches informed by the work of Dr. Bruce Perry. The Neurosequential Model of Therapeutics demonstrates how important it is to understand the dysregulation in the brain so that appropriate interventions can be targeted to regain self-regulation. Perry (2020) recommends the "3 Rs: Regulate, Relate, and Reason." Regulation refers to managing emotions and behavior in response to the environment. When children are regulated, they can stay calm and focused and are better able to learn and develop. Strategies that promote regulation include providing structure and routine, creating a calm and predictable environment, and using mindfulness techniques. Relationships are essential for healthy child development. Positive relationships with caregivers, peers, and other adults help children feel safe, secure, and supported and promote the development of social and emotional skills. Strategies that promote positive relationships include creating a nurturing and responsive caregiving environment, building strong bonds with children, and providing opportunities for social interaction and connection. Reasoning refers to the ability to understand cause-and-effect relationships and make logical decisions. When children can reason, they are better able to solve problems and make good decisions. Strategies that promote reasoning include providing opportunities for problem-solving and decision-making, encouraging curiosity and exploration, and helping children develop critical thinking skills.

PLAY THERAPY TREATMENT CONTINUUM

Play therapy is not just the introduction of board games and stories into therapy practice. The Association for Play Therapy describes it as the methodical application of a theoretical framework to create an interpersonal process in which licensed play therapists assist patients in preventing or resolving psychosocial challenges and achieving optimal growth and development (APT, 2023). Generally speaking, play therapy has an underlying process that builds on skills and strategies across a continuum to ensure optimal treatment outcomes. The beginning phase of play therapy treatment has been called the "warm-up stage" (Cochran et al., 2022), where play is contained and non-threatening. The focus is exploring the playroom and building a solid therapeutic alliance with positive attachment and trust between the client and the play therapist. The middle phase of play therapy has also been called the "aggressive" or "regressive" stage (Cochran et al., 2022). During the intermediate phase of treatment, play becomes exploratory. As the child or adolescent engages in play, they naturally move out of their comfort zone into "unsafe" play, where they can have a more profound emotional expression that allows for catharsis. A more profound vulnerability is present as the child or adolescent works through the presenting problems and issues. Resistance and adverse reactions are managed through play and therapeutic relationship. Play behavior in this phase utilizes re-enactment, imagination, and often symbolism to go beyond words to a deeper level of healing and transformation through the power of play. The final phase in the play therapy treatment continuum is often called the "termination" or "mastery" stage (Cochran et al., 2022), where the focus is on closure and resolution. Play behavior

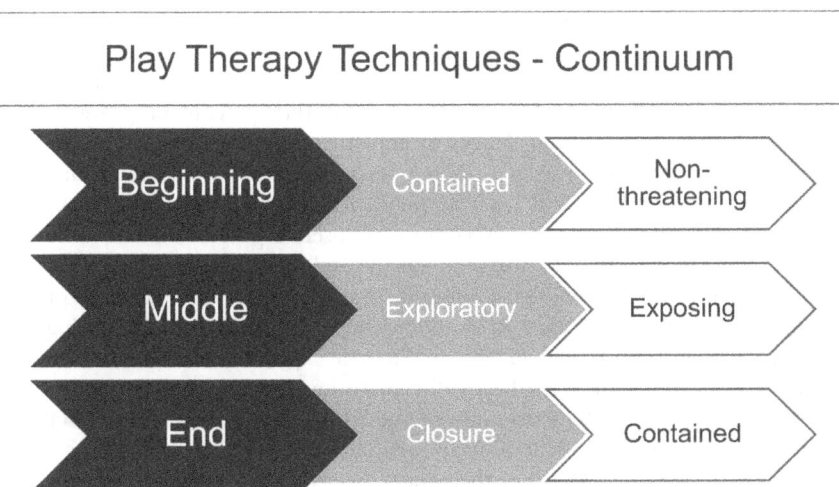

Figure 7.1 Play Therapy Continuum

Source: © 2019 Baker, L. & Cross, M. R. *ALL RIGHTS RESERVED.* Cross, M. R. & Baker L. (2019, October) Play Therapy Continuum [Conference Presentation] Healing Traumatic Grief & Loss Through Play Therapy: A Bottom-Up Approach. Association for Play Therapy International Conference, Little Rock. AK.

in this phase consistently shows developmentally and emotionally appropriate behaviors and interpersonal interactions. The play contains and demonstrates an integration of the therapeutic work that has taken place.

SUMMARY OF RESEARCH-BASED THEORIES FOR TREATMENT

In treating suicide, a multi-modal approach is recommended for effective and individualized treatment planning (Drewes et al., 2011). Interventions for risk factors, warning signs, and protective factors will be explored in what follows. Integrative Expressive Play-Based Therapy assists children and adolescents in managing emotional distress by allowing them to communicate their feelings through play. Integrated into play therapy are interactive, experience-based strategies that leverage multi-sensory experiences to facilitate self-discovery, personal expression, developmental goals, social interaction, and emotional healing. They utilize visual arts, dance movements, and drama performances within a therapeutic context (Malchiodi & Crenshaw, 2014). Integrative Expressive Play-Based Therapy integrates play that examines and encourages healthy sensory-motor functioning, emotion identification and regulation, behavioral regulation, and attachment play (Green & Drewes, 2013).

Research on the efficacy of play therapy treatment has been extensive and has covered many populations (Ray, 2015). As noted previously, Bratton et al. (2005) conducted a meta-analysis of play therapy research in response to criticism that there is insufficient evidence to show that play therapy works. Conclusions from the research study found that play therapy is efficacious in various settings with diverse populations and across different theoretical models and that non-directive models like CPPT are very effective. In other research, it was noted that CCPT was explored most of the time within the body of play therapy research as opposed to different theoretical approaches (Ray, 2015).

A child's natural language is play. The school environment provides a natural and ideal setting for students of all ages to learn and grow; play therapy can complement the process. Of course, there are some challenges in implementing play therapy in schools. One such challenge is a reluctance to see play therapy as a preventive or responsive intervention. Research by Trice-Black et al. (2013) recommended that play therapy be a dynamic part of a comprehensive and developmentally-aware counseling program. Many school-based counseling programs have seen the subject of suicide and STB through a crisis management model rather than a thorough understanding of the assessment and treatment of STB in youth. Another challenge for school-based counseling programs when addressing STB in students is that teachers, who have the most face-to-face exposure to students, are not mental health practitioners and often do not have sufficient training to identify STB accurately. This can lead to underestimating the seriousness of the STB that may be present. Sheftall et al. (2016) noted that teachers and school personnel often turnover quickly, leading to poorly trained staff who are not fully aware of the education environment. Hence, minimizing and denying symptoms is not uncommon.

The efficacy of using CCPT in schools has been researched by Ray et al. (2014), showing that there is quantitative and promising qualitative support for using CCPT in the school setting. Schools inherently work to establish relationships. As in play therapy, schools must create a warm and emotionally safe learning environment to achieve optimum learning or psychological outcomes.

Cognitive Behavioral Play Therapy (CBPT) is based on theories of emotional development, which are sensitive to the individual and incorporate thinking/feeling interventions with the play-based paradigm. Cognitive Behavior Play Therapy focuses treatment interventions on thought-stopping and restructuring thoughts and affirmations, refocusing beliefs, and changing behaviors. Studies have determined that Thought Suppression (TS) or "Thought Stopping" is a distinct method of inhibiting thoughts. While generic thought suppression can have varied and modest effects on mental conditions, TS can significantly improve a person's ability to manage stress when applied appropriately within a Cognitive Behavioral Therapy (CBT) framework. This effect surpasses any potential simultaneous reduction of habituation impacts during exposure therapy (Bakker, 2009). *The Stop & Calm Intervention* (Baker, 2019) helps with the thought-stopping and downregulation of youth coping with suicidal ideation. The therapist and youth collaborate to develop a list of suicidal thoughts that plague the child or adolescent.

The supply list to create the *Stop & Calm Intervention* includes red construction paper (folded in half), scissors, one black permanent marker, a glue stick, clear tape, a wooden craft stick, and a 4"×4" calming picture either hand-drawn or clipped from a magazine.

Create a STOP sign using scissors; cut the folded red paper (fold is on top) into the shape of a STOP sign. On one side, write **STOP** with the black permanent marker. On the other side of the STOP sign, cut and paste the picture to match the STOP sign shape. Then, insert the popsicle stick into the bottom of the open fold. Attach the stick with clear tape. You now have the *Stop & Calm* tool. Working from the list of suicidal thoughts, one can practice *Stop & Calm* by thinking about a negative thought, then looking at the STOP sign and saying **"STOP."** Then, turn the STOP sign over to the *Calming Side* of the sign.

Dialectical Behavioral Therapy (DBT) is a flexible method that comprises elements of behavior therapy, cognitive behavior therapy, and mindfulness, and it incorporates

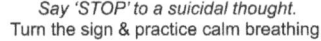

Example CBT Play Therapy – Stop & Calm

Supplies

- A Calming Picture
- Craft stick
- Red construction paper (folded in ½)
- Glue Stick & Tape
- Pair of Scissors
- Colored Marker

Directions

1. Create a Stop Sign by cutting the red paper with the fold on top.

2. Glue the two sides, with the craft stick at the bottom, use tape to secure the craft stick. On one side write the word STOP with marker. Tape a calm drawing on other side.

Say 'STOP' to a suicidal thought.
Turn the sign & practice calm breathing.

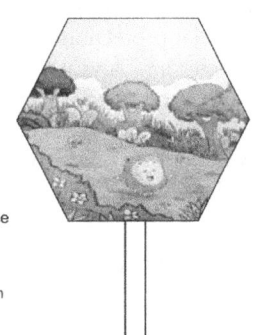

Figure 7.2 Stop & Calm Intervention

interventions within the play-based paradigm. DBT-A has been adapted for adolescents and DBT for children has been shown to be effective with children especially when parents and caregivers are involved in learning the DBT tools adapted for children (Perepletchikova et al., 2010). Integrative Expressive Play Therapy blends theory, technique, and common factors. Play therapy, Cognitive Behavioral Therapy (CBT), and Dialectical Behavioral Therapy (DBT) afford research-based theory and interventions. Dialectical Behavior Therapy (DBT) focuses treatment interventions on mindfulness and meditation, behavioral chain analysis, and coping skills. The following is an example of Paced Breathing to downregulate and calm oneself in DBT.

Paced Breathing (Linehan, 2014) is a DBT intervention for downregulating emotions inside the youth. It involves deliberately slowing down the exhalation part of the breathing cycle, stimulating the parasympathetic nervous system (PNS). The activation of the PNS can induce a calming and soothing effect, helping youth feel more rooted, mindful, and less agitated. The adolescent should breathe slowly and deeply from the belly. This is called diaphragmatic breathing. Next, the adolescent would slow the pace of their breathing to one breath every 12 seconds. Lastly, the adolescent exhale should be longer than their inhale; for example, for a ten-second exhale, the inhale would be five seconds, and the exhale would be seven seconds (Linehan, 2014) children. Deep breaths for younger children can be facilitated by asking the child to choose a stuffed animal, lie down, and place it on their belly, and as they breathe in deeply, they can feel and watch the stuffed animal rise and fall to their breaths.

Applying the Prescriptive Play Therapy model to the assessment and treatment of suicide in children and adolescents allows the play therapist to incorporate interventions and techniques from such evidence-based protocols as Expressive Play Therapy, Cognitive

Behavioral Play Therapy, and Dialectical Behavior Therapy (Malchiodi & Crenshaw, 2014). An individual or family play therapy intervention from a Prescriptive Therapy model may include interventions selected from Integrative Expressive Play-based Therapy, CBT, and DBT to meet the needs of youth or families coping with STB. It requires increasing emotional protection against the negativity that can permeate youth and families' thinking, behaviors, and negative self-talk with suicidal ideation. For many individuals, suicidal thoughts and behaviors can seem to stack up and feel confusing. To help the child or adolescent examine these complex issues, the play therapist or school counselor can utilize the *Deconstruct to Reconstruct* (Baker, 2023a) intervention. This intervention incorporates key CBT and Expressive Play-based Theory constructs to facilitate learning and growth.

DECONSTRUCT TO RECONSTRUCT

Intervention: For a child or adolescent struggling with Suicidal Ideation (SI), a play therapist, school-based play therapist, or clinician invites the youth to build a block stack or a block creation. Each block color is assigned to a question about SI. The blocks are a metaphor for how suicidal thoughts block the child and adolescent from feeling free to think what they would like to think. SI does not allow their minds to think freely without suicidal ideation (Baker, 2023a).

Supplies: A piece of lined paper, 1–2 pieces of watercolor paper, a set of colored blocks, magazines, scissors, decoupage glue, watercolor pens or brush and watercolor paints, and a thin permanent marker if the youth chooses to write any of their SI answer words onto their art paper.

Once built, the client points to or plucks a block from their creation and then answers the question on the block (or related to that block). For example, Red blocks– How often do you experience suicidal thoughts? Green blocks: What does your suicidal thinking say? Blue blocks: How does your suicidal do suicidal thoughts make you feel? And Yellow blocks: What would you like to say back to your suicidal thoughts? A clinician can add to or create a list of questions tailored to the SI of a particular child or adolescent. Deconstructing SI can assist youth in more deeply understanding their own SI, where and why they may be feeling suicidal, and what they might like to say about their suicidal thoughts (Baker, 2023b).

Reconstruction comes through reforming their SI into a new vision expressed by the child or adolescent. The youth's deconstruction of SI is now reconstructed into a new self-created image that holds a new understanding of their SI. The client can write their answers onto lined paper, or the clinician can transcribe them. Once the block activity has yielded some possible answers, the youth can use their own words or the transcribed words from the clinician to assist in developing their expressive play-based project. If a youth combines these into their project, words can be written using a thin permanent marker or cut out from magazines and glued with decoupage glue onto the watercolor paper. Watercolor pens express, mix, or amplify the youth's expressions. The watercolors with brushes can also be added or used instead of watercolor pens. Some words will fade or will be more amplified depending on the colors chosen. This activity moves from the containment of blocks to identifying suicidal thoughts, allowing for a sense of control. Then, the youth advances into the less controllable media of watercolors. Youth may choose not to draw words from the block intervention and instead use only colors to express and explore their suicidal thoughts and feelings flowing with their creation (Baker, 2023b).

When treating a child or adolescent with suicidal ideation, the clinician must use all available resources in an individualized treatment plan to authoritatively assess for risk factors, protective factors, and warning signs that might be or could be put in place to improve safety matching needs of the client with interventions that heal and protect.

FAMILY PLAY THERAPY

General Family Systems theory is a conceptual framework that examines family relationships and interactions as an integrated whole rather than focusing on individual members in isolation. It views a family as a complex system where each member has a role that influences the behavior and emotions of the other members. Changes or actions taken by one individual can have a ripple effect throughout the system (Johnson & Ray, 2016).

Family Play Therapy allows families to join together to build trust and stop focusing on one person in the family as the identified patient. Family play therapy involves engaging with children and their families, where significance is derived from actions and behaviors. Play is a remarkably innovative method to reveal meaning through activities, often the preferred communication channel for children. Using play is an impactful way to interact with families, presenting therapists and family members with various practical techniques. These can range from family art therapy to puppet-based family interviews to impromptu and deeply meaningful storytelling. The rhythm of therapy, both throughout the session and in specific moments, can be significantly enhanced by this method. Through the lens of play, one can delve into new meanings tied to actions and explore novel activities associated with different interpretations (Trotter, 2013). The research underscores the significance of involving caregivers in the process to enhance the outcomes for children (Bratton et al., 2005). Family play therapy has the potential to alter fixed views that family members may hold about each other. For example, a parent can engage with a child using a Virtual Augmented (AR) coloring page, such as Quivervision coloring packs like Quiver Masks (Quivervision, 2022). Both parent and child color a Mask page together, hold up their cell phones with the AR application, and watch the coloring page come to life with their faces behind the Masks. The child's eyes become expressive, and the parent softens and sees themselves as a child when they are young, being surprised for the first time. This experience builds empathy with their child over a playful experience and new knowledge in family play therapy.

FAMILY VALUES

To increase protection against emotional negativity for youth and families, highlighting values in affirmations can be helpful. In a groundbreaking study of value-based affirmations by Cohen et al. (2006), consisting of a double-blind, randomized controlled trial, the researchers explored whether psychological threats could be mitigated by prompting students to reaffirm their sense of self-worth or "self-integrity."

Middle-to-low-income seventh graders in a multicultural school were given a list of 12 values (e.g., relationships with friends/family, having a particular skill, religion) and randomly assigned to one of two groups. Students in the experimental group were asked to select the two or three values most important to them and write a paragraph on their significance in their lives. In contrast, students in the control group chose their least important values and wrote about why someone else might find them necessary (Cohen et al., 2006).

The study revealed that this short in-class writing task substantially improved the grades of Black students in the experimental group, shrinking the achievement gap by 40%. The affirmation exercise did not affect the grades of White students, indicating that self-affirmation may have reduced stereotype threat among Black students or reinforced aspects of their self-esteem that helped alleviate stress levels, thereby enhancing performance (Cohen et al., 2006). One technique to assist families in uncovering their values is the "Click Down Technique" developed by Dave Logan (2011) in his book *Tribal Leadership*.

Finding the family or personal core value steps:

1. Begin by posing a broad inquiry, such as "What truly brings me joy?"
2. Delve deeper by following up your initial response with a "why" question to understand the underlying reasons.
3. When you notice the responses begin to echo previous answers, you have reached the fundamental value.
4. Continue to "click down" until you have no more answers, or you are repeating the same answer.

Example:

1. "What truly brings me joy?" Family and Friends
2. Why? The connection we share.
3. Why? Connection means Love; Love is security.
4. Why? It's just Safe.

For this person, feeling safe in the family is a core value.

Understanding one's values is connected to affirmations for self-worth. In a family setting, developing an understanding of the family's values can also assist the family in creating a positive outlook to be proud of and follow.

The intervention *The Family Values Affirmation Quilt* (Baker, 2013) can assist families in identifying their core values. Materials include foam core with adhesive back sheets cut into 3"x4" long strips, one sheet of foam core without adhesive, permanent color markers to write words on the foam core, foam core stickers, glue sticks, and other adhesive decorations such as stickers, jewels, and glue sticks. The intervention process is to ask the family to look at a list of values and to choose the values each family member feels are essential to them. Be sure to leave blank spaces on the values sheet so families can consider their specific values that may not be on the values list. Each family member or youth can write their value into one of the foam core strips. Family members write an affirmation based on their values on another foam core strip. This affirmation is a statement to themself about their positive value to reinforce the positive values about themselves and their family. Lastly, the youth and family members write at least three values and affirmations on the foam core strips. The family can then decorate their strips and stick their value and affirmation strips to the larger foam core to create a large *Family Values Affirmation Quilt*.

The *Family Values Affirmation Quilt* was inspired by the following question: If suicide is a threat to a youth and family, can identifying their values, writing, and talking about those

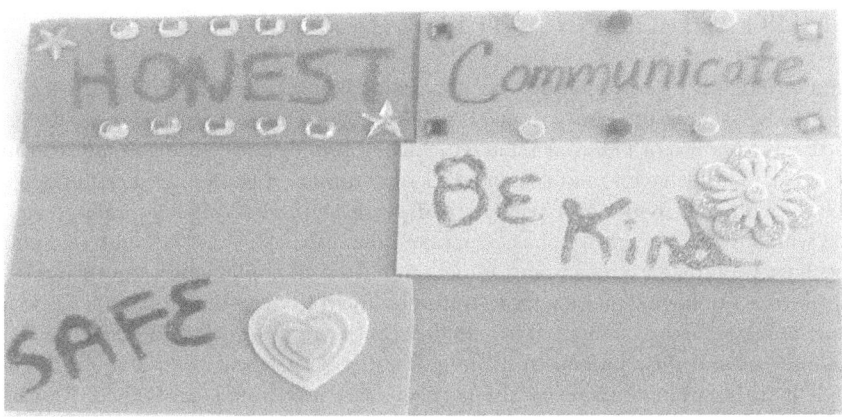

Figure 7.3 Family Values Affirmation Quilt

Source: Baker, L. (2013, May). The Family Values and Affirmation Quilt. [Conference Presentation]. "Sexting," Texting, Mobility & Porn – Family Play Therapy Techniques for Children & Teens. 8th Annual Sothern California Regional Association for Play Therapy Conference, Orange County, CA.

values provide some protection against the stress families face against suicide? More research is necessary.

Family cohesiveness plays a primary role in many communities. For the Lakota Nation, kinship holds significant importance in the structure of the tiyóśpaye, or extended family. It embodies principles of harmonious living, belonging, viewing relationships as a primary form of wealth, and valuing trust in others. These values are integral to the functioning of the tiyóśpaye (*Seven Lakota Values*, 2022).

From the Lakota perspective, the accurate measure of one's wealth is one's family. This unit provides a safety net, offering support during good and challenging times. A person becomes part of a tiyóśpaye through birth, marriage, or adoption, extending family ties to their tribe and the entire Lakota nation. This vast familial network ensures they can anticipate a warm welcome and support wherever they travel as if they were among their immediate family (*Seven Lakota Values*, 2022).

Another intervention is called the *Bag of Marbles* (Rodrigues, 2011). Material includes many colored marbles, some larger to represent parents or caregivers, some smaller marbles to represent other family members and tribal peoples, and a cloth bag with a tie to hold the chosen marbles. The intervention is for the youth to select the marbles that represent the family of the youth so they can carry their family with them as a daily reminder of the youth's connection to their family. The bag of marbles also represents a sense of belonging to their family and reminds them of the power of being a part of their tribe and the Lakota Nation. The youth can play with the marbles to self-soothe and also look at the marbles as they represent their family and their Lakota tribe and Nation.

In Chapter 2, we examined some unique aspects of working with suicide. Gaming Addiction and assisting families in managing their time with technology are two other issues to consider in treating suicide.

GAMING ADDICTION AND TECHNOLOGY

Gaming Addiction is now identified as a "Gaming Disorder" by the (*Gaming Disorder*, 2024). The 11th Revision of the International Classification of Diseases (ICD-11) describes gaming disorder as a pattern of behavior related to "digital gaming" or "video gaming" (*Gaming Disorder*, 2024). This behavior manifests as a lack of control over gaming, giving it undue importance over other activities and pursuits and persisting or intensifying gaming even when faced with adverse outcomes. It has been noted that many play and school-based play therapists have been diagnosing gaming addiction in their clinics, practices, and schools. Youth may overreact to having parents try to transition them from gaming to another activity, like eating, going to bed, or school. This conflict can become so desperate between the child or adolescent and their parents and caregivers that it can escalate to a youth threatening suicide if their gaming or Internet use is taken away, moderated, or stopped. Research has shown that youth and their families can be treated in therapy to address gambling addiction through play therapy.

Combined findings from four studies suggest that CBT could be the top treatment to reduce internet use and boost self-awareness among users. Specifically, after a short CBT course, 54 teenagers aged between 9 and 19 (with 16.7% classified as Internet addicts) demonstrated a notable reduction in the time they spent online, along with a decrease in emotional and physical repercussions linked to their Internet use (Szász-Janocha et al., 2021). Cognitive Behavioral Play Therapy (CBPT) combined with Expressive Play-Based Therapy can also effectively treat gaming addiction. Kim et al. (2018) conducted a combined CBT and music therapy program for adolescents with excessive Internet use. The findings revealed that, after a one-month group intervention, participants displayed reduced scores in gaming addiction, depression, and anxiety (Kim et al., 2018).

Many youth use extensive media, often obsessing over several sites to maintain peer connections. This behavior leads to chronic sleep deprivation and has a negative impact on cognitive functioning, academic success, and social-emotional functioning (Abi-Jaoude et al., 2020). After a systematic review of the current literature, it was found that prolonged use of smartphones and social media sites – more than one to two hours a day – deteriorates mental health (Abi-Jaoude et al., 2020). It was further recommended that families work with their youth and mental health professionals to review the risks of emotional distress from social media and smartphone use. When families are involved in educating and solving these concerns with their child or adolescent, they must maintain an atmosphere of open communication free from judgment (Abi-Jaoude et al., 2020). For example, the *Techno Home Activity Board* can assist a play therapist and a school-based play therapist in working with families to strategize ways to communicate their concerns and develop new ways to relate to social media and technology use in the home.

FAMILY INTERVENTION FOR TECHNOLOGY

Techno Home Activity Board (THAB) (Baker, 2015) enables families to benefit cooperatively by increasing awareness of technology use time. With the THAB, a family can co-create alternative ways to use technology in their home. Supplies include one mini tri-fold board, rooms of your choice (free clipart for personal use only), Art Skill Pre-Cut Poster Shapes 1 Package (available @ Education Stores), create family faces cards to represent those who live in the home (free clip art faces for personal use only). Technology cards can be created by drawing or using free clip art of cell phones, laptops, desktops, tablets, TVs, game players, VR headsets, AR glasses, or headsets to be used as game pieces. Design the cards with glue sticks, scissors, and felt pens – one piece of 9.5"×11" cardstock. A family can create the *Techno Home Activity Board* using the materials. With a glue stick and scissors, create the rooms in their home. Include kitchens and bathrooms. These are rooms or areas where any family uses technology in their home. Some play therapists and school-based play therapists make one game board and use it with all their families. Making one board is more cost-effective and less time-consuming. It is the clinician's choice to decide the best approach for their way of working.

Directions:

- Place the *Techno Home Activity Board* on the table or floor with Families.
- Place Face cards and the Technology cards on the Technology Home Board.
- Begin with the youngest family member and let them choose a Face card to represent each family member.
- Have them choose a Technology card and place the Face card and the Tech card into the room they feel each family member is most often in when using that technology. The goal here is for each person to identify their personal experience with their family members regarding their perception of technology use in their family. For example, a child may perceive that Dad is always on his laptop in his office. The child would place his dad's Face card and a Laptop card into the home office or area his dad uses. When it is Dad's turn, he can put his son's Face card and the technology in the appropriate room. By this method, both parties become aware of their habits regarding technology and its effect on their relationship. They can work together to increase awareness and decrease conflict.
- Have each family member repeat the process, allowing them to explore their perception of technology use in the family.

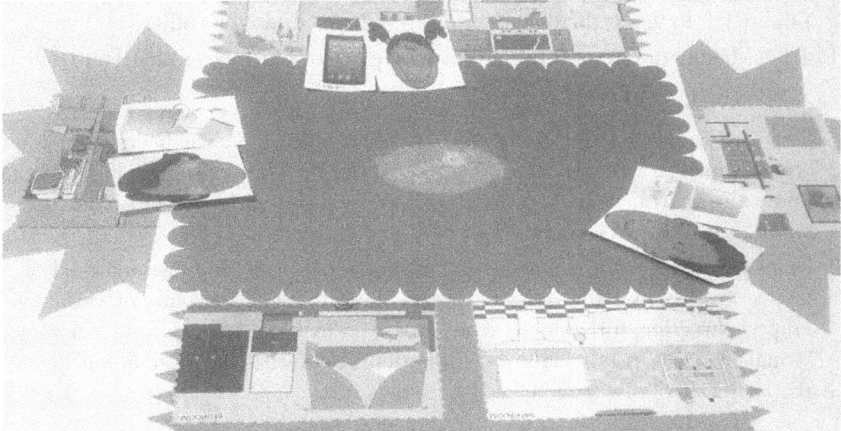

Figure 7.4 Techno House Board Game Diagram

Source: Baker, L. (2015, May). Techno Home Activity Board [Conference Presentation]. Tech Gone Wild! Sexting, Porn, and Cyberbullying in Treatment. Expressive Therapies Summit, New York, NY.

- After each family member has taken a turn, photograph each board. The pictures can be used for another session to process further.
- At the next session, families can refer to printed pictures placed on the table or floor as a discussion opportunity for each family member to consider how technology affects their relationships. Family members can provide positive feedback and support for each other while working to reduce and change their technology use.
- Parents must assess their use of technology and that of their children and adolescents. The family working together promotes a greater sense of fairness among all members, a sense of "we are all in this together" to solve this issue.

FAMILY EXPRESSIVE PLAY-BASED INTERVENTIONS FOR FAMILIES IN PLAY THERAPY

A leading authority in Family Play Therapy, Dr. Eliana Gil, recommends an integrated approach for engaging the entire family in treatment. An example of one of her integrated interventions is the Family Aquarium Project (Gil, 2015).

Family Aquarium Project (FAP)

This expressive play-based intervention usually takes two to three sessions to complete.

Materials: poster board (can choose blue to represent water – also can use white and let client[s] select the color of the "environment"), various color cardstock or construction paper, markers, crayons, glitter, sequins, feathers, other decorative material, glue, and scissors.

Directions:

Task 1 – This may take one entire session: Each family member draws a picture of a fish. Decorate the fish; some art and crafts materials should be made available. The fish are left to dry at the play therapist or school counselor's office.

Task 2 – Making the Aquarium – Use a large piece of blue poster board (or white poster board).

Give the following directions to the family: "This blue poster will become an aquarium where your fish will coexist. Your job is to decide what kind of living environment you want for your fish. You decide where the fish will go vis-a-vis your needs and wants. Find the place you like."

Processing: Consider the aquarium as an individual projective task followed by a collective task. Notice the unique aspects of each fish. Environment variables: full/empty, nurturing, threatening. The fish are co-existing. How do they negotiate individual/systemic needs? Humor? Bountiful? Impoverished? Relational issues: conflict, enmeshed, disengaged?

Wonder what it is like to live here? Wonder if these fish (or your fish) need anything else to live here? Wonder what these fish (or your fish) might be saying to the other fish?

Witnessing the Family Aquarium Project, play therapists and school counselors get a glimpse into the family dynamics. Witnessing the process of creating the FAP allows clinicians to observe how the family works together and may provide insight into a family's inner workings (Gil, 2015).

Bottom Up Interventions

In supporting the 3 R's, the sequence of engagement from Dr. Bruce Perry (Perry, 2009), these upcoming interventions focus on **r**egulating a child or adolescent to allow for **r**elating with the youth, and, finally, **r**easoning can become available.

Snug and Rug and the 'No Good Very Bad Thing': A Story of Coping, Calming & Courage for Children (Baker & Cross, 2019b) include two interventions that assist youth with calming and comfort. In the first intervention, the child or adolescent creates a *Blanket with Fringe*, assisted by the clinician and family members. Choose 1.5 yards of double-sided anti-pill fleece material, cut a 4"×4" inch square from each corner to allow for knot tying, and begin to cut 1" to 2" strips around the edges of the fleece. Help from caregivers will build bonds and connections. Once the strips are cut, it is a mindful practice to tie a knot at the bottom of each strip. Again, this project joins the parent or caregiver with the youth as they work together. Once the blanket is complete, the parent or caregiver suggests wrapping the youth securely, like a burrito. The youth is "Safe in a hug by a bug!" If you prefer to snuggle in the blanket, that works too. We would ask, before this step, modeling with the youth, the practice of having the parent or caregiver ask to approach to wrap the blanket with fringe or to have the parent or caregiver show the child or adolescent how to wrap themselves up in the blanket with fringe.

Scarf with Fringe Intervention (Baker & Cross, 2019a) is an adaptation that is smaller and uses less fabric. Cut a strip of fleece the length suitable for a scarf, and at each end, cut 1" to 2" strips at the top and bottom of the fleece that covers the size of the short side of the scarf's edge. Choose a material in fleece that brings the client comfort. The scarf is worn thick or thin and can be a calming reminder to relax and breathe. Again, this can be done with a parent or caregiver. In this adaptation, the parent/caregiver can create their scarf with the youth, demonstrating an attachment theory known as mirroring based on self-psychology by Heinz Kohut. Explained in therapeutic contexts, "mirroring" refers to the therapist's act of reflecting where they praise, commend, recognize, and appreciate the client's feelings of accomplishment and pride.

Additionally, "twinship" can arise when the therapist and client recognize shared experiences, humor, and interests or engage in a light-hearted philosophical conversation (Finlay, 2015); for example, a youth and their therapist like the same fabric or a parent/caregiver chooses the same fleece fabric.

Another adaptation, *Comfort Tagalong* by Cross (2022), created for mini comfort and as a transitional object, calls for finding a character you love on fleece fabric and purchasing only enough to cut out that image entirely. For example, an owl is on fleece fabric. Cut out the owl. You can cut a small hole in the top, add a tie (ribbon or string), and tie it inside your purse, bag, or backpack. Simply rubbing that small fleece object can bring comfort in a pinch. One can even tuck that little fleece image in their pocket. Ready for a soothing rub right there in one's pocket!

Snug and Rug and the 'No Good Very Bad Thing': A Story of Coping, Calming & Courage for Children (Baker & Cross, 2019b) also includes a *coloring book* with black and white coloring pages. A parent can copy a coloring page from the book with crayons or felt pens. Coloring is a calming, relaxing, and mindfulness practice for youth and adults alike.

SHORT BRIEF IN-HOSPITAL TREATMENTS

The Attempted Suicide Short Intervention Program

The Attempted Suicide Short Intervention Program (ASSIP), originating in Switzerland, operates on the premise that understanding the unique journey leading to a suicide attempt is crucial in crafting effective prevention strategies. ASSIP centralizes the patient's story and views a suicide attempt as an action aimed at achieving a specific goal – often the cessation of unbearable emotional pain – rather than merely a symptom of mental illness (Gysin-Maillart et al., 2016).

Gysin-Maillart et al. (2016) describe ASSIP as an innovative brief therapy grounded in a patient-centric model of suicidal behavior, emphasizing the early establishment of a therapeutic alliance. The process unfolds over three sessions. In the first session, patients narrate their self-harm journey while being video recorded. The second session involves a joint review of the recorded narrative by the patient and the ASSIP-trained therapist. The third session focuses on creating safety planning strategies to deter future suicidal behavior. This collected information, summarizing the individual's case and safety plans, is shared with the patient, their family (if the patient agrees), and other healthcare providers. The ASSIP serves as a blueprint to mitigate future risks within the community. Additionally, therapists send "caring contact" letters for several months after the in-person sessions. The manual provides detailed guidelines for this highly structured treatment, including checklists, educational materials, and standard letters for healthcare professionals in diverse clinical environments (Gysin-Maillart et al., 2016).

A Swiss study involving 120 recent suicide attempt survivors divided participants into two groups. Half received standard therapy (control group), while the others underwent ASSIP. After two years, results indicated that the ASSIP group had roughly 80% fewer suicide attempts and over 70% fewer hospitalization days than the control group (Gysin-Maillart et al., 2016).

COLLABORATIVE ASSESSMENT AND MANAGEMENT OF SUICIDE

The Collaborative Assessment and Management of Suicide (CAMS) is a clinically validated method that has evolved substantially over a quarter-century of dedicated research in the field. CAMS, a psychotherapeutic structure created by David Jobes, is a semi-structured therapeutic model. It emphasizes the significance of an active collaboration between the patient and therapist. It aims to evaluate and address the individual underlying elements or triggers of suicidal tendencies. Furthermore, CAMS is constructed to foster a robust clinical alliance that enhances the patient's will to live (Ryberg et al., 2016).

Central to the CAMS approach is the use of the Suicide Status Form (SSF), a multipurpose clinical assessment, treatment planning, tracking, and outcome tool. The original development of CAMS was rooted mainly in SSF-based quantitative and qualitative assessment of suicidal risk. As this line of research progressed, CAMS emerged as a problem-focused clinical intervention designed to target and treat suicidal "drivers" and ultimately eliminate suicidal coping (Jobes, 2012).

Blossom et al. (2022) stated that in response to the escalating rates of adolescent suicide, CAMS had evolved a specific version tailored to this demographic, known as the

Collaborative Assessment and Management of Suicide for Adolescents (CAMS-4Teens). It incorporates a new element, the CAMS Parent Report Form (CAMS PRF), to involve parents effectively and efficiently in the treatment process. CAMS has been with adolescents and children (CAMS-4Kids) as young as 4. Clinicians are encouraged to consider parental characteristics with empathy, enabling patient- and family-centric decisions. This nonjudgemental and empathetic evaluation of parents facilitates their involvement. It ensures that treatment and discharge plans take into account the strengths and needs of the parents, as well as the preferences and priorities of the patients (Blossom et al., 2022).

CAMS is widely utilized in various healthcare settings, including clinics and hospitals, as a one-off intervention or short-term strategy during inpatient stays and even as a continued treatment in intensive outpatient programs. It is integrated into the evaluation process of Mobile Crisis Response Teams in several states and local organizations, aiding decisions about disposition and treatment options for individuals in crisis. CAMS is also applied by Military Behavioral Health providers and Veterans Affairs' inpatient and outpatient services. Its successful implementation extends to Sovereign Nations and Tribes, and it has been a crucial component of Zero Suicide initiatives both domestically in the U.S. and globally (Tarallo & Lucas, 2021).

THE TEACHABLE MOMENT BRIEF INTERVENTION

The Teachable Moment Brief Intervention (TMBI) draws from two evidence-based strategies for suicide prevention: a) the therapeutic philosophy of the Collaborative Assessment and Management of Suicide (CAMS) (Jobes, 2012) and b) Dialectical Behavior Therapy's (DBT) functional analysis of self-directed violence (Linehan et al., 2006). CAMS' therapeutic philosophy is built on creating a cooperative relationship with the patient and addressing the unique factors connected to their suicidal thoughts. DBT's functional analysis of self-directed violence aims to acknowledge and validate the internal and external triggers leading to a suicide attempt while recognizing that the ultimate wish might not solely have been death. The collaboration-centric approach of this intervention directs the therapist to guide the patient in uncovering the specific elements leading to their suicide attempt during the functional analysis, contrasting with a psychoeducational approach where the therapist, as an expert, explains general reasons behind suicide attempts.

The TMBI's focus on cooperation and functional analysis aims to take advantage of and enhance the heightened willingness to change that typically arises during the "teachable moment" window, an effect triggered by significant events. More research is needed, but this brief approach, mainly for hospital use, is a hopeful addition to brief suicide interventions.

These short hospitalization brief interventions are crucial to the goal of Zero suicide (*Zero Suicide*, 2022). Although play therapists and school counselors may work more often in outpatient settings, they must still be aware of these interventions and ask if a youth comes from any settings noted previously to provide the most appropriate postvention and follow-up care.

PARENTS AND CAREGIVERS IN TREATMENT

In the initial stages of childhood, kids usually form strong attachments to their parents and develop a trusting bond. This trust extends to the outside world, viewing it as a secure environment conducive to growth. This developmental journey is most intense during the teenage years. Adolescents grapple with fast-paced, physical changes, navigating between the values of parents and peers, forming emotional and physical connections with the opposite sex, and uncertainties about future career paths. While these "developmental challenges" can be stressful, most young individuals navigate them smoothly without significant hurdles. Then there are those young individuals who struggle with life stressors and developmental challenges that can lead to feeling like they are a burden or lack a sense of belongingness. A lack of feeling that one belongs can lead to STB.

Parents and caregivers are challenged when working with youth afflicted with STB. A parent's instinct to protect their child or adolescent can be deactivated by a lack of awareness of risk factors and warning signs, which could cause the parent to dismiss or minimize the youth's presentation of STB. Once STB has been identified, there is also the parent's individual emotional experience of trying to grasp how their child or adolescent can even be contemplating suicide, let alone acting out self-harm behaviors. The high prevalence of parental unawareness and adolescent denial of suicidal thoughts found in research by Jones et al. (2019) suggests that many adolescents at risk for suicide may go undetected. This has important clinical implications for pediatric settings, including the need for a multi-informed approach to suicide screening and a personalized approach to assessment based on empirical data (Jones et al., 2019). Play therapy research has found that including parents and caregivers in the treatment process improves outcomes (LeBlanc & Ritchie, 1999, 2001). In a study by Conner et al. (2014), there was compelling data that the perceived connectedness the child or adolescent has to the father was associated with a lower risk for STB and suicide plans and attempts.

Interestingly, the research also noted that this connection to the father did not lower the frequency of *thinking* about death and dying. This information can lead to better prevention strategies that include the family system. Trying to detect and identify STBs is challenging, even when one has training. For parents and caregivers, breaking down the denial of STB through greater awareness of risk factors and warning signs of STB is essential.

Parents, caregivers, and professionals can sometimes be held back from acting because a youth's STB may appear to be manipulation. Regardless of whether a young person's suicidal intent seems "authentic," play therapists, school counselors, parents, and caregivers must treat every suicidal indication with utmost seriousness. Never downplay such threats. Often, these warnings signal a plea for help, expressing, "I'm struggling." Overlooking this can lead the individual to act on their words. It's always better to err on the side of caution (*What Can Parents Do to Prevent Youth Suicide*, n.d.). Jones et al. (2019) advise using a multi-informed method in clinical settings.

Play therapists or school counselors must understand the family dynamics to identify strengths and potential family obstacles that might hinder STB detection. Research indicates that students who felt they received minimal parental support in the past were at a greater risk of contemplating suicide (Macalli et al., 2018). Macalli et al. (2018) advocate for examining perceptions of parental support to evaluate the risk of suicide and, if necessary, implementing prevention strategies. Family dynamics can impact treatment outcomes (Frey & Hunt, 2017). When it comes to prevention, all eyes must be open to detecting and identifying warning signs to decrease suicide risk factors and warning signs. Resilience factors can reduce the likelihood that risk factors and warning signs will result in suicidal thoughts and actions. When a young person is deemed at risk, schools, families, and peers must cultivate the following protective elements in their environment:

- Support and unity within the family, along with open dialogue
- Support from friends and a tight-knit social circle

- A strong relationship with schools and the broader community
- Cultural or religious faith-based beliefs that endorse a healthy lifestyle
- Strong coping mechanisms and skills for solving problems, including handling conflicts
- A positive outlook on life, high self-worth, and a clear sense of direction
- Accessibility of quality medical and mental health services

(National Association of School Psychologists (NASP), 2015)

ROLE IN ACCESSING SERVICES

It is crucial to understand how parents and caregivers manage a suicidal crisis with their adolescent, how this impacts them as parents/caregivers, how they cope after identification of STB, and how accessing/maintaining services to completion of treatment reflects on the parent/caregivers. The conclusions drawn from an analysis of 22 research articles affirm previous studies, indicating that parents face deteriorating well-being and mental health when their adolescent is experiencing suicidal tendencies. Three time-related themes were pinpointed: the initial recognition of the suicidal behavior, the period of managing the behavior, and the phase following the cessation of the suicidal phenomena (Rheinberger et al., 2023). Although research shows that parents look for assistance from a diverse range of services such as mental health experts, hospital personnel, school mental well-being staff, and peer networks, many studies highlight the difficulties parents encounter in securing support while their child is experiencing suicidal tendencies (Rheinberger et al., 2023). This research goes further by pinpointing the specific challenges parents face in these circumstances and elaborating on the support they seek for themselves and their adolescent child (Rheinberger et al., 2023). The experience of having a teenage child involved in suicidal behavior affects the mental health of parents/caregivers, with significantly heightened levels of emotional distress such as anxiety, depression, guilt, and worry. Although research shows that parents look for assistance from a diverse range of services such as mental health experts, hospital personnel, school mental well-being staff, and peer networks, many studies highlight the difficulties parents encounter in securing support while their child is experiencing suicidal tendencies (Rheinberger et al., 2023). The availability of professional mental health services is routinely affected by expensive costs, extended wait periods, and lengthy referral processes, as noted in studies by Corscadden et al., 2019 and Tristiana et al. Access to services needs to improve for both youth with STB and their parents/caregivers.

In a recent review of research with youth who were in grief from suicide loss, it has been shown that bereavement can lead to a rupture of stability and homeostasis within the family system (Krysinska & Andriessen, 2022). Parents, caregivers, and youth have unique experiences of loss, and their coping strategies can also vary. Child and adolescent grief and loss experiences can lead to more disruption within the family system from misunderstanding the shared experience or not feeling in sync with each other's emotional response (Krysinska & Andriessen, 2022).

An intervention that can aid families in processing their feelings of bereavement after suicide loss and give a visual image that represents the family's ever-changing stability (instability) is the *Grief Sculpture Mobile* (Cross, 2023).

Supplies: 3–4 thin wooden dowels approximately 12" long, yarn, ribbon or string, scissors, blank stickers, and two different colors of permanent markers.

Procedure: Invite the family members to think about the changes due to the loss by suicide. Discuss how each family has a sense of stability within the homeostasis system. When there has been a rupture in the stability, families can feel shaken up in ways they had not anticipated. Ask each family member to use the blank stickers to write down a word or brief phrase that shows how they have felt shaken up by the suicide loss. Once completed, have them tie the dowels together at the apex, creating an X. Add additional dowels like spokes on a wheel. Fasten a length of ribbon (yarn or string) to each end of the dowels. Each family member then attaches their sticker(s) to the end of the ribbon. If there are many stickers, ribbons can be affixed to other parts of the dowel to accommodate the number of stickers used. Attach a string length to the top of the sculpture to hang down, like a mobile over a baby's bed.

Have each family member take turns putting their stickers on the end of the ribbons. One color is for reactions to the suicide loss, and one color is for what might be needed to regain stability (homeostasis). For example, a reaction might be that one of the siblings is isolated from the rest of the family. To regain stability, everyone in the family has dinner together, even if it is just for a few minutes. It is important to note that when a new feeling or trigger is added, homeostasis changes to a new stable point. This new stable point may be one the family does not necessarily like. Once the sculpture is finished, demonstrate how one event can shake everything up by tapping one of the dowels and showing how everything else also begins to move. Families are encouraged to take their sculpture home and find a suitable place to hang it to remind them of all they have been through and that they can recover with time.

SUICIDE PREVENTION WITH PARENTS AND CAREGIVERS IN PLAY THERAPY

Research by Velasco et al. (2020) regarding barriers to prevention services and help-seeking behaviors found two major themes that impede accessibility: stigma and negative beliefs about mental health services and professionals. In other research by Braun et al. (2021), what was found to be most beneficial in promoting willingness to seek help in youth ages 15–24 was to view suicide prevention videos that shared personal stories of peers who struggled with suicidal ideation and help-seeking. Significantly lowered suicidal ideation was reported.

The overriding goal is to keep the children and adolescents safe from harm. How we do this is based on therapeutic play. It is not just the individual who is involved when suicide is present. Families, school personnel, and other allied professionals are all part of the system for preventing suicide. Prevention utilizing expressive play-based interventions helps clients with STBs before becoming critical. When play therapy is combined with phase-based treatment, clinicians may be able to offer more supportive interventions that encourage safety, the resolution of traumatic material, and a smooth transition to the future (Green & Myrick, 2014). The *Questions, Cautions, and Warnings Box* (Cross & Baker, 2022) intervention utilizes phase one of a three-phase model for treating complex trauma, focusing on establishing safety and stabilization (Green & Myrick, 2014). The first phase of treatment addresses having control over the symptoms, building skills to improve emotional and impulse regulation, psychoeducation, having a positive therapeutic relationship, and understanding the role of trauma in self-destructive behaviors. As the child or adolescent explores their suicidal thoughts, feelings, and behaviors, they can improve their overall understanding of what is happening and strategize ways to improve safety and feel more stable. The child and parents (or other family members) are given a cigar box, shoe box, or another craft box with an attached lid to decorate with collage materials and other craft supplies. They are then asked to use small slips of paper to write any questions, cautions, or warnings related to the child's suicidal thoughts or behaviors. For example, one of the questions might be, "What can I do to help you when you feel sad?" or "Why is it so hard to feel better?" A caution might be, "I need to go to bed at a regular time to feel rested and not upset." An example of a warning might be, "When I am not sleeping well, I get scared and overwhelmed." The players can also write amusing questions, cautions, or warnings. For example, "Can you use a funny voice to sing the Happy Birthday Song?" It is important to note that creating many different slips to choose from makes for a more compelling game. Once finished, the slips of paper are put into the box. They are then given a die to play with the *Questions, Cautions, and Warnings Box* intervention (Cross & Baker, 2022). The child and family can set the rules, or the play therapist can suggest the following. Each person takes a turn to roll the dice. If it is an even number, the person who rolls the dice can choose one of the other players to select a slip of paper from the box to answer or discuss. If it is an odd number, the person who rolls the dice must choose a slip of paper from the box and answer or discuss what is written on the slip of paper. As an incentive, the family can choose to give a treat to each player who answers the questions. This intervention provides an opportunity to facilitate communication within the family system through indirect teaching and improving self-expression. It can also be applied within group counseling at school.

For many children and adolescents, suicidal ideation increases when they do not feel heard or seen; they have a sense of being invisible. The play-based intervention *It's All In The Bag: I Hear You; I See You!* (Cross & Baker, 2022) is designed to help the child or adolescent identify who will listen, validate their feelings, and increase self-awareness. Begin by having the child or adolescent list the people at school who would be good to share feelings with. Ask what makes these people suitable to share feelings with – what attributes do they have? Once the play therapist or school play therapist clearly understands what the child is looking for, the child or adolescent can be invited to create two paper bag puppets. One will be a character they make up who wants to be seen and heard but has difficulty making that happen. One is the character that will listen and see them. Have the child or adolescent use the art supplies to create it however they want. Then, ask them to identify which puppet they would like to be and which puppet they would like the educator/school counselor to be. Then, use puppet role-play to talk about and validate those feelings so that the child or adolescent feels seen and heard.

Parental support and understanding are crucial in preventing feelings of hopelessness and suicidal thoughts in young individuals. Staying attuned to a teenager's emotions is essential. Even if they do not openly express their feelings, they might still be anxious about significant upcoming events or deeply affected by personal setbacks. They desire comprehension from their parents. Empathizing and actively listening, coupled with relevant guidance or discussion, can be beneficial (*What Can Parents Do to Prevent Youth Suicide*, n.d.).

Family connection in *Questions, Cautions, and Warnings Box* intervention (Cross & Baker, 2022) and feeling heard and listened to in *It's All In The Bag: I Hear You; I See You!* intervention (Cross & Baker, 2022) assist youth with suicide prevention. Combining psychoeducation with

IT'S ALL IN THE BAG: I HEAR YOU; I SEE YOU!	

Supplies:
 	
 • 2 Paper lunch bags
 • Crayons, markers
 • Construction paper
 • Scissors
 • Glue
 • Googly eyes,
   pom poms, assorted stickers 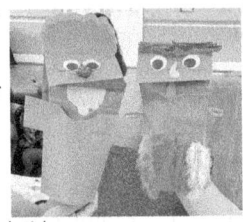
	Trust and Help-Seeking
	 List whom you feel safe sharing feelings with.
	 Invite the child to use the paper bag to make 2 puppets.
	
	 What attributes do they have?
	   1 - Will be a great listener for kids
	   2 - Has challenges in being seen & heard by others.
	 Child creates
	 Which puppet do they want to be?
	 Roleplay scenarios with the child.

Figure 7.5 It's All In The Bag: I Hear You; I See You! Intervention

Source: Cross, M. R. & Baker, L. (2022, October). It's All In The Bag: I See You, I hear You, I value You. [Conference Session]. Restoring Hope to Youth in Play Therapy: Suicide Assessment, Treatment and Prevention, Internal Association for Play Therapy Conference, St. Louis, MO.

Expressive Play-based play therapy allows parents and caregivers to work with their children and adolescents to develop strategies for preventing suicide. The *Handy Helping Hands* intervention (Baker & Cross, 2021a) assists families by creating a hand outline or using a hand-die cut shape (found in school supply stores). The goal is to encourage the youth and caregivers to brainstorm helpers if the youth is feeling overwhelmed, anxious, and having suicidal feelings and thoughts. With a felt pen, they use the handprint and write the names and phone numbers of the essential people on each finger of the *Handy Hands,* such as a supportive parent or caregiver, teacher, play therapist or school counselor, a safe adult or friend's parent. *The Handy Hands* can be decorated with art materials. The *Handy Hands* can be hung on a poster or photographed and kept on an adolescent's cell phone. Increasing a child's awareness that safe and trusted helpers will listen and genuinely care can be a significant step forward.

Another intervention for families to practice at home in a play therapy session or school-based play therapy is the *Circle of Hope Collage* intervention (Baker & Cross, 2021b). Supplies include three paper circles in descending sizes, which can be different colors or all one color. Each circle represents an area of the youth's life. The first circle, Prevention in the Community, includes access to services like regular medical and mental health services, faith-based spiritual care, interest groups, social, art, sporting events, or activities in the community that support youth. The next circle is Prevention with Families and Friends. It includes removing the means for youth, connecting with youth, and getting them involved in an activity together, like creating art, going to a park, kicking a ball, reading a book, or baking cookies. The term "quality time" is often thrown around in parenting guides and sometimes greeted with skepticism. However, a strong bond between young people and their parents requires shared moments. It is typical to hear of ongoing disagreements between parents and teenagers. With so much time invested in disputes, why not allocate some of it to enjoy each other's company (*What Can Parents Do to Prevent Youth Suicide,* n.d.)? The last circle

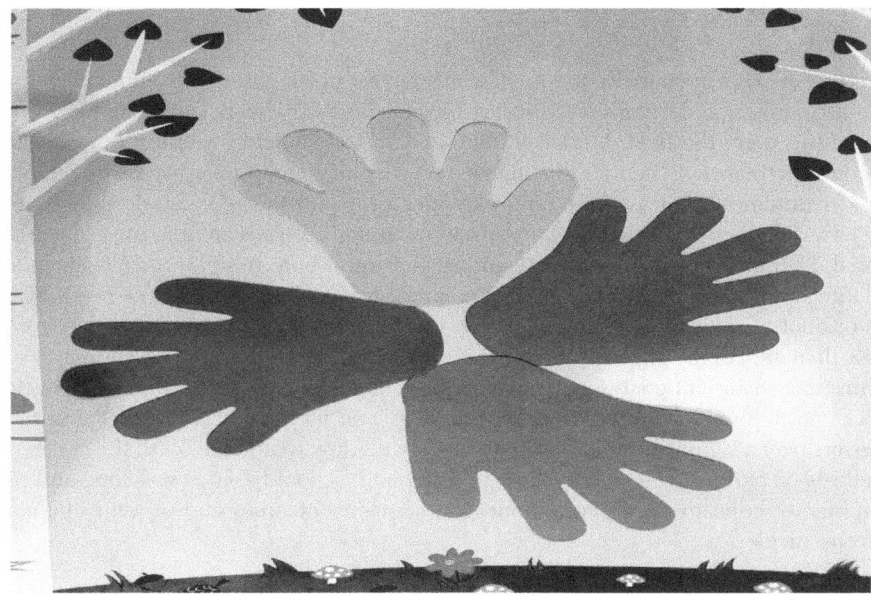

Figure 7.6 Helping Hands Intervention

Source: Baker, L. & Cross, M. R. (2021, October). The Circle of Hope. [Conference Presentation]. Suicide Assessment, Treatment and Prevention: Restoring Hope to Youth in Play Therapy, California Association for Play Therapy. Little Rock, AK.

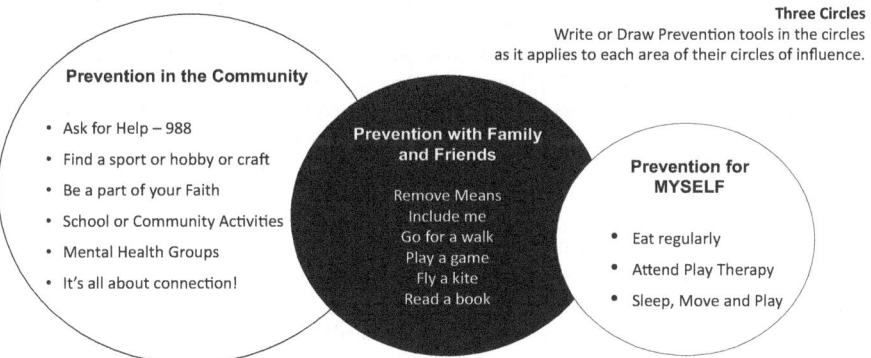

Figure 7.7 Circles of Hope Collage

Source: Baker, L. & Cross, M. R. (2021, October. The Circle of Hope. [Conference Presentation]. Suicide Assessment, Treatment and Prevention: Restoring Hope to Youth in Play Therapy, California Association for Play Therapy. Little Rock, AK.

is Prevention for Myself, which includes developing ideas for self-care. These can be eating regularly, having good sleep hygiene, and exercising. The youth can write words in each circle, draw pictures, or collage pictures from old magazines. This creates a three-circle poster that can be hung up as a reference for children and adolescents. It can also serve as a family reminder of how parents, caregivers, and family members can provide support.

CONCLUSION

Treatment of STB in children and adolescents requires collaboration from all allied professionals, parents, and caregivers to ensure the child's or adolescent's safety in the current crisis and to avert the next. Understanding and treating suicidal youth requires a firm foundation in treatment theories that inform the work for a comprehensive treatment plan. By understanding the play continuum, play therapists and school counselors can examine relevant themes that arise in play therapy treatment. It is essential to apply Neurosequential Therapeutics to treatment planning and use a bottom-up approach, including regulating, relating, and reasoning to create interventions that will meet the needs of the child or adolescent where the dysregulation is observationally centered. The recognized themes then inform the play therapy process by using evidence-based interventions to support meeting treatment goals for suicidal children and adolescents. Treatment of suicidal youth requires family involvement to ensure safety and increase prevention. Parents and caregivers play a significant role in successful play therapy treatment. With the collaborative efforts of parents, caregivers, allied professionals, school-based counselors, and play therapists, we hope to significantly improve treatment outcomes and prevent one more loss from suicide.

REFERENCES

Abi-Jaoude, E., Naylor, K. T., & Pignatiello, A. (2020). Smartphones, social media use, and youth mental health. *Canadian Medical Association Journal, 192*(6), E136–E141. https://doi.org/10.1503/cmaj.190434

Association for Play Therapy. (2023). *Association for Play Therapy*. www.A4PT.org. Retrieved April 6, 2023, from www.a4pt.org/page/Research

Baker, L. (2013, May). *The family values and affirmation quilt* [Conference Presentation]. "Sexting," Texting, Mobility & Porn – Family Play Therapy Techniques for Children & Teens. 8th Annual Sothern California Regional Association for Play Therapy Conference, Orange County, CA.

Baker, L. (2015, May). *Techno home activity board* [Conference Presentation]. Tech Gone Wild! Sexting, Porn, and Cyberbullying in Treatment. Expressive Therapies Summit, New York, NY.

Baker, L. (2018). *Minirock box adapted sandtray for schools* [Intervention] [Unpublished].

Baker, L. (2019). *The stop & calm intervention* [Conference Session]. Suicide Prevention, Assessment & Treatment of Traumatic Grief for Children & Teens in Play Therapy. International Association of Play Therapy Conference, Dallas, TX.

Baker, L. (2023a). *Deconstruct and reconstruct* [Intervention] [Unpublished].

Baker, L. (2023b). *Squish and smash* [Intervention] [Unpublished].

Baker, L., & Cross, M. R. (2019a). Blanket with fringe and scarf with fringe [Intervention]. Snug and rug and the "no good very bad thing" a story of coping, calming & courage for children. *Therapy2Thrive*. www.amazon.com/Snug-Rug-Good-Very-Thing/dp/1733464905

Baker, L., & Cross, M. R. (2019b). Snug and rug and the "no good very bad thing": A story of coping, calming & courage for children. *Therapy2Thrive*. www.amazon.com/Snug-Rug-Good-Very-Thing/dp/1733464905

Baker, L., & Cross, M. R. (2021a, February). *Handy hands* [Conference Presentation]. Suicide Assessment, Treatment and Prevention: Restoring Hope to Youth in Play Therapy, California Association for Play Therapy, San Diego, CA.

Baker, L., & Cross, M. R. (2021b, February). *The circle of hope* [Conference Presentation]. Suicide Assessment, Treatment and Prevention: Restoring Hope to Youth in Play Therapy, California Association for Play Therapy, San Diego, CA.

Bakker, G. M. (2009). In defense of thought stopping. *Clinical Psychologist, 13*(2), 59–68. https://doi.org/10.1080/13284200902810452

Blossom, J. B., Ridge-Anderson, A., Adrian, M., & Jobes, D. A. (2022). A developmentally informed approach to the Collaborative Assessment and Management of Suicide (CAMS) for adolescents (CAMS-4Teens) and engaging parents in treatment. *Practice Innovations, 7*(4), 303–312. https://doi.org/10.1037/pri0000189

Bratton, S. C., & Lin, Y. D. (2015). *The evidence base for play therapy: Does it exist? —And if it does, how do I use it?* [PowerPoint Slides]. Association for Play Therapy Annual Conference, Atlanta, GA. http://evidencebasedchildtherapy.com/am_cms_media/uploaded/a/0e4598521_1444832764_apt-2015pt-researchupdated10-8-2015.pdf

Bratton, S. C., Ray, D. C., Rhine, T., & Jones, L. (2005). The efficacy of play therapy with children: A meta-analytic review of treatment outcomes. *Professional Psychology: Research and Practice, 36*(4), 376–390. https://doi.org/10.1037/0735-7028.36.4.376

Braun, M., Till, B., Pirkis, J., & Niederkrotenthaler, T. (2021). Effects of suicide prevention videos developed by and targeting adolescents: A randomized controlled trial. *European Child & Adolescent Psychiatry, 32*(5), 847–857. https://doi.org/10.1007/s00787-021-01911-6

Cochran, N. H., Nordling, W. J., & Cochran, J. L. (2022). *Child-centered play therapy.* Routledge eBooks. https://doi.org/10.4324/9781003260431

Cohen, G. L., Garcia, J. H., Apfel, N., & Master, A. (2006). Reducing the racial achievement gap: A social-psychological intervention. *Science, 313*(5791), 1307–1310. https://doi.org/10.1126/science.1128317

Conner, K. R., Wyman, P. A., Goldston, D. B., Bossarte, R. M., Lu, N., Kaukeinen, K., Tu, X., Houston, R. J., Lamis, D. A., Chan, G., Bucholz, K. K., & Hesselbrock, V. (2014). Two studies of connectedness to parents and suicidal thoughts and behavior in children and adolescents. *Journal of Clinical Child and Adolescent Psychology, 45*(2), 129–140. https://doi.org/10.1080/15374416.2014.952009

Corscadden, L., Callander, E., & Topp, S. M. (2019). Who experiences unmet need for mental health services and what other barriers to accessing health care do they face? Findings from Australia and Canada. *International Journal of Health Planning and Management, 34*(2), 761–772. https://doi.org/10.1002/hpm.2733

Cronholm, P. F., Forke, C. M., Wade, R., Bair-Merritt, M. H., Davis, M., Harkins-Schwarz, M., Pachter, L. M., & Fein, J. A. (2015). Adverse childhood experiences: Expanding the concept of adversity. *American Journal of Preventative Medicine, 49*(3), 354–361. https://doi.org/10.1016/j.amepre.2015.02.001

Cross, M. R. (2022, October). *Comfort tagalong* [Conference Session]. Restoring Hop to Youth in Play Therapy: Suicide Assessment, Treatment and Prevention, International Association for Play Therapy Conference, St. Louis, MO.

Cross, M. R. (2023). *Grief sculpture mobile* [Intervention] [Unpublished].

Cross, M. R., & Baker L. (2019, October). *Play therapy continuum* [Conference Presentation]. Healing Traumatic Grief & Loss Through Play Therapy: A Bottom-Up Approach. Association for Play Therapy International Conference, Little Rock, AK.

Cross, M. R., & Baker, L. (2022, October). *It's all in the bag: I see you, I hear you, I value you* [Conference Session]. Restoring Hope to Youth in Play Therapy: Suicide Assessment, Treatment and Prevention, International Association for Play Therapy Conference, St. Louis, MO.

DBT-RU: DBT Skills from Experts. (2020, April 10). *TIP skills: Paced breathing* [Video]. YouTube. www.youtube.com/watch?v=y4ElmnxNuT8

Drewes, A. A., Bratton, S. C., & Schaefer, C. E. (2011). *Integrative play therapy.* John Wiley & Sons.

Drewes, A. A., & Schaefer, C. E. (2015). *The therapeutic powers of play* (eBooks, pp. 35–60). John Wiley & Sons, Inc. https://doi.org/10.1002/9781119140467.ch3

Dye, H. A. (2018). The impact and long-term effects of childhood trauma. *Journal of Human Behavior in the Social Environment, 28*(3), 381–392. https://doi.org/10.1080/10911359.2018.1435328

Finlay, L. (2015). *Relational integrative psychotherapy: Process and theory in practice.* Wiley.

Frey, L. M., & Hunt, Q. A. (2017). Treatment for suicidal thoughts and behavior: A review of family-based interventions. *Journal of Marital and Family Therapy*, *44*(1), 107–124. https://doi.org/10.1111/jmft.12234

Gaming Disorder. (2024). World Health Organization. Retrieved March 30, 2024, from https://www.who.int/standards/classifications/frequently-asked-questions/gaming-disorder

Gaskill, R. G., & Perry, B. P. (2014). The neurobiological power of play: Using the neurosequential model of therapeutics to guide play in the healing process. In C. A. Malchiodi & D. C. Crenshaw (Eds.), *Creative arts and play therapy for attachment problems* (pp. 178–194). Guilford Publications.

Gaskill, R. G., & Perry, B. P. (2017). A neurosequential therapeutics approach to guided play, play therapy, activities for children who won't talk. In C. A. Malchiodi & D. C. Crenshaw (Eds.), *What to do when children clam up in psychotherapy. Interventions to facilitate communication* (1st ed., pp. 38–66). Guilford Publications.

Gil, E. (2015). *Play in family therapy* (2nd ed.). Guilford Press.

Green, E. J., & Drewes, A. A. (2013). *Integrating expressive arts and play therapy with children and adolescents.* John Wiley & Sons.

Green, E. D., & Myrick, A. C. (2014). Treating complex trauma in adolescents: A phase-based, integrative approach for play therapists. *International Journal of Play Therapy*, *23*(3), 131–145. https://doi.org/10.1037/a0036679

Gur, R. E., Moore, T. M., Rosen, A. F., Barzilay, R., Roalf, D. R., Calkins, M. E., Ruparel, K., Scott, J. F., Almasy, L., Satterthwaite, T. D., Shinohara, R. T., & Gur, R. C. (2019). Burden of environmental adversity associated with psychopathology, maturation, and brain behavior parameters in youths. *JAMA Psychiatry*, *76*(9), 966. https://doi.org/10.1001/jamapsychiatry.2019.0943

Gysin-Maillart, A., Schwab, S., Soravia, L. M., Megert, M., & Michel, K. (2016). A novel brief therapy for patients who attempt suicide: A 24-months follow-up randomized controlled study of the Attempted Suicide Short Intervention Program (ASSIP). *PLOS Medicine*, *13*(3), e1001968. https://doi.org/10.1371/journal.pmed.1001968

Hambrick, E. P., Brawner, T. W., Perry, B. D., Brandt, K., Hofmeister, C., & Collins, J. M. (2019). Beyond the ACE score: Examining relationships between timing of developmental adversity, relational health and developmental outcomes in children. *Archives of Psychiatric Nursing*, *33*(3), 238–247. https://doi.org/10.1016/j.apnu.2018.11.001

Jobes, D. A. (2012). The Collaborative Assessment and Management of Suicide (CAMS): An evolving evidence-based clinical approach to suicidal risk. *Suicide and Life Threatening Behavior*, *42*(6), 640–653. https://doi.org/10.1111/j.1943-278x.2012.00119.x

Johnson, B. D., & Ray, W. A. (2016). Family systems theory. *Encyclopedia of Family Studies*, 1–5. https://doi.org/10.1002/9781119085621.wbefs130

Jones, J. D., Boyd, R. C., Calkins, M. E., Ahmed, A., Moore, T. M., Barzilay, R., Benton, T. D., & Gur, R. E. (2019). Parent-adolescent agreement about adolescents' suicidal thoughts. *Pediatrics*, *143*(2). https://doi.org/10.1542/peds.2018-1771

Kim, S., Yim, H., Jo, S., Jung, K., Lee, K., & Park, M. H. (2018). The effects of group cognitive behavioral therapy on the improvement of depression and anxiety in adolescents with problematic internet use. *Soa.Cheongsonyeonjeongsinuihak, Journal of Korean Academy of Child and Adolescent Psychiatry*, *29*(2), 73–79. https://doi.org/10.5765/jkacap.2018.29.2.73

Kottman, T. (2014). Positive emotions. In A. A. Drewes & C. E. Schaefer (Eds.), *The therapeutic powers of play* (pp. 103–120). John Wiley & Sons, Inc.

Krysinska, K., & Andriessen, K. (2022). Perspectives on family-based suicide prevention and postvention. *British Journal of Psychiatry Open*, *8*(4). https://doi.org/10.1192/bjo.2022.532

LeBlanc, M., & Ritchie, M. H. (1999). Predictors of play therapy outcomes. *International Journal of Play Therapy*, *8*(2), 19–34. https://doi.org/10.1037/h0089429

LeBlanc, M., & Ritchie, M. H. (2001). A meta-analysis of play therapy outcomes. *Counseling Psychology Quarterly*, *14*(2), 149–163. https://doi.org/10.1080/09515070110059142

Linehan, M. (2014). *DBT? Skills training manual* (Second edition). Guilford Publications.

Logan, D., King, J., & Fischer-Wright, H. (2011). *Tribal leadership: Leveraging natural groups to build a thriving organization.* HarperBusiness.

Lowenfeld, M. (1993). *Understanding children's Sandplay: Lowenfeld's world technique.* Margaret Lowenfeld Trust.

Macalli, M., Tournier, M., Galéra, C., Montagni, I., Soumaré, A., Côté, S. M., & Tzourio, C. (2018). Perceived parental support in childhood and adolescence and suicidal ideation in young adults: A cross-sectional analysis of the i-Share study. *BMC Psychiatry, 18*(1). https://doi.org/10.1186/s12888-018-1957-7

Malchiodi, C. A., & Crenshaw, D. A. (2014). *Creative arts and play therapy for attachment problems.* Guilford Publications.

Maughan, B., Collishaw, S., & Stringaris, A. (2013). *Depression in childhood and adolescence.* PubMed. https://pubmed.ncbi.nlm.nih.gov/23390431

National Association of School Psychologists (NASP). (2015). *National Association of School Psychologists (NASP).* Retrieved August 21, 2023, from www.nasponline.org/

Opiola, K. K., & Bratton, S. C. (2018). The efficacy of child parent relationship therapy for adoptive families: A replication study. *Journal of Counseling and Development, 96*(2), 155–166. https://doi.org/10.1002/jcad.12189

Perepletchikova, F., Axelrod, S. R., Kaufman, J., Rounsaville, B. J., Douglas-Palumberi, H., & Miller, A. L. (2010). Adapting dialectical behaviour therapy for children: Towards a new research agenda for paediatric suicidal and non-suicidal self-injurious behaviours. *Child and Adolescent Mental Health, 16*(2), 116–121. https://doi.org/10.1111/j.1475-3588.2010.00583.x

Perry, B. D. (2009). Examining child maltreatment through a neurodevelopmental lens: Clinical applications of the neurosequential model of therapeutics. *Journal of Loss & Trauma, 14*(4), 240–255. https://doi.org/10.1080/15325020903004350

Perry, B. D. (2020, April 2). *4. Regulate, relate, reason (sequence of engagement): Neurosequential network stress & trauma series.* www.youtube.com/watch?v=LNuxy7FxEVk

Perry, B. D., Pollard, R., Blakley, T. L., Baker, W. L., & Vigilante, D. (1995). Childhood trauma, the neurobiology of adaptation, and "use-dependent" development of the brain: How "states" become "traits." *Infant Mental Health Journal, 16*(4), 271–291. https://doi.org/10.1002/1097-0355(199524)16:4

Quivervision. (2022). *Quivervision.* Retrieved August 9, 2023, from https://quivervision.com/

Ray, D. C. (2015). Research in play therapy: Empirical support for practice. In D. A. Crenshaw & A. L. Stewart (Eds.), *Play therapy: A comprehensive guide to theory and practice* (pp. 467–482). The Guilford Press.

Ray, D. C., Armstrong, S. C., Balkin, R. S., & Jayne, K. M. (2014). Child-centered play therapy in the schools: Review and meta-analysis. *Psychology in the Schools, 52*(2), 107–123. https://doi.org/10.1002/pits.2179

Rheinberger, D., Shand, F., McGillivray, L., McCallum, S., & Boydell, K. M. (2023). Parents of adolescents who experience suicidal phenomena – A scoping review of their experience. *International Journal of Environmental Research and Public Health, 20*(13), 6227. https://doi.org/10.3390/ijerph20136227

Rodrigues, A. (2011, October 17). Lakota sioux girl 'stands against the wind.' *ABC News.* https://abcnews.go.com/blogs/headlines/2011/10/lakota-sioux-girl-stands-against-the-wind

Rubin, L. C. (2006). *Using superheroes in counseling and play therapy.* www.amazon.com/Using-Superheroes-Counseling-Play-Therapy-ebook/dp/B0055FFAOG

Ryberg, W., Fosse, R., Zahl, P., Brorson, I., Møller, P., Landrø, N. I., & Jobes, D. A. (2016). Collaborative Assessment and Management of Suicidality (CAMS) compared to treatment as usual (TAU) for suicidal patients: Study protocol for a randomized controlled trial. *Trials, 17*(1). https://doi.org/10.1186/s13063-016-1602-z

Schaefer, C. E., & Drewes, A. A. (2014). *The therapeutic powers of play: 20 core agents of change* (2nd ed.). Wiley.

Sheftall, A. H., Asti, L., Horowitz, L. M., Felts, A., Fontanella, C. A., Campo, J. V., & Bridge, J. A. (2016). Suicide in elementary school-aged children and early adolescents. *Pediatrics, 138*(4). https://doi.org/10.1542/peds.2016-0436

St. Joseph's Indian School. (2022, April 27). *Seven Lakota values.* Aktá Lakota Museum & Cultural Center. https://aktalakota.stjo.org/lakota-culture/seven-lakota-values/

Szász-Janocha, C., Vonderlin, E., & Lindenberg, K. (2021). Treatment outcomes of a CBT-based group intervention for adolescents with Internet use disorders. *Journal of Behavioral Addictions*, *9*(4), 978–989. https://doi.org/10.1556/2006.2020.00089

Tarallo, J., & Lucas, A. (2021, October 20). *Suicide prevention clinical framework for organizations: CAMS-care*. CAMS. https://cams-care.com/about-cams/organizations/

Trice-Black, S., Bailey, C. L., & Riechel, M. E. K. (2013). Play therapy in school counseling. *Professional School Counseling*, *16*(5). https://doi.org/10.1177/2156759x1201600503

Trotter, K. (2013). Family play therapy. In N. R. Bowers (Ed.), *Play therapy with families: A collaborative approach to healing* (pp. 91–112). https://psycnet.apa.org/record/2014-01051-004

Velasco, A. A., Cruz, I. S. S., Billings, J., Jimenez, M., & Rowe, S. (2020). What are the barriers, facilitators, and interventions targeting help-seeking behaviors for common mental health problems in adolescents? A systematic review. *BMC Psychiatry*, *20*(1). https://doi.org/10.1186/s12888-020-02659-0

What can parents do to prevent youth suicide. (n.d.). https://suicideprevention.nv.gov/Youth/WhatYouCanDo

Wilson, B., & Ray, D. C. (2018). Child-centered play therapy: Aggression, empathy, and self-regulation. *Journal of Counseling and Development*, *96*(4), 399–409. https://doi.org/10.1002/jcad.12222

Zero Suicide (By Education Development Center). (2022). *Zerosuicide.edc.org*. Retrieved August 13, 2023, from https://zerosuicide.edc.org/

CHAPTER 8

IMPACTS OF DIVERSITY IN SUICIDE ASSESSMENT, TREATMENT, AND PREVENTION FOR CHILDREN AND ADOLESCENTS

8.1 Overview
   Rebekah Byrd and Yumiko Ogawa

8.2 Black American Children and Adolescents
   Althea T. Simpson

8.3 Hispanic/Latine Children and Adolescents
   Matthew Nicholas Schramm and Jose Luis Tapia-Fuselier, Jr.

8.4 Native American and Alaskan Native Children and Adolescents
   Ruben Colon

8.5 Asian Americans and Pacific Islander Children and Adolescents
   Yung-Wei Dennis Lin

8.6 Understanding Suicidality in LGBTQ Youth Through the Lens of Queer-PRYSM
   Leslie W. Baker

8.7 Autistic and Neurodivergent Children and Adolescents
   Robert Jason Grant

8.8 Summary
   Rebekah Byrd and Yumiko Ogawa

DOI: 10.4324/9781003358565-10

CHAPTER 8.1

OVERVIEW

Rebekah Byrd and Yumiko Ogawa

This chapter will examine suicide assessment, treatment, and prevention for children from historically and currently minoritized and oppressed communities. Children can internalize external and uncontrollable factors such as social injustice and start living with helplessness and hopelessness. Play therapists must provide culturally inclusive care for all clients, and understanding culture in suicide assessment is imperative.

The following information includes specific statistics on how Black, Latino/a, AAPI, LGBTQIA, Native American, and Alaskan Native fare when impacted by such internalized injustice and how this relates to suicidality. Assessment information, the importance of therapeutic relationships, culturally specific information from culture-specific risk factors, protective factors, warning signs, case examples, play therapist implications, and considerations for culturally sensitive practice.

Play therapy is effective with diverse cultural groups and marginalized children (Post et al., 2019). Play therapists are uniquely suited to practice from a place of cultural sensitivity, humility, and competency. Play therapists are also aware of their biases and how their identities and cultures impact practice. Self-awareness of cultural biases, values, and beliefs is the foundation for multicultural competence and social justice advocacy (Post et al., 2019). According to APT's Play Therapy Best Practices: Clinical, Professional, and Ethical Issues (2022):

> Play therapists ought to be cognizant of how their own identity (i.e., cultural, ethnic, racial, political, etc.) or biases may influence interventions, application of interventions, and therapeutic philosophy. Play therapists should make every effort to gain knowledge about diverse populations by increasing their understanding of multicultural counseling from a social context. Additionally, play therapists shall support and respect the culture, cultural identity, and unique experiences of their clients and families.
>
> (*Play Therapy Best Practices Clinical, Professional & Ethical Issues*, 2022 p. 4)

Play therapists recognize that we can only discuss and understand cultural competence by exploring and understanding social justice advocacy (Ceballos et al., 2021). Further, this quest for cultural competence and social justice advocacy is ongoing and far-reaching. "Counselors who are multicultural and social justice competent are in a constant state of developing attitudes and beliefs, knowledge, skills and action that allow them to effectively work with clients from a multicultural and social justice framework" (Ratts et al., 2016, para. 24). These concepts are essential when working with suicidality among children and adolescents of diverse backgrounds.

Many authors in this chapter address the importance of working with the systems in which children reside to alleviate the pain that leads to their suicidal thoughts and behaviors (STB). Those systems include but are not limited to family, educational, religious, and spiritual systems. In addition, when the root cause of minoritized youth's suicidal ideation, attempts, and completion is embedded in discrimination, oppression, capitalism, and the

DOI: 10.4324/9781003358565-11

absence of a sense of belonging, social justice advocacy competencies become crucial and urgent. Yet, at this point, few articles and studies discuss play therapists' social justice advocacy attitudes (Chase & Post, 2022; Ceballos et al., 2012; Elmadani, 2020; Parikh et al., 2013). By bravely and gravely confronting historical and multigenerational trauma caused by many forms of "-isms," play therapists can bring healing in individuals and initiate a collective healing process for the marginalized in their social justice advocacy mission.

This chapter discusses assessment, treatment, and suicide prevention information through the lens of specific cultural and diverse groups. Discussed are the impact of acculturation, bicultural aspects, and intersectionality for consideration as to how these factors impact mental health and wellness. Concerns such as belongingness and connection within and outside one's culture are integrated into risk and protective factors – peer relationships are necessary specifically for adolescents and their developmental stage. Clinicians should pay attention to peer relationships as these may, in some cases, contribute to suicidality when confusion and conflicts about identity and acculturation increase client stress.

Further, play therapists need to understand the role of historical trauma (Ehlers et al., 2022), intergenerational trauma (see Brave Heart et al., 2011), and discrimination among minoritized groups and how these can be associated with increased risk factors, including suicidal ideation and suicidal attempts (see Assari et al., 2017; Benner et al., 2018; Johns et al., 2020; Madubata et al., 2022; Oh et al., 2020; Perez-Rodriguez et al., 2014). "Racial and ethnic minority populations are thus disproportionately burdened by youth suicide risk, And yet, we know very little about how race-related or culture-specific experiences explain youth suicide risk" (Polanco-Roman, 2020, para. 2). For a play therapist to recognize and detect both warning signs and protective factors of diverse children and adolescents, there must be a thorough yet distinct knowledge of the individual, their culture, their traditions, their ability status, their identity, and the many ways in which these factors present and intersect. The client's culture and characteristics must be central to understanding warning signs and protective factors, and the play therapist is careful not to evaluate based on their own culture, characteristics, or presentation.

Warning signs and assessments will be discussed as well. Risk factors and warning signs specific to varying cultural groups are not well documented due in part to a lack of representation in studies examining suicide (Cha et al., 2018). Additionally, "the need for additional population-based research into suicide attempts and ideation, as well as exploration of additional risk factors" (Kirby et al., 2019, p. 658). While mental health professionals understand overall warning signs, risk factors, and protective factors, it remains uncertain whether these apply to culturally diverse populations (Cha et al., 2018). "Nonetheless, despite the long-standing interest in culture and suicidal behaviors, there are few reports of effective culturally tailored or culturally sensitive interventions for suicidal adolescents" (Goldston et al., 2008, p. 14).

Cultural perceptions about mental health services can also be a barrier to seeking mental health services. Clinicians should consider the role of culture in the client or family's help-seeking behavior and contemplate the role of family shame, stigma, and guilt present in some cultural backgrounds. Expectations of one's culture and family are also important considerations when evaluating and assessing suicidality. Also significant to consider are disparities in access to and mental health care use. Despite well-documented disparities, despite attempts to ameliorate them, they remain to date (McGuire & Miranda, 2008; Mahajan et al., 2021). Due to inequalities, mistrust in mental health services among diverse populations is another significant disparity to consider (Henderson et al., 2015). Play therapists respect substantiated apprehension and work to build trust with minoritized communities while respecting cultural boundaries and beliefs.

Although there are no research studies on the effectiveness of play therapy with minoritized children with suicidality, play therapy is considered an effective intervention to work with children and adolescents with various issues. The metanalytic review by Lin and Bratton (2015) examined the 52 controlled outcome studies (a total of 1,848 child participants) completed between 1995 and 2010 to explore the effectiveness of Child-Centered Play Therapy (CCPT). Among the results, they reported statistically significant and higher mean effect size for CCPT studies mainly recruiting non-White children than CCPT studies mainly recruiting white children. This result indicates the racial diversity and inclusion inherent in play therapy intervention.

The chapter's authors discuss one of the therapeutic powers in play therapy that is particularly effective in working with minoritized children with suicidality: "storytelling." Therapeutic powers of play are core agents of change inherent to all play therapy approaches, and therapeutic powers "transcend culture, language, age and gender" (Drewes & Schaefer, 2014, p. 1). By facilitating children's freedom of self-expression in play therapy while battling suicidal thoughts, play therapists are helping them activate the self-healing part of the brain (Badenoch, 2008) and reducing the sense of despair, hopelessness, and helplessness.

CHAPTER 8.2

BLACK AMERICAN CHILDREN AND ADOLESCENTS

Althea T. Simpson

Mental health disorders are associated with increased mortality, mainly through suicide, morbidity, and loss of productivity (World Health Organization, 2024). Statistics reflect a dramatic increase in the rates of suicidality among Black children and adolescents. Studies by Klingenbjerg (2017), Lindsey et al. (2019), and Sheftall et al. (2016) indicate that elementary school-age children (5 to 11) are the tenth most likely age group to die by suicide. Black males in this age group have even higher rates and are more likely to die by strangulation in a home environment after an argument with friends or family. These decedents died without leaving a suicide note and had a prior history of mental health concerns with higher rates of attention deficit hyperactivity disorder than depression (Sheftall et al., 2016). Comparably, adolescents are more likely to display depressive symptoms and die by suicide after arguments with a boyfriend or girlfriend. Subsequently, studies have found that Black male youths aged 15–19 years old have the steepest rates of suicide (Joe, 2006) and may require medical attention for injuries related to lethal methods of suicide (Lindsey et al., 2019). Of note, studies show that from 2001 to 2017, Black girls' suicide completion increased by 182%.

Being Black is often viewed as synonymous with strength and confidence, so if a child or adolescent struggles psychologically or emotionally, they may need to carry it around to avoid being burdensome to their family. Therefore, Black children and adolescents are less likely to receive mental health assessments and treatment, contributing to the perpetuation of suicidal behaviors or death by suicide. Emotional or psychological problems among Black adolescents are almost exclusively discussed with their families, who respond with messages consistent with not talking to "outsiders" about their mental health problems (Congressional Black Caucus, 2019).

RISK AND PROTECTIVE FACTORS

Black people are disparaged based on their race. They consistently endure experiences that convey "I do not matter." They are constantly faced with society's devaluation of Black lives. This is not an exhaustive list of stressors; however, risk factors and suicidality in Black children and adolescents were found to include depression, delinquent behavior, history of abuse/neglect (Joe, 2008), alienation, hopelessness, despair (Joe, 2006) previous suicide attempts, suicidal ideation, mood, anxiety, substance use (Merchant et al., 2009), sexual victimization, bullying (Fitzpatrick et al., 2008), and sexual and gender minority status (Opara et al., 2020). In addition, at varying degrees, family adversity (Anghel, 2020), socio-economic disadvantage, adolescent parenthood, parental separation, parental mental health problems, and stressful family life events can increase their likelihood of developing mental health difficulties. These experiences range from being stressful to overriding their ability to cope. Some children have an internal locus of control that forges inherent learned resilience, fostering more positive outcomes despite struggling with multiple risks and adversities (Anghel, 2020).

DOI: 10.4324/9781003358565-12

While familial risk factors do not singularly perpetuate suicidality in the Black community, it is essential to understand the protective role of community, religion, and religious participation (Fitzpatrick et al., 2008) in reducing risk and increasing their overall health and well-being. Of greatest importance, Black people value strong family connections, which are substantially relevant to their cultural identity and belief system.

CONCEPTUAL FRAMEWORK

Two theories show promise in guiding clinicians to offer effective treatment interventions to this population:

- Ecosystemic play therapy (EPT) integrates a variety of techniques and theories to create a single model that "addresses the total child within the context of the child's ecosystem" (Boyer, 2010), incorporating key elements of the analytic, child-centered, and cognitive-behavioral models of play therapy (O'Connor, 2001).
- Ecosocial Theory (Anderson, 2004), a multilevel theory of disease distribution that links social and biological processes with a dynamic, historical, and ecological perspective, addresses population distributions of disease and social inequalities in health.

O'Connor (2001) posits that the play therapist's primary role is to help reorganize cognitive or expedient core beliefs. Two specific components of this model may be helpful and make Black youth and their families more receptive to play therapy treatment. The first

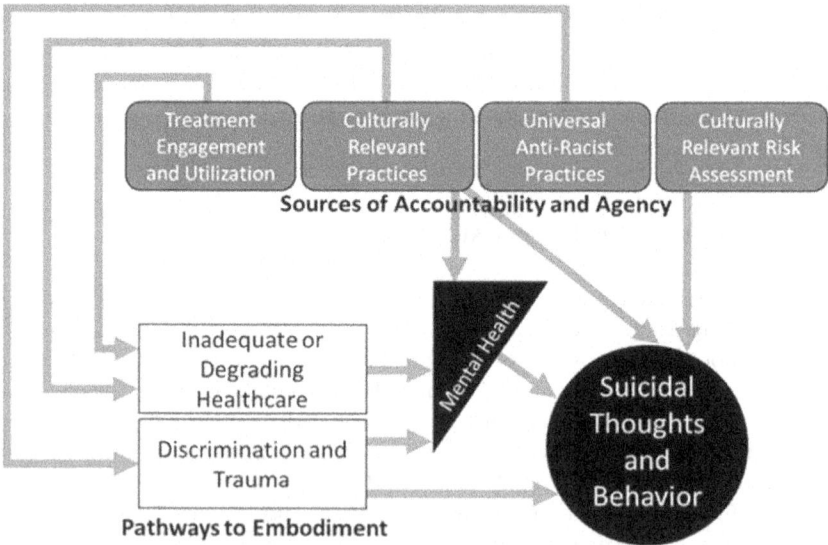

Figure 8.1 Ecosocial Framework for Suicide Prevention among Black Youth

Source: Ecosocial Framework For Suicide Prevention Among Black Youth. Cohen, D. R., Lindsey, M. A., & Lochman, J. E. (2021). Applying an ecosocial framework to address racial disparities in suicide risk among black youth. Psychology in the Schools, 59(12), 2405–2421. Pp. 2408 https://doi.org/10.1002/pits.22588

is the personality concept, defined as the "sum of intra-and interpersonal characteristics, attributes, cognition, beliefs, values, and so forth that make a person unique" (Boyer, 2010, p. 203). The personality concept is based on two drives: maximizing reward and minimizing punishment to meet one's needs while avoiding pain, stress, and unpleasantness. Early attachments fall within the second drive in which children attach to primary caregivers or connect socially, thus seeing others as emotionally supportive (Boyer, 2010). The other component is phenomenology, as its primary goal is to capture the essence of the lived experiences of individuals related to a specific phenomenon without interpreting, explaining, or theorizing (van Manen, 2017); hence, storytelling would allow children and families to share their lived experiences from their perspective, which is as valid as any outsider's perception of their situation (O'Connor, 2001).

Cohen et al. (2021) argue that the elements presented in the Ecosocial Framework offer practical strategies as suicide-preventative measures in multiple environments. Figure 8.1 illustrates the pathways to embodiment that degrade mental health and increase the risk for suicidal thoughts and behavior. Furthermore, it indicates that mental health can be improved, and suicide risk can decrease through accountability and agency, subsequently diminishing pathways to embodiment.

PSYCHOEDUCATION TO COMBAT MENTAL HEALTH STIGMA

The stigma of having a mental health problem becomes a barrier that can lead to delay, avoidance, or disengagement from mental health treatment (Alvidrez et al., 2009). Trying to have conversations in the Black community about the rise of suicidality and death by suicide among Black children and adolescents, despite research findings and statistical evidence, tends to be chalked up to the devil being sent to steal, kill, and destroy the Black community through their children. Psychoeducation, typically an underutilized intervention, can be beneficial. The American Psychiatric Association (Akena et al., 2021) contends psychoeducation improves knowledge in a specific subject area that serves the goals of treatment and is defined as "an approach that combines educational, psychotherapeutic, and experiential components" (Alvidrez et al., 2009). Thus, using psychoeducation in play therapy as an intervention with Black youth and their families can enhance mental health knowledge and improve outcomes and self-efficacy.

INDIVIDUAL PLAY THERAPY TREATMENT

Play therapy allows individuals to solve complex problems through the power of purposeful play. Play therapy strategies that address emotional regulation can help children and adolescents find and recognize emotions other than sadness, thus increasing emotional states (Leigh, 2017). Clinicians need to understand the intersecting factors (Opara et al., 2020) that may contribute to their risk and differentiate between varying suicidal expressions (Romanelli et al., 2022). As they understand the risks of suicidal thoughts and behaviors, they can effectively screen, assess, and implement play therapy strategies, including teaching emotional regulation and cognitive restructuring in response to maladaptive thinking and behaviors.

CASE EXAMPLE

Anton is an 8-year-old Black male referred to play therapy treatment because of his suicidal thoughts and increased expressions of not wanting to be alive. Anton's parents sought treatment services after multiple calls from the school expressing concern over Anton's suicidality. His assessment and subsequent play therapy treatment were delivered virtually. Case conceptualization was employed with the parents to identify the scope of Anton's presenting issues.

During the assessment, Anton's parents denied any mental health concerns on either side of their family. Parent sessions revealed that the family was under extreme stress, including financial stress and the stress related to their middle child with special needs. Anton is the oldest of three children and was tasked to pick up the slack of cleaning the house and helping with his two younger siblings. Anton also had to endure physical aggression from siblings with special needs. His parents reported disrespectful and aggressive behaviors at home and expressed frustration with Anton entering their room each night because of nightmares. There appeared to be multiple interpersonal and family factors contributing to Anton's suicidality.

Throughout the therapeutic process, a therapeutic check-in was done at the beginning of sessions to assess for safety and to explore difficulties Anton struggled with since our previous session. We ended each session with mindful breathing and felt sense activities to increase internal strengthening. The beginning phase of treatment focused on building a therapeutic rapport with Anton and his parents and psychoeducation around childhood mental health concerns and suicidality. Expressive art-based activities focused on identifying, expressing, and communicating emotions. We created fictitious characters each week and engaged in mutual storytelling about the child's problems. Anton would tell a story, and then I would tell the same story with a different ending focused on solving the child's problems.

After about 12 weeks, suicidality was no longer present, but Anton still experienced depressive symptoms and high levels of anxiety with poor frustration tolerance. His treatment goals were outlined as we moved into the middle phase of treatment. We identified three treatment goals to address depressive symptoms, frustration tolerance, and anxiety. Partialization, a strategy for helping clients manage multiple presenting problems, was used not to overwhelm Anton but to address the most urgent problems. Resourcing continued to help Anton tolerate emotions as we moved into processing. In addition to being a Registered Play Therapist-Supervisor™, I am a Certified LEGO® SERIOUS PLAY® Facilitator and have adapted this innovative method as a psychotherapeutic tool. Intentionally integrating LEGO® into play therapy practice can increase emotional intelligence and develop problem-solving capabilities.

Anton was given a range of LEGO® build activities using a directive play therapy approach. After building the LEGO® model, he shared stories, and then we reflected on what was shared.

Good affect expression starts with the play therapist eliciting feelings the child already knows (Deblinger et al., 2015) and expanding his vocabulary with bibliotherapy or expressive activities. Each session, Anton was invited to close his eyes and take a few slow, long breaths in through his nose, breathing in calm, peace, compassion, etc., and exhaling stress, worry, sadness, etc. He was then asked to use his imagination to visualize himself in a chosen scenario. Anton was asked to watch his thoughts come and go, whether by the beach, in a peaceful room, in a cave, or wherever. After doing his best to imagine himself in that scene, he was asked to become aware of his thoughts and observe whatever was coming up, no matter what those thoughts were. He was asked not to try to stop his thoughts and do his best not to criticize himself for any of his thoughts. He was instructed that when he was ready, he would take a deep breath in through his nose and out through his mouth and open his eyes. Hands-on bricks, Anton was asked to create an individual LEGO® model that could contain his unhelpful emotions and thoughts. Anton was then asked to share and reflect on his models and encouraged to describe his actual feelings related to the experience, including intensity. As a part of activity processing, the play therapist should be curious about the youth's LEGO® models and aspects of their stories that lead back to lived experiences that may contribute to the suicide of any youth.

The use of metaphors and storytelling remained the central interventions as Anton moved through the phases of treatment. This approach allowed Anton to normalize and minimize the intensity of his emotions. Much work had been done individually with Anton through family and parental sessions, and after ten months, we entered the final phase of treatment.

During this phase, we reviewed treatment goals, therapeutic gains, and how to access support. Research indicates a strong correlation between parents' levels of distress and how that influences how children react and respond to distressing situations (Cohen et al., 2006). Thus, involving Anton's parents throughout the play therapy treatment process was necessary, although they were not the direct clients. This was also an opportunity to assess their ability to be a secure base, provide support, and model behavior to help improve Anton's overall emotional and behavioral functioning.

CONCLUSION

In recent years, suicide attempts among Black children and adolescents have frequently grown, irrespective of gender (Lindsey et al., 2019). Black children and adolescents are a high-risk group for suicidality, and further culturally specific research is needed to develop suicide prevention and treatment interventions. The Black community often places many expectations on themselves, so allowing themselves permission to feel a full range of emotions without judgment may be difficult. Culturally responsive spaces are needed that allow "Black Pain" into sessions without being dismissed or unacknowledged by the clinician. Clinicians must move from a state of cultural competence to cultural responsiveness that includes meeting Black children, adolescents, and their families with humility, compassion, and consideration respective of their experiences.

CHAPTER 8.3

HISPANIC/LATINE CHILDREN AND ADOLESCENTS

Matthew Nicholas Schramm and Jose Luis Tapia-Fuselier, Jr.

INTRODUCTION

The Hispanic/Latine (H/L) population within the United States (U.S.) is 62.1 million people (Pew Research Center, n.d.) and is growing rapidly, raising the possibility of increased mental health issues and incidences of suicide (Germán et al., 2015). Suicide is the third leading cause of death for H/L children between 10 and 14 and the second leading cause for ages 15 to 24 (Jimenez-Colon & Duarte-Velez, 2022; Price & Khubchandani, 2022). According to the Youth Behavior Risk Surveillance System, 21% of H/L adolescent females considered suicide, while 14% engaged in at least one attempt (Germán et al., 2015). Assessments and interventions must address cultural considerations within the H/L community to effectively treat this high-risk group. This chapter will explore assessments and prevention through a culturally responsive lens.

Cultural identities must be considered when exploring the suicidal thoughts and behaviors (STB) and non-suicidal self-injury (NSSI) of H/L children and adolescents. H/L children who experience high levels of discrimination have 2.4 times more suicidal thoughts and behaviors than H/L children exposed to lower levels of discrimination (Price & Khubchandani, 2022). The use of mental health services by H/L youth is half that of non-Hispanic children (Caplan, 2019). From a cultural and religious context, H/L families are less apt to utilize mental health services due to potential shame, stigma, and guilt (Caplan, 2019). The youth's or family's citizenship status may cause fear of government identification and deportation. H/L families experience many challenges that vary according to their time in the U.S. Immersing into a new culture and language impacts the entire family system of recent arrivals. Different generations of youth will have different experiences as they navigate multiple assimilation processes and stressors (Jimenez-Colon & Duarte-Velez, 2022). Depending on the family composition, H/L youth may become bicultural (i.e., maintain the values of both cultures) to minimize risk and increase protection. Moreover, culturally and linguistically responsive mental health care is limited due to various factors such as geographical region, training and linguistic skills of therapists, access to healthcare, family finances, and other limitations. These limitations result in H/L populations being less likely to receive adequate mental health services (Llamas & Alvarado, 2022).

The low mental health research available for this population is an indicator of economic, cultural, and structural barriers. It limits the clinician's ability to include relevant data in the treatment process. This puts Latine individuals at a higher risk of mental health disorders. H/L teenagers are more likely to attempt suicide than any other group of teenagers; this youth population also had the highest rate of drug use. (Llamas & Alvarado, 2022). Understanding the intersections of culture, identity, and suicide, identifying risk and protective factors, and creating assessments will be discussed in the next section.

DOI: 10.4324/9781003358565-13

SUICIDE AND ASSESSMENT

The H/L population faces significant challenges when seeking mental health services. Much of this stems from Latine families facing a higher risk of poverty and other financial distress due to educational gaps (Wamser-Nanney & Steinzor, 2016). It is evident that there is a high correlation between financial anguish and the struggle to access mental health resources amongst the H/L population, creating high rates of STB and NSSI. It is essential to distinguish between NSSI and suicidal ideations. NSSI may manifest as self-tattooing, piercing, pulling out hair, and allowing or inviting others to induce pain. The risk factors contributing to NSSI are neglect or parental indifference, family violence, and separation and loss. NSSI is utilized as a coping strategy to self-regulate and socially regulate. Youths experiencing hopelessness, isolation, and loneliness may engage in NSSI. Manifestation in H/L youth varies depending on the family system, cultural identity, gender, sexual orientation, disability, etc. H/L youth may experience extreme hopelessness, isolation, and loneliness due to their parent's immigration status, deportation, limited English fluency, or culture shock. The gender identity of the H/L youth is also important to consider regarding their form of expression of NSSI. Cultural dynamics within the family system are also important: the response of parents/caregivers, who might themselves be experiencing feelings of distress, may be invalidating, minimizing, or critical.

H/L youth's dominant methods to complete suicide are hanging, suffocation, and strangulation (Price & Khubchandani, 2022). Risk indicators for H/L youth are prior suicide attempts, alcohol and drug use, mood and anxiety disorders, and access to lethal means (Suicide Prevention Resource Center, n.d.). As mentioned, H/L youth may navigate different cultural dynamics depending on their family's time in the U.S. Experiences that contribute to STB are alienation, acculturated stress, hopelessness, and discrimination (Suicide Prevention Resource Center, n.d.). Serving H/L youth requires conceptualizing their intersectional identities to their presenting problem in particular contexts.

The makeup of the populations studied must be considered when evaluating assessments of STB and NSSI. While specific assessments may present as common and best practice for NSSI and STB, caution should be taken when interpreting results and utilizing them for recommendations, safety, and treatment planning for H/L youth. Standardized assessments only sometimes reflect the concerns, living conditions, etc., experienced by H/L youth.

For H/L children who demonstrate STB, the clinician must provide an environment that does not heighten feelings of guilt or shame. Conceptualizing STB from a culturally responsive lens requires the clinician to be aware of contributing factors. The child may be unable to answer specific questions based on their developmental level and age. The *Fairy Tale Test* can support a clinician working with a H/L child between the ages of 4 and 10. While its original design was a projective test, the *Fairy Tale Test* has been modified to explore the child's thoughts, feelings, and reactions to STB (Orbach et al., 1983). Due to their storytelling nature, puppets and other expressive toys can be utilized to facilitate this assessment. Storytelling is often part of the H/L culture and can be a bridge to the child's inner world. Here are the steps to facilitate the assessment:

- Have the child draw a fairy or pick a puppet or a miniature figure. Be sure to have a variety of fairies to represent your client's identities.
- Ask the child to tell you a story by creating a world with the fairy they drew or selected.

- The story should contain the fairy's best friend who is going through something difficult. Based on the information the clinician has about the child's presenting concerns, the best friend would be dealing with the same issues. Have the child draw or select a toy to represent the best friend. Allow the child to name their best friend.
- Invite the child to enter a fairy world where they are playing with their best friend. The clinician then co-creates a story, taking the role of the best friend dealing with something difficult. The clinician observes the child's response verbally and non-verbally.
- By observation and interpretation, the clinician gains insight into the child's attraction to life, attraction to death, repulsion of death, and repulsion of life.
- Do not ask direct questions. Utilize Child-Centered Play Therapy (CCPT) skills and techniques to facilitate depth in the child's engagement with the Fairy Tale Story.

(Orbach et al., 1983)

Once the child has completed their Fairy Tale Story, the clinician assesses the themes of the child's story to determine if further standardized assessments are needed. In working with the family, the clinician would only share themes of the assessment and gather more details to support the conceptualization. Limiting the discussion to themes and not sharing explicit details of the session allows the clinician to protect the youth's confidentiality.

CASE EXAMPLE

Juan (he/him/his) is a 6-year-old H/L student in first grade and recently began to state that he wants to die. He has been drawing buildings far off to the corner of the paper's right side with a stick figure hanging on a tree. His mood appears to be depressed, and he has not been engaging in typical developmental play. The teacher contacts the school counselor (SC) to provide an assessment in their office. The SC conducts a Fairy Tale Story assessment with Juan. Juan picked a fairy for himself and named his best friend Carlos. He acted out Carlos having a hard time at home by stating, "Me quiero morir" ("I want to die"). The SC explored this through Carlos and reflected on his feelings. Juan continued to share Carlos's feelings that no one liked him and that he was alone. The SC reflected on his feelings and responded in a calm, empathic tone. The SC joined the play by responding directly to Carlos and offering comfort and care. The SC planted seeds of possibility, and Carlos felt he was not alone. After the assessment, it was clear that Juan was demonstrating themes of attraction to death. Through the Fairy Tale Story, the SC facilitates depth and connection without using open-ended questions that might not result in clear answers. This assessment tool offers a relationship that empowers the student to open up in an accepting and non-judgmental space. Suppose Carlos verbalizes serious attraction to death and repulsion to life. In that case, the SC will move to other formal standardized suicide assessments to determine the following steps to protect the student, such as the Columbia Suicide Severity Rating Scale for young children.

FAMILY SYSTEMS

H/L adolescents within the family system encounter challenges in learning to interact with parents and peers. In many cases, it is difficult for H/L youth and families to distinguish between separate cultures. (Zayas et al., 2010). This creates difficulties for H/L adolescents trying to separate their family life from their school and personal life. Many H/L individuals rebelled against their families to fit their peers' new norms. This caused an increase in tension, thereby creating more frequency in STB as a way of coping with their negative frame of mind (Germán et al., 2015). Many H/L parents, having a stigmatized view, invalidate their teen's STB. This behavior often leads H/L teens to shut down, to feel misunderstood and shamed, and it causes emotional dysregulation (Germán et al., 2015; Zayas et al., 2010). Suicide often stems from family conflict due to recent arguments, leading to overwhelming emotions and distress patterns (Zayas et al., 2010). The severity of adolescents' emotions escalates when their problems are negatively received.

Understanding the H/L population's family system and traditions is essential to creating adequate counseling-responsive practices. According to Ceballos et al., the counselor must work with the adolescent's parent or guardian by consistently communicating about what treatment looks like and taking the initiative to learn more about their culture (2020). Including the caregiver in treatment may alleviate anxiety (Ceballos et al., 2020). It is also said that H/L families are more likely to stay in therapy when a therapeutic purpose and an end goal are expressly defined (Wamser-Nanney & Steinzor, 2016). Therefore, establishing guidelines at the beginning is essential when working around the Latine family system.

PLAY THERAPY/ACTIVITY THERAPY/SCHOOL-BASED INTERVENTIONS

Within the H/L adolescent population, there is a positive connection between the impact of Child-Centered Play Therapy (CCPT) and students' self-esteem compared to students who didn't receive CCPT throughout the school year (Post et al., 2019). When working with predominately low-income H/L individuals, CCPT was vital in lowering behaviors and reducing externalizing behaviors (Post et al., 2019). The culturally responsive qualities of CCPT were beneficial to H/L students. CCPT focuses heavily on a multicultural lens as children communicate their needs and cultural values through play. (Post et al., 2019). For this reason, CCPT creates comfort in H/L children and adolescents when expressing the different value systems within their lives. Being relation-based rather than directive, CCPT benefits H/L students subjected to adverse childhood experiences. Resiliency within H/L adolescents is built through relationships where the counselor is a consistent helper for that adolescent. H/L adolescents need to feel safe from judgment to allow vulnerability (Post et al., 2019). H/L adolescents need to feel secure to express themselves, and counselors must look within a multicultural lens to develop greater competency when working with diverse populations. The result will be greater empathy between the counselor and the client/family systems.

RECOMMENDATIONS

Play therapists must be culturally aware as they work with minoritized children. This includes socioeconomic status and the developmental needs of these children who live in a diverse society (Post et al., 2019). As a mental health professional, incorporating primary language and culturally nostalgic games in therapy can create a warmer environment for these individuals. This builds significantly more rapport while meeting the needs of the client. It also creates a space where clients feel comfortable discussing topics related to their culture (Llamas & Alvarado, 2022). The following interventions are recommended to support H/L children, youth, and families: Child-Centered Play Therapy (CCPT) and Socio-Cognitive Behavioral Therapy for Suicidal Behaviors (SCBT-SB) (Jimenez-Colon & Duarte-Velez, 2022). Families should be directly involved in treatment for children and youth with suicidal behaviors or non-suicidal self-injury. Integrating family with treatment is critical to assessing protective and risk factors, evaluating parental/caregiver support, and establishing safety plans with all involved.

CHAPTER 8.4

NATIVE AMERICAN AND ALASKAN NATIVE CHILDREN AND ADOLESCENTS

Ruben Colon

INTRODUCTION

Native American communities are diverse tribal nations, and the rates of suicide vary from one community to the next. In many Native communities, suicide has only recently emerged after the 1960s (O'Keefe et al., 2022). In 2019, suicide was the second leading cause of death for Native American/Alaska Natives (NA/AN) between the ages of 10 and 34 (Allen et al., 2021). Risk factors of suicide for NA and AN youth are closely linked to the challenges tribal communities regularly face, such as substance abuse, suicide clusters, poor mental health, depression, oppression, poverty, and historical trauma (CDC, 2023; Weniger et al., 2020).

ASSESSMENT

Warning signs for the NA/AN communities mirror those for the general population. An effective intervention will require the therapist to possess in-depth knowledge of the client's tribal environment, such as the culture, the financial situation, and the interactivity within the tribe, as well as many other factors. Without this information, the therapist may find it challenging to establish a relationship that the client will find trustworthy and safe (Thomason, 2011).

The therapist must know how the dominant social culture's values, beliefs, and norms in the dominant social culture may not align with those in tribal communities. The following areas must be considered when assessing NA and AN youth: whether or not there were ceremonial or social gatherings during the mother's pregnancy or labor that welcomed the baby and had spiritual significance (SAMHSA, 2022). For many NA and AN youth, stigma and embarrassment have often become a barrier to discussing thoughts of suicide (Freedenthal & Stiffman, 2007). Clinicians are also advised to ask about any involvement in the youth's cultural or spiritual practices. Studies have shown that participation in spiritual activities generally reduces the risk of suicide (National Indian Child Welfare Association & Sahota, 2019). Many NA and AN have had to learn to navigate between two very different social environments: "white" and "native." It may be important to explore whether the youth's life experiences relate more to a rural or urban lifestyle. Clinicians might be able to demonstrate cultural sensitivity and regard during the suicide assessment process by asking about connections to culture, family, land, and nature and by inquiring about any existing strengths in bonds and meaningful traditions. For those youth who have mainly had rural life experiences in reservation settings, it may be difficult for them to navigate in "white" urban settings, which can lead to stressors. Lastly, it is important to ask about conflicts with gender and sexual identity that might be causing distress.

DOI: 10.4324/9781003358565-14

ESTABLISHING A THERAPEUTIC RELATIONSHIP

Trust is needed to elicit an accurate assessment of the individual. This is built through the interviewer's expression of genuine care and concern. Families might be apprehensive about establishing an open, trusting relationship with a therapist among NA and AN communities. Parents may understand whether the professionals view their work as a career they entered simply to make a living or a calling where they strive to fulfill a life purpose inspired by a higher power. Suppose a therapist can demonstrate a person-centered approach that shows caring concern and unconditional positive regard. In that case, it is more likely that the client will perceive that the therapist is genuine in their efforts to support them with life stressors.

In many clinics that serve native populations, the clinical staff are often not permanent and instead tend to serve the specific community for a set period. This temporary nature of their roles in a person's life may cause hesitation to divulge and fully express themselves in confidence due to the impending end of the therapeutic relationship. Another challenge in obtaining a truthful and honest answer when asking questions about suicidal ideation may be the interviewee's apprehension about the potential effects of disclosing thoughts of suicide, which may result in involuntary hospitalization and cause further isolation and separation from families and natural support systems. Psychiatric facilities may be distant from rural areas. The Indian Health Services *(Indian Health Service (IHS), n.d.)* website recommends compassionate and attuned directness that demonstrates an openness for the true experience of the youth: "Be willing to listen and allow emotional expression. Don't panic, talk openly, recognize that the situation is serious, don't pass judgment, reassure that help is available, don't promise secrecy, and don't leave the person alone." Abeysundera and Khanna (2022) note that some tribal groups believe that by directly discussing the topic of suicide, one may expose themselves to allowing "ghost spirits" to enter their being and cause illness or suicidal ideation.

The Rogerian approach of creating a close and empathetic relationship may also result in the helping professional being viewed more as an extended relative. This notion of joining the family as a helping professional also involves establishing proper boundaries in the therapeutic relationship and awareness of helpful/unhelpful countertransference.

CULTURALLY SPECIFIC COUNTERTRANSFERENCE CONCERNS

The therapist should resist any urge to share personally experienced trauma. Shared experiences of personal or historically relevant trauma are believed to impact an individual's physical and psychological well-being negatively. They can lead to mental health stressors or psychiatric disorders (Brave Heart et al., 2011).

PROTECTIVE FACTORS

As with risk factors and warning signs, protective factors that mitigate suicidal thinking and behavior are best seen through the culture of NA and AN youth (Weniger et al., 2020). The following protective factors have been known to help address suicide in NA and AN youth: developing strengths in the native language and identity, kinship and community, and engagement in cultural and spiritual practices.

Studies have shown that participation in spiritual activities generally reduces the risk of suicide (National Indian Child Welfare Association & Sahota, 2019). Whether Native youth participated in Native-based spiritual practices or church-related activities, both were shown to be protective factors against suicide and substance abuse. A study by Yu and Stiffman (2007) noted that attending general cultural activities (i.e., feasts, pow-wows/dances, and community events) was positively associated with alcohol use. Still, participation in spiritually related activities (i.e., sweat lodges, rites of passage, naming ceremonies, and talking circles) was negatively correlated with alcohol use. It is important to note that healing practices and spiritual rituals vary significantly among NA and AN youth.

There is power in the words we choose. If the interventions are referred to as "protective factors," they will likely be perceived as less stigmatizing and more acceptable among Native communities. One new study (Allen et al., 2021) has observed that promoting protective factors demonstrates better outcomes than focusing on reducing risk factors. This new model integrates indigenous beliefs, knowledge, culture, and community collaboration.

CULTURALLY APPROPRIATE TREATMENT

Narrative Therapy, Expressive Play-based Therapy, and Cognitive Behavioral Therapy, as integrated within traditional native practices, have been demonstrated to achieve effective treatment outcomes (McDonald et al., 2019; Graham, 2013; Mehl-Madrona & Mainguy, 2020) due to the traditional storytelling that is common for many tribal communities. Play Therapy and Sandtray Therapy are effective because they encourage clients to tell their "story" their way. Since storytelling is a traditional method among NA and AN peoples, narrative therapy provides an excellent approach to integrating culturally specific ways of helping youth tell their stories (Mehl-Madrona & Mainguy, 2020). One method formally adopted for NA and AN children and youth is Trauma-Focused Cognitive Behavioral Therapy (TF-CBT). Evidence-based practice for NA and AN youth, using the interventions of Honoring Children, the Mending the Circle program (Big Foot & Schmidt, 2010), has been vital in addressing trauma for NA and AN children and families. This method strives to consider Native belief systems by identifying indigenous practices that bring healing, identifying Native ways of interpreting the world and how things happen, using traditional ways of making sense of things gone wrong, the method of finding balance and harmony between the self and sacred elements; identifying paths or roads toward healing and wellness. Some culturally specific adaptations to the models may include demonstrating honor toward the child, incorporating tribal-specific teachings, storytelling, use of humor, ceremonies, smudging, and cleansing rituals (I Love Ancestry, 2014).

PREVENTION FOR SUICIDAL CHILDREN AND ADOLESCENTS

Effective suicide prevention strategies for NA and AN youth include native parenting programs, camps, activities, cultural and spiritual practices, and indigenous and adapted therapy approaches. For children of younger ages, Family Spirit is a program designed to provide a pathway to good mental health prevention services across the lifespan. This model focused on home visitations and was specifically designed for Native Americans by Native Americans (Begay & Johns Hopkins Center for American Indian Health, 2019). In the study by Allen et al. (2021), a vital element of this method is working to prevent suicide at both the individual and community levels. The framework strives to collaborate with communities and promote the use of cultural and community-specific resources to address contributing factors that increase suicide risks for the person and society at large.

CASE EXAMPLE

Amy is a 15-year-old female whose father is a full-blooded Native American with Muscogee (Mvskoke/Creek) tribal, Caucasian American. A teacher became concerned when Amy was observed crying in the cafeteria and running to the restroom. Amy's teacher referred her to the school counselor to privately express her feelings and thoughts in a supportive environment. Amy was hospitalized due to her disclosure to a school counselor that she planned to take a lethal dose and die by suicide during the weekend.

Initially, Amy was guarded and said she was only upset because she was being called derogatory names and teased by some classmates. The school counselor noticed a sense of hopelessness and helplessness when Amy expressed frustration about her inability to cope with feelings related to aggression toward indigenous people. She further stated that she struggled to leave the house, had difficulty sleeping, had nightmares, and had crying spells several times a day. Amy mentioned that she had been bullied throughout the time she attended middle school and high school. Classmates ridiculed Amy for her weight, disheveled appearance, and poor hygiene. On one occasion, four girls physically assaulted her during her first year and posted a video of the assault on social media.

Amy disclosed to the school psychologist that she was feeling depressed and that she had daily thoughts of wishing she was dead. Amy thought that killing herself would be the revenge she sought on those who bullied her. Amy had a deep sense of perceived burdensomeness. The school counselor and Amy agreed that she would not be safe at home, so she was placed on an involuntary hospital hold due to her suicidal ideation and depression. Amy was referred to an Intensive Outpatient Program (IOP) upon discharge from the hospital. Amy's father insisted that the IOP therapist have the specific cultural awareness to integrate Amy's Native background with sound medical practice. During the first 16 weeks of therapy, Amy could tell her story about her traumatic bullying experiences in the school environment. The therapist used the Native American-specific Trauma Focused Cognitive Behavioral Model Honoring Children and Mending the Circle to help Amy tell the story of her difficulties coping with abuse at school. After completing the trauma-based therapy, Amy continued to attend therapy sessions to expand and reinforce her repertoire of coping skills to deal with anxiety and depression.

During the process, the therapist integrated expressive play therapy and Native American wellness concepts to help teach Amy strategies to cope with her difficulties. The three art projects were constructing a dream catcher to help learn ways to manage and regulate emotions and creating a medicine wheel pendant to learn and practice ways to self-monitor and regulate balance in life. The beading of a hair barrette with tribal-specific colors and symbols reinforces a healthy sense of identity.

The art projects allowed Amy to personalize her creations with colors, symbols, and materials that signified her paternal ties to the Muscogee Nation. Along the way, she connected more closely with her father. She learned about their tribal affiliation when he helped her look into ways she could symbolize their heritage in her expressive art therapy projects.

Each art project helped Amy integrate robust coping strategies with her unique Native background.

Amy's case manager aided in educational advocacy, coordination of services, and connection to community-based resources. The case manager helped Amy's parents understand how to request an evaluation for special education eligibility and advocate for a safe school environment. Once Amy was found eligible for services based on her mental health and academic declines, the case manager helped her parents learn how to participate effectively in meetings related to Amy's education and offered information regarding services and support at school. The case manager also connected Amy and her family to a local agency that provides social services to Native American families. Amy enjoyed attending social gatherings and art classes three to four times monthly. Her parents were also matched with elder mentors who helped Amy learn to bond with her mother during activities such as hair braiding and with her father by creating Native art projects together. To further prevent crisis and hospitalization, the case manager could also assist by coordinating meetings with clinic staff and linking the family to additional support services.

Throughout the therapy process, the clinician adapted principles of CBT, such as recognizing how healthy core beliefs rooted in indigenous wellness principles can positively influence thoughts, feelings, and behaviors. The three previous art projects strived to encourage the natural process of play and creativity to heal and promote a strong sense of identity.

Amy received academic support services, established positive connections at school, and graduated with her senior class. By the time she finished high school, she was no longer experiencing suicidal ideation and aspired to continue her education by attending college. Amy was able to use her clinical support services to improve her ability to cope with anxiety, increasing her confidence and reducing her level of depression. Amy continued to seek ways to connect with her cultural heritage and practice Native American wellness concepts in her everyday life.

CHAPTER 8.5

ASIAN AMERICANS AND PACIFIC ISLANDER CHILDREN AND ADOLESCENTS

Yung-Wei Dennis Lin

There is a general myth that Asian Americans and Pacific Islanders (AAPI), including children and adolescents, have higher suicide rates compared with other ethnic groups (Hijioka & Wong, 2012). Although the official statistics have shown that the suicide rates among Asian Americans are lower than the U.S. national suicide rates across all age groups, the rates of suicidal ideation and attempts among AAPI youth are very similar to the rates of the overall youth in the U.S. (Suicide Prevention Resource Center, 2020). Suicide recently became the leading cause of death among AAPI youth aged between 10 and 14 and the second leading cause of death among those between 15 and 24 years old (Centers for Disease Control and Prevention, 2021).

SUICIDE RISK FACTORS

It is generally believed that adverse childhood experiences (ACEs) are typical risk factors among child and adolescent suicides. Past research has shown a high association between ACEs and premature death, including suicide (Brown et al., 2009; Perez et al., 2016). Particularly, every additional ACE may increase the odds of attempted suicide two to five times (Dube et al., 2001). In addition to the common adverse experiences/risk factors, unique cultural heritages and conflicts experienced by AAPI youth may also be considered risk factors.

ACCULTURATION

Acculturation among immigrants has been widely discussed and researched in terms of its impact on their mental health and wellness, including suicidality. The impact of acculturation appears more complicated and significant to the second generation of immigrant families, especially the AAPI youth (Lau et al., 2002). Joiner's (2005) interpersonal psychological theory emphasizes belongingness as a protective factor against suicide risk for the general population. Still, due to the complex acculturation among AAPI youth, this theoretical framework may not be completely applicable.

According to Joiner's theory, family relationships are generally believed to be one significant type of social connection (or belongingness). However, Wong and Maffini (2011) suggested that family relationships may no longer be a protective factor against suicide behaviors among AAPI youth who are highly acculturated. AAPI youth typically experience significant cultural differences within and outside of their families, in which their parents (or

DOI: 10.4324/9781003358565-15

grandparents) may hold their Asian cultural values, such as collectivism, filial piety, harmony, etc., strictly, while they gradually embrace individualism, equity, advocacy, etc. through their acculturation process. Therefore, the stronger their connection with their families, the greater the cultural conflicts they may experience. AAPI youth who experience such cultural conflicts in their families may develop a high suicide risk due to a strong sense of helplessness and hopelessness when they are constantly forced to obey their parents.

Peer relationships are another vital form of social connection and belongingness and may be extremely critical to adolescents. Similar to family relationships, peer relationships may not follow Joiner's theory as a protective factor toward suicide behaviors among AAPI youth. Wong and Maffini (2011) also suggested that AAPI youth with a lower level of acculturation may experience peer relationships as a risk factor for their suicide behaviors. For example, AAPI adolescents who have deep connections with their peers may experience stronger confusion about their self-identity. They may sense great difficulty culturally identifying with their parents and, at the same time, recognize their cultural differences from their peers. When they mainly hang out with other AAPI peers, they may become even more aware of themselves being culturally marginalized, which may further increase their stress of acculturation.

HELP-SEEKING STIGMA AND FAMILY SHAME

Stigma toward mental health concerns is a common barrier to help-seeking behaviors among some populations, particularly AAPIs, due to their traditional Asian culture (Kim & Zane, 2016). In many AAPI families, family reputation or fame is much more highly protected than personal values, and mental health concerns are generally considered a personal weakness (or inability to control one's behaviors). Thus, seeking mental health services is often perceived as a shame to the person and the whole family (Lee et al., 2009). Although filial piety highly emphasizes children's obedience to parents, Confucianism in traditional Asian culture also strictly holds parents accountable for children's behavioral problems. In other words, children's mental health concerns, including suicide, are generally viewed as parents' failure in their parenting. Parents may feel extremely shameful and guilty when considering mental health services for their children, and children may also choose to hide their suicidal ideations due to such stigma and family stress.

ACADEMIC STRESS

There is an old saying in Chinese culture: "Academic pursuit is more valuable than anything else." This old saying reveals the strong emphasis on academic performance in many Asian families, including AAPI families. Due to this cultural value, AAPI parents tend to have very high educational expectations (Goyette & Xie, 1999) and pressure their children significantly. Past research has also shown that AAPI youth tend to choose college majors with better future salaries and careers that require more education and bring higher average incomes

(Xie & Goyette, 2003) due to parental expectations, persuasion, or pressure. Such high academic stress may be a unique suicide risk factor for AAPI youth. It has been repeatedly reported that AAPI adolescents chose to end their own lives immediately after they fulfilled their parents' expectations with college admissions.

RACISM AND DISCRIMINATION

Racial discrimination is not new to Asian populations in the U.S., and past research has demonstrated a significant association between discrimination and suicide risk (Lee, 2019; Yip, 2015). Some factors in school settings may aggravate racial discrimination experiences among AAPI youth. For example, growing up in Asian families, they may have learned from their parents to act as a "model minority" (Choi et al., 2022). Their diligent, quiet, and compliant dispositions may be easily perceived as nerdy, socially awkward, and highly tolerant of bullying. Some AAPI youth may even be told by their parents to tolerate or ignore discrimination because their parents do not know how to respond or firmly believe in the model minority principle. Unfortunately, reoccurring racial discrimination will likely worsen their mental health and suicide risk.

WARNING SIGNS AND SUICIDE ASSESSMENT

Suicide warning signs and assessments specifically for AAPI youth have not been adequately researched. Suicidology experts and clinicians typically follow the same principles when informally assessing youth suicide across racial/ethnic populations. Suicidology literature has suggested specific youth warning signs (Barrio, 2007); however, it is highly recommended that clinicians and caregivers keep a high multicultural sensitivity when working with AAPI youth. For example, a sudden academic performance fall might be a warning sign for this population. Social disconnection, isolation, and physical complaints might be warning signs ignored easily by caregivers. Also, researchers recently suggested that suicide notes among AAPIs, especially youth, tend to contain themes such as apologies and interpersonal conflicts (Wong et al., 2022).

Suicide prevention and intervention among AAPI youth, similar to suicide assessment, has not yet been researched much, so there is no unique prevention and intervention program or model for this population.

However, I highly recommend Applied Suicide Intervention Skills Training (ASIST) for clinicians and caregivers. ASIST is a 14-hour, two-day, internationally recognized training model that equips trainees (either professionals or nonprofessionals) with intervention skills to respond to suicidal situations. ASIST has been widely recognized and used by many organizations, including the Centers for Disease Control and Prevention (CDC), multiple state governments, branches of the Armed Forces, and many crisis centers. The training effects of ASIST on enhancing clinicians' intervention skills and readiness to intervene have been well-researched in a variety of settings (Illich, 2004; McAuliffe & Perry, 2007; Shannonhouse et al., 2018), particularly in K-12 schools (Shannonhouse et al., 2017). The following case example demonstrates how to utilize *Pathway for Assisting Life* (PAL), the unique immediate intervention model taught in ASIST (Lang et al., 2013), to respond to an AAPI youth suicide situation.

CASE EXAMPLE

Amy (pseudonym) is a 14-year-old high school student who moved to the U.S. with her parents when she was 4 years old. Amy's father is a senior biochemical engineer in a large pharmaceutical company, and her mother is a senior data analyst in a large information technology company. Amy's parents came to the U.S. from an East Asian country for better job opportunities. During Amy's first year in middle school, she became isolated and appeared anxious about her academic performance. She often worked on her school assignments or studied for tests until late at night and maintained a 4.0 GPA. Since Amy's first semester in high school, her grades have dropped significantly, and she often complained about headaches and stomachaches. The pediatrician diagnosed Amy's headache and stomachache as psychological, not physical. Amy's parents felt disappointed and further blamed Amy for using physical symptoms as excuses for her grade drop. Recently, Amy thought of suicide but only told the school counselor that she could never meet her parents' expectations and always felt lonely and sad. Amy's parents came to the U.S. from an East Asian country for better job opportunities.

PAL MODEL PHASE I: CONNECTING

In responding to Amy's sadness and assessing her suicide risk, I recommend first carefully identifying Amy's risk factors and suicide warning signs. Amy's struggles with her academic performance, somatic symptoms, loneliness, sadness, and hopelessness toward her parents' high expectations are clear warning signs. After gathering these warning signs from Amy, I would take the initiative and ask her the direct suicide question, such as "Amy, you sound very sad and stressed by your parents' expectations. I also feel a sense of hopelessness in your voice. I am wondering if suicide has been in your mind." Working with young individuals like Amy, it would be critical to confirm their suicidal ideations early and provide a healthy source for them to talk about their suicidal thoughts rather than letting them hide their suicidal thoughts in mind and reach out to their peers or inappropriate online resources.

PAL MODEL PHASE II: UNDERSTANDING

Now that Amy has affirmed that she is thinking about suicide, I move into phase two of the PAL model with Amy. In this second phase, my goal is to learn more about her experiences and the psychological pains behind her suicidal thoughts. People at risk of suicide need and want someone to understand their psychological pain. Children or adolescents like Amy most likely want their parents to understand them. Unfortunately, Amy's parents have not yet been able to meet her needs. As an immediate intervention provider, I must help Amy vent her emotions and pains and communicate my empathic understanding of her reasons for suicide. Amy may feel relieved through this catharsis process and gradually reveal her uncertainty about suicide. This kind of uncertainty may be expressed as a wish, "I wish my parents could understand me more," or "I don't know how to tell my parents my true feelings." For some adolescents who have difficulties directly verbalizing their emotions or thoughts, I might try sandtray or expressive art techniques to help them vent. Such techniques may be highly beneficial for AAPI youth because the culture in most AAPI families tends to promote tolerance and discourage emotional expression. After identifying Amy's uncertainty about suicide, I would further invite Amy to commit to her current safety so that together, we can work on how to help her communicate with her parents and get her needs met.

PAL MODEL PHASE III: ASSISTING

Even after at-risk people in phase three have committed to their personal safety, they may still need help making healthy decisions that discourage suicidal tendencies. Thus, in PAL Model Phase III, I aim to work with Amy to develop a plan to keep her safe. This plan should not just come from me since I have a limited understanding of Amy's life and family. In the process of developing this safety plan, I need to continue assessing Amy's suicide risk by exploring her plan and method of suicide. As mentioned previously, acculturation may moderate the effect of family or peer connections and further increase suicide risk to AAPI youth. Thus, It is critical to explore Amy's acculturalization, her perception of conflict, and her identification with her peers and her family or other students' families. Informing parents about students' suicidal ideation is usually required in suicide response protocols in school settings. Developing a safety plan in Phase III also allows me to assess Amy's readiness for talking with her parents about her stress and suicidal thoughts. When parents are invited to the school, it will be critical for me to facilitate the conversation and further advocate for Amy. Another essential task in the conversation with Amy's parents is to invite them to form a team so that together, we can keep Amy safe and free of suicidal inclinations. During the conversation with Amy's parents, I carefully assessed both Amy's and her parents' commitment to follow through with Amy's safety plan.

CONCLUSION

Suicide intervention is never easy with AAPI youth due to this population's unique and complicated cultures. Working with Amy's parents, I need to constantly assess their emotional status, attitude, and perspective toward Amy's suicide risk to determine their involvement level in Amy's safety plan. Also, their knowledge and knowledge of and attitude toward mental health may be critical to Amy's postvention. Suicide postvention usually includes long-term mental health care and coping strategies that can continue to promote individuals' wellness. Now Amy is committed to her current safety plan after the PAL model, appropriate long-term support for Amy's wellness is needed to continue her movement away from suicide. Psychoeducation may be necessary to improve parents' attitudes and knowledge toward long-term mental health services. The selection of mental health services should be based on Amy's needs and preferences. Individual counseling, sandtray or expressive art therapy, small group counseling, or even parenting programs for parent-child relationship improvement are all possible and beneficial options. With Amy's commitment to her current safety and appropriate long-term support, I am hopeful that all mental health professionals, paraprofessionals, and Amy's parents can continue enhancing Amy's wellness and, together, prevent her from turning back to the route of suicide.

CHAPTER 8.6

UNDERSTANDING SUICIDALITY IN LGBTQ YOUTH THROUGH THE LENS OF QUEER-PRYSM

Leslie W. Baker

Children and adolescents who practice or identify with non-traditional modes of gender and sexuality face unique challenges that put them at a higher risk for suicide than their heterosexual and cisgender peers. According to the Trevor Project, a national organization that provides crisis intervention and suicide prevention services, over 50% of these individuals have reported having suicidal thoughts; one in five transgender and nonbinary youth have attempted suicide; and LGBTQ youth of color are even more likely to have done so (The Trevor Project, 2022).

Increased awareness and swift interventions that promote enduring stability are urgently needed to support this community. The recent rash of transphobic legislation throughout the US and UK is an obstacle to preventing suicide in LGBTQIA+ youth. Such legislation severely limits how local communities, critical to a child's development, can accommodate their queer children (Whitten & Thomas, 2023). As a queer community advocate who has worked with children for 11 years, Megan Carmody (personal communication, January 25, 2023) explained,

> It's one thing to be afraid of your family because of your existence, another to be a danger to your family (no matter how accepting and supportive they are) because of your existence. This fear is more trans-focused, but history has shown that trans rights are the proverbial canary in the coal mine for broader queer rights.

WARNING SIGNS

Clinicians working with LGBTQ youth must be sensitive to behaviors and statements indicating a young person is considering or planning suicide. Non-traditional lifestyles or appearances can result in bullying and violence victimization, poor mental health, alcohol and other drug use, and poor academic performance (Gower et al., 2018). Minority stress, interpersonal constructs, partner violence, homelessness, and lack of family support can accompany higher rates of suicidal ideation/attempts/completion (WestEd et al., 2019). In addition, exposure to SOGICE (Sexual Orientation and Gender Identity Change Efforts), a program commonly referred to as "conversion therapy," which attempts to "cure" the client by altering their sense of identity and gender preferences, can be very harmful. Green et al (2022, para. 34) noted, "Young LGBTQ respondents who had undergone SOGICE experienced dramatically higher levels of suicidality than their LGBTQ peers not exposed to such experiences."

Parents, caregivers, and educators should be aware of warning signs that may indicate an LGBTQ child or adolescent is at risk of suicide. These include:

- Increased social isolation or withdrawal from friends and family.
- Changes in eating or sleeping habits.

DOI: 10.4324/9781003358565-16

- Increased use of drugs or alcohol.
- A decline in academic performance.
- Expressions of hopelessness or helplessness.
- Engagement in self-harm behaviors.
- Speech referencing suicide or a desire to die.
- Experience discrimination, harassment, or bullying based on sexual orientation or gender identity.

(The Trevor Project, 2022; Diamond et al., 2021)

PROTECTIVE FACTORS

Several protective factors can help reduce the risk of suicidal behavior among LGBTQ children and adolescents. Research has shown that using correct pronouns and access to facilities matching gender identity decreases suicide ideation and suicide attempts while improving educational performance (Olson et al., 2016). The National Survey on LGBTQ Youth in China noted that "having a more inclusive school climate and more school resources, especially a positive LGBTQ role model, were significantly associated with the reduction of LGBTQ students' suicidal ideation" (Wei & Liu, 2019). School programs and educators are about recognizing individuals and creating an environment where every gender can thrive. Schools and educators must include those who align with traditional or adaptable binary views and those who reject gender norms altogether (Mayo, 2022).

In an alternative lifestyle, youth who are accepted and supported by their families, schools, and communities have a lower risk of suicide and better mental health. With its unique challenges, access to mental health resources and services is vital to this population. Connection to the larger LGBTQ community can provide a sense of belonging and social support, reducing the impact of minority stress on at-risk populations.

EVIDENCE-BASED TREATMENT FOR LGBTQ YOUTH

Trauma-Focused Cognitive Behavioral Therapy (TF-CBT) develops coping skills to manage the emotions and behaviors of adolescents who have experienced a traumatic event (Cohen et al., 2018). TF-CBT, structured to include both individual and family therapy, works to reduce symptoms such as anxiety, depression, and post-traumatic stress disorder (PTSD) and improve the individual's overall functioning (Thielemann et al., 2022) TF-CBT can be adapted to include the Family Acceptance Project (FAP™), which, as its name implies, works to increase family support and understanding of LGBTQ youth (Cohen & Acsw, 2022) through educational workshops, support groups, and counseling services. In addition, TF-CBT has created a specific adaption manual, TF-CBT LGBT, for trauma-impacted LGBTQ youth (Cohen et al., 2018).

The Queer Prevention of Youth Suicidality Model (Queer PRYSM) integrates four theoretical frameworks into a comprehensive approach to support LGBTQ youth at risk of or coping with suicidality (Williams et al., 2022).

The four frameworks of Queer PRYSM:

1. Minority Stress Theory (MST), developed by Ilan Meyer in the late 1990s, explains the high rates of mental health problems among LGBTQ individuals (Meyer, 1995).
2. Person-in-Environment and Risk and Resilience (PIE-R&R) emphasizes the dynamic interplay between individuals and their environments (Hatzenbuehler, 2011).

    a. The Interpersonal-Psychological Theory of Suicide (IPTS), developed in 2005 by Thomas Joiner, explains suicidal ideation and behavior by highlighting the role of social disconnection, perceived burdensomeness, and acquired capability for suicide (Fulginiti et al., 2020; Joiner, 2007).

3. Intersectionality, first introduced by legal scholar Kimberlé Crenshaw in 1989, examines how various social identities, such as race, gender, class, sexual orientation, and ability, intersect and interact to produce oscillating hierarchies of oppression and privilege (Williams et al., 2022).
4. Prevention.

As is often the case with health issues, prevention is critical. Queer-PRYSM offers support groups that provide a safe space for LGBTQIA+ youths. This opportunity for empathy and understanding from peers, essential to a population that already feels stigmatized and disenfranchised, may serve as an alternative to hospitalization (Williams et al., 2022). Queer youth displaying signs of suicidality, such as suicidal thoughts and behaviors, need immediate services to prevent suicide. Those experiencing these severe psychological challenges may benefit from various interventions, including developing a safety plan, access to mental health treatment, and fostering supportive and affirming interpersonal connections (Williams et al., 2022). Even when hospitalization is required, positive communication will be essential during the outpatient therapy phase. Another source of preventive intervention can be prioritizing Gender and Sexuality Alliances and universal bullying prevention programs at schools (Marraccini et al., 2022). Safe, inclusive, and welcoming environments for LGBTQ students can help individuals achieve a better quality of life by building a positive self-concept and overcoming internalized stigma (Mezzalira et al., 2022).

CASE EXAMPLE AND TREATMENT

After the 11-year-old boy, Jack, came to his parents with thoughts of suicide stemming from the bullying he had received at school and online, they sought counseling for him. Jack, who insisted that the play therapist call him "Red," disclosed that they were non-binary and feared the reaction of their conservative Catholic family should they find out. The play therapist, using the TF-CBT LGBT (Insalaco, 2019), introduced Red to an intervention called *How Do I Identify* (Baker, 2021). The play therapist traced Red's body on paper to create their body shape. The body shape is then glued onto another piece of paper, allowing for a background around the body shape. The client can decorate the body shape in any way they desire, with paint, glitter, watercolors, and pastels to express themselves. Red chose to decorate their body shape with various pastels and acrylic paints, commenting on the freedom of this experience. In the following session, personal descriptives are written onto sticky notes and then stuck to the body shape with a glue stick, representing the client. Red began describing positive attributes such as "I am tall," posting the sticky note above the image's head; "I am smart," posting the sticky note on the head; and "I am non-binary," posting the sticky note at the heart. The clinician began to see Red making more positive references to themselves over time.

The play therapist then transferred the therapy focus to a downregulation intervention called Progressive Muscle Relaxation (PMR) (Toussaint et al. 2021). Before moving into TF-CBT LGBT, it is vital that a child feels relaxed. The play therapist showed Red how to use PMR by tensing and releasing their body parts (arms, hands, legs, shoulders, head, stomach, neck, and back). The play therapist includes breathing in as they tense for about three seconds, then breathing out, releasing their tensed body part. The play therapist also adds a guided imagery component, such as having them imagine a bubble passing through their limbs and body parts, deepening relaxation as they exhale. Once the youth has completed the PMR with deep breathing and guided imagery, the child is often relaxed and ready to begin TF-CBT LGBT. Toussaint et al. (2021) study noted that deep breathing is important for relaxation; however, achieving physiological states of relaxation is more strongly induced by PMR and guided imagery. Once Red felt relaxed, they could begin writing their narrative of both the first bullying incident they had experienced and the worst bullying incident. They reviewed and rewrote the stories with their play therapist to correct any cognitive errors that might perpetuate the trauma state.

As the intensity of Red's trauma lessened, they began to discuss their fears regarding their parents, who, to this point, had regarded them as their gender-binary son, and by integrating TC-CBT LGBT with FAP™, the play therapist combined trauma recovery with family acceptance interventions to bridge the gulf that Red feared. The parents engaged in psychoeducation that offered definitions of how they identified and helped them develop a basic understanding of what a non-binary youth might need from their family. They began to understand the model that gender identity is not a choice but is related to biology, development, and environmental factors, and by working with FAP™ and within TF-CBT LGBT, the team of Red, their parents, and their play therapist built components of family acceptance that reaffirmed the child's sense of belonging (Cohen & Acsw, 2022).

The father found a computer application called *Pronouns/Minus18* (n.d.), which he and the mother used to familiarize themselves with *they/their* pronouns that Red had requested. Becoming aware of the severe bullying Red had endured at the private Catholic school, the family located a local public school that offered an LGBTQ community, including a faculty-supported club for youth. The treatment dramatically and positively affected Red: "Hearing my parents refer to me by my correct pronouns because they found an app they had never heard of before, I knew things were moving in the right direction with them!" The parents also found support in finding a Catholic-based church open to diversity where they felt comfortable practicing their faith while maintaining the ability to love Red openly.

CONCLUSION

Sadly, not all families can find common ground, even with therapeutic intervention. Red and their family had access to programs that not all LGBTQ youths have. The goal is not only to highlight the critical nature of STB in LGBTQ children and adolescents but also to encourage more research to focus on these diverse populations. Integrating theories like Queer-PRYSM to address specific needs will improve mental health levels and ultimately help reduce the risk of suicidality (Williams et al., 2022). They are integrating treatments like TF-CBT LGBT with FAPTM to provide comprehensive treatment for the trauma many LGBTQ youth experience in schools, communities, and homes where they face bullying, lack of acceptance, loneliness, and rejection from faith organizations. TF-CBT LGBT has a manual developed specifically for the LGBT community, which considers the issues and needs of this population (Cohen & Acsw, 2022). Both TF-CBT LGBT and FAPTM work with families to assist with trauma education and the development of a base of protection for children and adolescents. Family acceptance, feeling safe within their environment, and the ability to develop social connections will promote stability and personal growth for LGBTQ youth (Katz-Wise et al., 2016). Schools have a role in developing school safety and creating an atmosphere of positive sexual and gender identity support programs (Mayo, 2022). Lastly, communities must provide access to high-quality, culturally appropriate, and LGBTQ-affirming mental health treatment and improved diagnostics.

CHAPTER 8.7

AUTISTIC AND NEURODIVERGENT CHILDREN AND ADOLESCENTS

Robert Jason Grant

INTRODUCTION

Walker (2022) stated that neurodiversity is the diversity of human minds, the infinite variation in neurocognitive functioning within our species. Neurodiversity is a biological fact. It's not a perspective, an approach, a belief, or a political position. A great deal of scientific evidence shows considerable variation among human brains; thus, neurodiversity can be thought of as the variance of human neurotypes. Walker furthered that the neurodiversity paradigm is a specific perspective on neurodiversity – a perspective or approach that boils down to these fundamental principles:

1. Neurodiversity is a natural and valuable form of human diversity.
2. The idea that there is one "normal" or "healthy" type of brain or mind or one "right" style of neurocognitive functioning is culturally constructed fiction.
3. The social dynamics regarding neurodiversity are similar to those of other forms of human diversity (e.g., diversity of ethnicity, gender, or culture).

Silverman (2015) shared that one way to understand neurodiversity is to think about human operating systems instead of diagnostic labels such as autism, dyslexia, and ADHD. The brain is, above all, a marvelous adaptive organism, adept at maximizing its chance of success even in the face of limitations. Just because a computer is not running Windows does not mean it's broken. Not all features of a neurodivergent operating system are bugs. Different is just different; it does not have to be pathologized.

Chapman and Botha (2022) stated that the neurodiversity movement is a social movement that emerged among autistic self-advocates. It has since spread and has been joined by many with diagnoses of attention-deficit/hyperactivity disorder, learning differences, sensory differences, and developmental coordination disorder, among others. By reconceptualizing neurodiversity as part of biodiversity, neurodiversity proponents emphasize the need to develop a society that supports the conservation of neurominorities through the construction of accepting and appreciating differences and thus making space for all. This is an alternative to the drive to eliminate diversity through attempts to "treat" or "cure" neurodivergence.

Underneath the "umbrella" of neurodiversity exist the labels of neurodivergent and neurotypical. Neurodivergent, sometimes abbreviated as ND, means having a mind that functions in ways that diverge significantly from the dominant societal standards of "normal." Being neurodivergent does not have to include a formal diagnosis, but neurodivergent identification often aligns with certain diagnoses such as autism, ADHD, learning differences, sensory differences, etc. Neurotypical, often abbreviated as NT, means having a style

DOI: 10.4324/9781003358565-17

of neurocognitive functioning that falls within the dominant societal standards of what is viewed as normal (Grant, 2023b).

Grant (2021) defined neurodiversity affirmation as a belief and an action. It is the application of the neurodiversity paradigm and movement. Neurodiversity affirmation is a belief and commitment in approach, which means valuing and respecting the different ways a neurodivergent client may process, feel, respond, communicate, and play. It means allowing the child to be themselves and not trying to change them to fit a neurotypical standard. Further, it means giving the client a voice in the decision-making process regarding their therapy and their life.

O'Halloran et al. (2022) proposed that uncertainties about the factors involved in suicidality in autistic and other neurodivergent children and adolescents are likely to be confounded by issues related to diagnostic overshadowing, masking, misunderstanding, and stigmatization that is characteristic of navigating neurodivergent life. For the best understanding of suicide issues and neurodivergence, key considerations must include a knowledge of the following terms/issues related to neurodivergence:

Masking – This usually involves purposefully suppressing, hiding, or trying to eliminate certain neurodivergent-related behaviors for fear of social rejection, displeasure, or prejudice.

Alexithymia – This is typically characterized by the inability to identify and describe emotions experienced by oneself.

The Double Empathy Problem – When people with very different experiences of the world interact, they will struggle to empathize with each other – for example, a neurotypical person interacting with a neurodivergent person.

Ableism – The discrimination and social prejudice against people with disabilities based on the belief that typical abilities are superior.

AUTISTIC AND NEURODIVERGENT RESEARCH AND STATISTICAL INFORMATION

It is challenging to fully conceptualize the statistical information for the neurodivergent population related to suicide. Neurodivergence covers a wide variety of individual experiences and diagnoses. With this limitation in mind, studies have identified statistical information risks for neurominority populations. Studies have shown that individuals with ADHD have a higher risk of suicidal thoughts and suicidal behavior. A few studies have investigated the role of psychological factors such as executive functioning and perfectionism as potential factors that may be associated with vulnerability to suicide (Balazs, 2017; Taylor et al., 2014; Impey, 2012).

Giupponi et al. (2018) proposed that many studies indicate an association between ADHD and suicidal behavior. Still, controversy exists as to whether the relationship is causal or instead an increased prevalence of pre-existing comorbid conditions and individual and family dysfunctional factors. O'Halloran et al. (2022) put forth that the incidence of suicidality (i.e., suicidal ideation, suicide acts, and attempts) among autistic children and adolescents is of particular concern. Autistic youth are six times more likely to attempt suicide and twice more likely to die by suicide (Kirby et al., 2019) – and at a significantly younger age – compared to their non-autistic peers. Suicide is a leading cause of premature death among autistic people.

Sarris (2022) stated that several studies published in the last ten years have examined suicide risk in autistic people. One study published in 2020 stands out for its size. In Sweden, researchers identified 54,000 autistic people using medical records from 1987 through 2013 and compared them to 271,000 non-autistic people. Researchers compare statistics between control groups and the general population (the comparison group) to determine whether having a particular condition increases the likelihood of incidence. In the Swedish study, researchers also included thousands of people who have a relative with autism, along with more than 1 million people who do not have autistic family members. Researchers found the highest rate of suicide attempts and death by suicide occurred among autistic people with no intellectual disability. Within that group, autistic people with attention deficit hyperactivity disorder (ADHD) had the highest rate. About one in ten had attempted suicide, a rate seven times higher than the comparison group. Autistic people with intellectual disability disorder also had a higher risk of suicide attempts, about double the risk of the comparison group. The study findings were startling for girls and women. One in five females who had both autism and ADHD (but not intellectual disability) had attempted suicide at least once.

Richa et al. (2014) proposed that clinical samples suggest suicide occurs more frequently in autistic individuals with low support needs. Physical and sexual abuse, bullying, and changes in routine are precipitating events associated with suicide risk. Sarris (2022) reported that autistic children are bullied more than their peers. Research shows that bullies and their victims have a higher risk of suicidal thoughts and behaviors. Autistic people have higher rates of underemployment or unemployment than the general population. Children and adults on the autism spectrum have higher rates of mental health conditions, such as depression, bipolar disorder, schizophrenia, anxiety, and ADHD, than neurotypical individuals.

Autistic people are subject to risk factors inherent to their diagnosis (differences in expression of feelings and thoughts) and risk factors common to the general population (abuse, depression, anxiety, etc.). The differences (from a neurotypical perspective and expectation) in autistic and neurodivergent children and adolescents in expressing emotions and thoughts make diagnosing suicidal ideation difficult and demand significant adjustments to traditional psychotherapeutic interventions (Richa et al., 2014).

WARNING SIGNS AND PROTECTIVE FACTORS

It is challenging to identify warning signs in neurodivergent children and adolescents because of constructs such as masking, alexithymia, double empathy problems, etc. A neurodivergent child may be masking how they are feeling and experiencing alexithymia and unable to notice or communicate a feeling the way the therapist expects to see or hear it. There also exists a great misunderstanding and mislabeling of neurodivergent children by neurotypical individuals. For the therapist to assess suicide-related warning signs and protective factors requires a deep understanding of neurodivergence itself – the spectrum of presentation and the many manifestations and how this can be a different experience of living from the neurotypical standard.

ASSESSMENT

To accurately assess possible suicide-related issues, the therapist would first need to understand the spectrum of presentation of the neurodivergent child or adolescent. Grant (2023b) outlined a neurodivergent spectrum of presentation summary sheet implemented in the intake and assessment phase of AutPlay® Therapy, which allows the therapist to indicate specific information about the neurodivergent child in the areas of identity awareness and acceptance, understanding emotions, special interests, depression, anxiety, perception, regulation, stimming, communication style, need for routine, self-advocacy, executive functioning, relationship development, sensory differences, play preferences, and social navigation.

It is critical to have assessment processes like the AutPlay® Neurodivergent Spectrum of Presentation before forming conclusions about possible suicide issues. Once the therapist understands the child's neurotype and neurodivergent presentation, knowing how the child communicates, expresses emotion, and manages executive functioning becomes much more accessible. The therapist can then better gauge possible suicide issues, protective factors, and therapy processes.

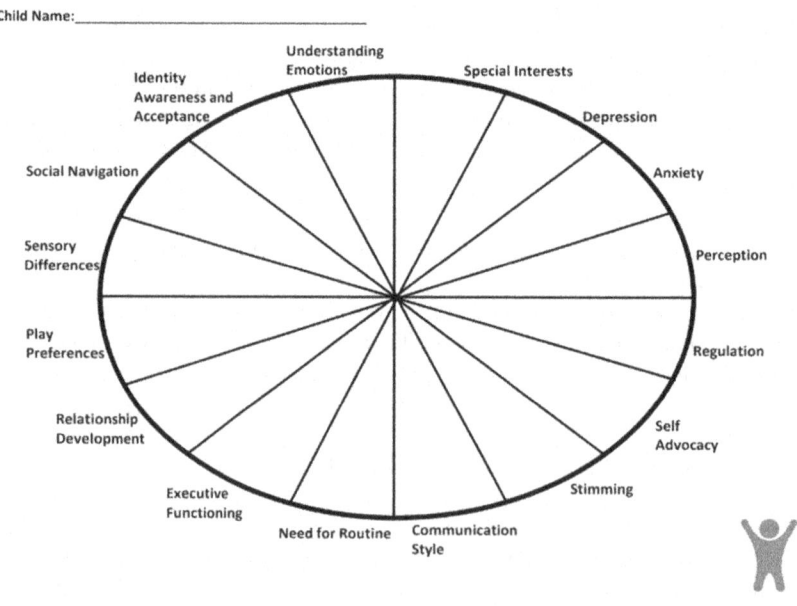

©Robert Jason Grant Ed.D · www.autplaytherapy.com

Figure 8.2 AutPlay Neurodivergent Spectrum of Presentation – Overview of Child

Source: AutPlay Neurodivergent Spectrum of Presentation – Overview of Child. Grant, R. J. (2023a) Neurodivergent Spectrum of Presentation [Graphic] [Unpublished]

CULTURALLY APPROPRIATE PREVENTION AND THERAPY

Providing culturally appropriate prevention and therapy for neurodivergent children is directly related to avoiding ableist processes and implementing neurodiversity-affirming practices. Kidd (2022) offered several tips for suicide prevention and treatment with autistic and neurodivergent clients. The following has been adapted for a complete neurodiversity-affirming approach:

1. Increase recognition and understanding of the neurodiversity paradigm and neurodivergent children (including more internalized presentations) in medical and mental health training.

2. Understand appropriate assessment of anxiety and depression symptoms and suicide risk when they co-occur with neurodivergence. There is currently a lack of measurement tools for mental health status and suicide risk that have been validated for autistic and neurodivergent children.

3. Increase awareness and acceptance of neurodivergence more generally within schools, universities, workplaces, and the community. For too long, society has focused on how neurodivergent individuals can change, but the focus needs to shift to how non-autistics can genuinely accept and be inclusive of neurodivergence. This will likely reduce feelings of rejection and suicide ideation for neurodivergent people.

4. Identify and pay attention to known risk factors – e.g., anxiety, depression, bullying, social challenges, ADHD, and gender-diverse. Monitor changes in anxiety and depression levels and reduce alexithymia.

5. Check in regularly with neurodivergent children and adolescents, as changes in behavior may not be noticeable.

6. Focus on increasing interoception, overall sensory awareness, and accommodating the individual's sensory needs to reduce sensory overload.

7. Provide concrete and visual examples when formulating a safety plan.

8. Include parents/supporting adults in the safety plan if possible and appropriate.

9. Help build protective factors such as social connections/friendships, a positive sense of self, self-advocacy, and effective ways to access support.

10. Modify mental health therapy to suit the child's cognitive and communication profile.

CASE EXAMPLE

Tyler entered therapy as a 15-year-old male diagnosed with autism spectrum disorder (autistic) and attention deficit hyperactivity disorder (ADHD). Tyler's parents brought him to therapy, and Tyler had also indicated that he wanted treatment. Tyler and his parents stated that he would become "highly emotional." They described social situations as a struggle (bullying and peer rejection). Tyler had low self-worth and was often critical and negative about himself. Tyler's presentation indicated low support needs. He attended public school and was active in the community. It was discovered as therapy progressed that Tyler did not like being involved in the community and did not want to attend school. These issues were complex for him, but his parents often downplayed the struggles and did not listen to Tyler's opinion.

The therapist proceeded through the AutPlay® Therapy intake and assessment phase. The therapist completed a Neurodivergent Spectrum of Presentation assessment on Tyler, which revealed he struggled with depression and anxiety, was not comfortable with his identity as an autistic or neurodivergent person (internalized ableism), possessed solid verbal ability, seemed to do a lot of masking, appeared to have some alexithymia issues, and had a particular interest and play preference in technology. Initially, therapy goals addressed regulation struggles, problematic peer situations, and improving Tyler's self-worth. As therapy progressed and a therapeutic relationship was established (Tyler felt safer as the relationship and therapy process progressed), he began to talk about thoughts and feelings of dying, ending his life, and not wanting to be "here" anymore.

As Tyler's suicide ideation increased, he began to talk about a plan, which, at one point, he seemed to try; typical safety procedures and preventative measures were put into place. Tyler's parents were involved, and the therapist and parents would consult each time Tyler referenced anything related to suicide. He was referred to a psychiatrist for a medication evaluation, and safety plans were implemented at home and school. It was challenging to say how relevant suicide was for Tyler as his alexithymia issues resulted in him recognizing and experiencing emotions differently from a neurotypical presentation. Typically, suicide ideation would emerge in highly stressful situations. In therapy sessions, Tyler would talk about "killing himself" as a venting or stress relief response, and midway through the session, he would feel calmer and regulated. At that point, he retracted from any suicide ideation. Regardless, with Tyler, as with any neurodivergent child, the assessment accuracy can be a struggle but must still be taken seriously.

As therapy shifted to a more intentional focus on suicide ideation, interventions were implemented to help address these issues. Interventions focused on autistic and neurodivergent identity, strengthening identity and self-worth, and addressing internalized ableism (the state of being heavily influenced by the stereotypes, misconceptions, and discrimination against autistic/neurodivergent people, to the point that such people believe that their neurodivergence makes them inferior). Interventions also focused on emotion recognition and regulation needs.

One intervention implemented, titled *A Look at My Strengths*, focused on helping Tyler recognize the strengths of his neurodivergent identity and improve his self-worth. In the intervention, the client is asked to cut out several pieces of colored construction paper. The client can cut them out in different shapes. On each shape, the client writes a strength, something they do well, or something positive about themselves. Printing off a list of positive traits or strengths online is sometimes helpful in helping the client identify their strengths. The therapist can also help the client by sharing strengths they have observed. Once the strengths have been identified, the shapes are taped onto the client – their arms, chest, etc. The therapist and client look in a mirror and go through each strength, discussing how they are a part of the client. The therapist then takes a photo of the client "wearing" their strengths and sends it to the client and parent as a visual to keep and access, reminding the client of their strengths.

Through interventions focused on helping Tyler become aware and appreciate his neurodivergent identity and decreasing his internalized ableism, Tyler stopped commenting about wanting to kill himself. The suicide ideation decreased, and he stopped commenting negatively about himself. Therapy also focused on helping him develop coping skills to help him regulate when he was having strong emotions/sensations. Because of Tyler's interest in technology, we incorporated Digital Play Therapy™. Tyler learned two apps on his tablet (*Breath2Relax* and *Fluid*) that he used for regulation. *Breath2Relax* is a guided deep breathing app that creates a strong visual to follow and allows the child to adjust the rhythm and length of breathing. *Fluid* is a sensory-based app that displays a liquid-like substance on the screen that moves and changes form and color with the child's fingers. It can also include a musical element. Tyler also participated in some cognitive exercises, such as implementing positive self-talk and creating affirmations. Tyler's suicidal ideation was managed, but he remained in therapy to address social navigation needs and continue strengthening his neurodivergent identity.

CONCLUSION

O'Halloran et al. (2022) stated that findings clearly show that autistic and neurodivergent children and adolescents are at a greater suicide risk than the general population, irrespective of age (i.e., younger children and older adolescents are at-risk) or sex (i.e., boys and girls are at-risk). Child and play therapists should actively inquire about suicide when working with autistic, ADHD, and other neurodivergent children, remembering that risk identification is crucial to prevention.

As play therapists move forward in greater awareness, assessment, and prevention of suicide-related issues in neurodivergent children and adolescents, they must commit to greater awareness and acceptance of the neurodiversity paradigm and affirming practices. Chapman and Botha (2022) proposed that first, there must be a reconceptualization of dysfunction as relational rather than an individual. Second, there must be a commitment to neurodivergence acceptance and pride and a disability community and culture to emancipate neurodivergent people from neuro-normativity. Third, therapists need to cultivate a relational epistemic humility regarding different experiences of neurodivergence and disablement.

As the risk of suicide in neurodivergent children and adolescents has repeatedly been shown to be higher than in their neurotypical peers, it is more imperative than ever that child and play therapists commit to a complete understanding of neurodivergent individuals to prevent suicide ideation, attempts, and death by suicide.

CHAPTER 8.8

SUMMARY

Rebekah Byrd and Yumiko Ogawa

Suicide is, in general, in part driven by an individual's experiences of extremely overwhelming personal distress. Such experiences intensify when individuals' exposure to larger sociological stressors such as racial inequality, systemic socioeconomic disparity, and oppression is ever present, not often acknowledged, and, if recognized, slow to change. In the meantime, we know that child development is a socially mediated process because children acquire cultural values, beliefs, and practices through exposure to their environment, including community, society, and culture. Those two facts show that minoritized children may consolidate the internalized injustice into their identity, leading to a higher risk of suicidality. Play therapy can be an effective means to understand children's internalized systemic oppression and the associated feelings of helplessness and hopelessness. In the meantime, play therapy can facilitate their inner resources and strengths to battle such despair through the therapeutic relationship with play therapists and school counselors.

Play therapists and school counselors are uniquely positioned to provide therapeutic services from a place of cultural sensitivity, humility, and competency – our call as professionals to ongoing advocacy, social justice, and multicultural initiatives. By boldly and sternly opposing historical and multigenerational trauma caused by many forms of "-isms," play therapists can cultivate healing in individuals and communities.

REFERENCES

Abeysundera, H., & Khanna, H. (2022). "Ghost on the coast": Persistent hallucinations through the prism of cultural concepts of distress. *Industrial Psychiatry Journal*. https://doi.org/10.4103/ipj.ipj_103_21

Akena, D., Kiguba, R., Muhwezi, W. W., Kwesiga, B., Kigozi, G., Nakasujja, N., & Lukwata, H. (2021). The effectiveness of a psycho-education intervention on mental health literacy in communities affected by the COVID-19 pandemic – a cluster randomized trial of 24 villages in central Uganda – a research protocol. *Current Controlled Trials in Cardiovascular Medicine, 22*(1), 446–446. https://doi.org/10.1186/s13063-021-05391-6

Alvidrez, J., Snowden, L. R., Rao, S. M., & Boccellari, A. (2009). Psychoeducation to address stigma in Black adults referred for mental health treatment: A randomized pilot study. *Community Mental Health Journal, 45*(2), 127–136. https://doi.org/10.1007/s10597-008-9169-0

Allen, J., Wexler, L., & Rasmus, S. (2021). Protective factors as a unifying framework for strength-based intervention and culturally responsive American Indian and Alaska Native suicide prevention. *Prevention Science, 23*(1), 59–72. https://doi.org/10.1007/s11121-021-01265-0

Anderson, N. B. (Ed.). (2004). *Ecosocial theory* (Vols. 1–2). SAGE. https://dx.doi.org/10.4135/9781412952576

Anghel, R. E. (2020). Stress coping resilience. *Euromentor Journal, 11*(s), 113–117. https://www.proquest.com/openview/ca3a0dfcd435d9089c1911b9f5c6aa36/1?pq-origsite=gscholar&cbl=1316370

DOI: 10.4324/9781003358565-18

Assari, S., Lankarani, M. M., & Caldwell, C. H. (2017). Discrimination increases suicidal ideation in Black Adolescents regardless of ethnicity and gender. *Behavioral Sciences, 7*(4), 75. https://doi.org/10.3390/bs7040075

Badenoch, B. (2008). *Being a brain-wise therapist.* Norton.

Baker, L. (2021). *How do I identify* [Intervention] [Unpublished].

Balazs, J., & Kereszteny, A. (2017). Attention-deficit/hyperactivity disorder and suicide: A systematic review. *World Journal of Psychiatry, 7*(1), 44–59.

Barrio, C. A. (2007). Assessing suicide risk in children: Guidelines for developmentally appropriate interviewing. *Journal of Mental Health Counseling, 29*(1), 50–66. https://doi.org/10.17744/mehc.29.1.1x8qu2axd1v6rv3q

Begay, M., & Johns Hopkins Center for American Indian Health. (2019, December 12). CEBC Program › Family Spirit. *Family Spirit Program.* ihs.gov

Benner, A. D., Wang, Y., Shen, Y., Boyle, A. E., Polk, R., & Cheng, Y. (2018). Racial/ethnic discrimination and well-being during adolescence: A meta-analytic review. *American Psychologist, 73*(7), 855–883. https://doi.org/10.1037/amp0000204

Big Foot, D. S., & Schmidt, S. R. (2010). Honoring children, mending the circle: Cultural adaptation of trauma-focused cognitive-behavioral therapy for American Indian and Alaska Native children. *Journal of Clinical Psychology, 66*(8), 847–856. https://doi.org/10.1002/jclp.20707

Boyer, W. (2010). Getting to know O'Connor: Experiencing the ecosystemic play therapy model with urban first nations people. *The Family Journal, 18*(2), 202–207. https://doi.org/10.1177/1066480710364090

Brave Heart, M. Y. H. B., Chase, J., Elkins, J., & Altschul, D. (2011). Historical trauma among Indigenous peoples of the Americas: Concepts, research, and clinical considerations. *Journal of Psychoactive Drugs, 43*(4), 282–290. https://doi.org/10.1080/02791072.2011.628913

Brown, D. W., Anda, R. F., Tiemeier, H., Felitti, V. J., Edwards, V. J., Croft, J. B., & Giles, W. H. (2009). Adverse childhood experiences and the risk of premature mortality. *American Journal of Preventive Medicine, 37*(5), 389–396. https://doi.org/10.1016/j.amepre.2009.06.021

Caplan, S. (2019). The intersection of cultural and religious beliefs about mental health: Latinos in the faith-based settings. *Hispanic Health Care International, 17*(1), 4–10. https://doi.org/10.1177/1540415319828265

Ceballos, P. L., Bárcenas Jaimez, G., & Bratton, S. C. (2020). Considerations for play therapy research with Latino populations. *International Journal of Play Therapy, 29*(4), 213–222. https://doi.org/10.1037/pla0000122

Ceballos, P. L., Post, P., & Rodríguez, M. (2021). Practicing child-centered play therapy from a multicultural and social justice framework. In E. Gil & A. A. Drewes (Eds.), *Cultural issues in play therapy* (pp. 13–31). The Guilford Press.

Centers for Disease Control and Prevention. (2021). *1999–2020 wide-ranging online data for epidemiological research (WONDER), Multiple Cause of Death files [Data file].* http://wonder.cdc.gov/ucd-icd10.html

Centers for Disease Control and Prevention. (2023, February 13). YRBSS data summary & trends. *Centers for Disease Control and Prevention.* Retrieved February 20, 2023, from www.cdc.gov/healthyyouth/data/yrbs/yrbs_data_summary_and_trends.htm

Cha, C. B., Tezanos, K. M., Peros, O. M., Ng, M. Y., Ribeiro, J. D., Nock, M. K., & Franklin, J. C. (2018). Accounting for diversity in suicide research: Sampling and sample reporting practices in the United States. *Suicide and Life Threatening Behavior, 48*(2), 131–139. https://doi.org/10.1111/sltb.12344

Chase, L., & Post, P. (2022). Factors impacting play therapists' social justice advocacy attitudes. *International Journal of Play Therapy, 31*(4), 248–258. https://doi.org/10.1037/pla0000184

Chapman, R., & Botha, M. (2022). Neurodivergence-informed therapy. *Developmental Medicine & Child Neurology, 65*(3), 310–317.

Choi, Y., Jeong, E., & Park, M. (2022). Asian Americans' parent-child conflict and racial discrimination may explain mental distress. *Behavioral and Brain Sciences*, *9*(1), 18–26. https://doi.org/10.1177/3727322211068173

Cohen, J. A., & Acsw, C. R. P. (2022, March 23). The trauma-focused CBT and family acceptance project: An integrated framework for children and youth. *Psychiatric Times*. www.psychiatrictimes.com/view/the-trauma-focused-cbt-and-family-acceptance-project

Cohen, D. R., Lindsey, M. A., & Lochman, J. E. (2021). Applying an ecosocial framework to address racial disparities in suicide risk among black youth. *Psychology in the Schools*, *59*(12), 2405–2421. https://doi.org/10.1002/pits.22588

Cohen, J. A., Mannarino, A. P., & Staron, V. R. (2006). A pilot study of modified cognitive-behavioral therapy for childhood traumatic grief (CBT-CTG). *Journal of the American Academy of Child and Adolescent Psychiatry*, *45*(12), 1465–1473. https://doi.org/10.1097/01.chi.0000237705.43260.2c

Cohen, J. A., Mannarino, A. P., Wilson, K., & Zinny, A. (2018). *Trauma-focused cognitive behavioral therapy LGBTQ implementation manual*. Allegheny Health Network. https://tfcbt.org/tf-cbt-lgbtq-implementation-manual/

Congressional Black Caucus. (2019). *Ring the alarm: The crisis of Black youth suicide in America*. Emergency Taskforce on Black Youth Suicide and Mental Health.

Cuartero, M. E., & Vidal, J. F. C. (2018). Self-care behaviours and their relationship with Satisfaction and Compassion Fatigue levels among social workers. *Social Work in Health Care*, *58*(3), 274–290. https://doi.org/10.1080/00981389.2018.1558164

Deblinger, E., Mannarino, A. P., Cohen, J. A., Runyon, M. K., & Heflin, A. H. (2015). *Child sexual abuse: A primer for treating children, adolescents, and their nonoffending parents* (2nd ed.). Oxford University Press.

Diamond, G. S., Kodish, T., Ewing, E. S. K., Hunt, Q. A., & Russon, J. (2021). Family processes: Risk, protective, and treatment factors for youth at risk for suicide. *Aggression and Violent Behavior*, *64*, 101586. https://doi.org/10.1016/j.avb.2021.101586

Drewes, A., & Schaefer, C. (Eds.). (2014). *The therapeutic powers of play: 20 core agents of change*. Wiley.

Dube, S. R., Anda, R. F., Felitti, V. J., Chapman, D. P., Williamson, D. F., & Giles, W. H. (2001). Childhood abuse, household dysfunction, and the risk of attempted suicide throughout the life span: Findings from the adverse childhood experiences study. *Journal of the American Medical Association*, *286*(24), 3089–3096. https://doi.org/10.1001/jama.286.24.3089

Ehlers, C. L., Yehuda, R., Gilder, D. A., Bernert, R. A., & Karriker-Jaffe, K. J. (2022). Trauma, historical trauma, PTSD, and suicide in an American Indian community sample. *Journal of Psychiatric Research*, *156*, 214–220. https://doi.org/10.1016/j.jpsychires.2022.10.012

Elmadani, A. (2020). Investigating the relationship between race, attitude toward poverty, color-blind attitudes, and multicultural education in relation to social justice advocacy (Publication No. 28086837) [Doctoral dissertation, University of North Carolina at Charlotte]. ProQuest Dissertations Publishing.

Fitzpatrick, K. M., Piko, B. F., & Miller, E. (2008). Suicide ideation and attempts among low-income African American adolescents. *Suicide & Life-Threatening Behavior*, *38*(5), 552–563. https://doi.org/10.1521/suli.2008.38.5.552

Freedenthal, S., & Stiffman, A. R. (2007). "They might think I was crazy": Young American Indians' reasons for not seeking help when suicidal. *Journal of Adolescent Research*, *22*(1), 58–77. https://doi.org/10.1177/0743558406295969

Fulginiti, A., Goldbach, J. T., Mamey, M. R., Rusow, J. A., Srivastava, A., Rhoades, H., Schrager, S. M., Bond, D., & Marshal, M. P. (2020). Integrating minority stress theory and the interpersonal theory of suicide among sexual minority youth who engage crisis services. *Suicide and Life Threatening Behavior*, *50*(3), 601–616. https://doi.org/10.1111/sltb.12623

Germán, M., Smith, H. L., Rivera-Morales, C., González, G., Haliczer, L. A., Haaz, C., & Miller, A. L. (2015). Dialectical behavior therapy for suicidal Latina adolescents: Supplemental dialectical corollaries and treatment targets. *American Journal of Psychotherapy, 69*(2), 179–197. https://doi. org/10.1176/appi.psychotherapy.2015.69.2.179

Giupponi, G., Giordano, G., Maniscalco, I., Erbuto, D., Berardelli, I., Conca, A., Lester, D., Girardi, P., & Pompili, M. (2018). Suicide risk in attention-deficit/hyperactivity disorder. *Psychiatria Danubina, 30*(1), 2–10. https://doi.org/10.24869/psyd.2018.2

Goldston, D. B., Molock, S. D., Whitbeck, L. B., Murakami, J. M., Zayas, L. H., & Hall, G. C. N. (2008). Cultural considerations in adolescent suicide prevention and psychosocial treatment. *American Psychologist, 63*(1), 14–31. https://doi.org/10.1037/0003-066x.63.1.14

Gower, A. L., Rider, G. N., McMorris, B. J., & Eisenberg, M. E. (2018). Bullying victimization among LGBTQ youth: Critical issues and future directions. *Current Sexual Health Reports, 10*(4), 246–254. https://doi.org/10.1007/s11930-018-0169-y

Goyette, K., & Xie, Y. (1999). Educational expectations of Asian American youth: Determinants and ethnic differences. *Sociology of Education, 72*(1), 22–36. https://doi.org/10.2307/2673184

Graham, J. T. (2013). Expressive therapy as a treatment preference for aboriginal trauma. *Pimatisiwin: A Journal of Aboriginal and Indigenous Community Health, 2*(3).

Grant, R. J. (2021). *Understanding autism: A neurodiversity affirming guidebook for children and teens.* AutPlay Publishing.

Grant, R. J. (2023a). *Neurodivergent spectrum of presentation* [Graphic] [Unpublished].

Grant, R. J. (2023b). *The AutPlay therapy handbook: Integrative family play therapy with neurodivergent children.* Routledge.

Hanson, T., Zhang, G., Cerna, R., Stern, A., & Austin, G. (2019). Understanding the experiences of LGBTQ students in California. *ERIC* (No. ED601909). Ed.gov Institute of Education Sciences. Retrieved April 8, 2023, from https://eric.ed.gov/?id=ED601909

Hatzenbuehler, M. L. (2011). The social environment and suicide attempts in lesbian, gay, and bisexual youth. *Pediatrics, 127*(5), 896–903. https://doi.org/10.1542/peds.2010-3020

Henderson, R. C. W., Williams, P., Gabbidon, J., Farrelly, S., Schauman, O., Hatch, S. L., Thornicroft, G., Bhugra, D., & Clement, S. (2015). Mistrust of mental health services: Ethnicity, hospital admission, and unfair treatment. *Epidemiology and Psychiatric Sciences, 24*(3), 258–265. https://doi. org/10.1017/s2045796014000158

Hijioka, S., & Wong, J. (2012). *Suicide among Asian Americans.* www.apa.org/pi/oema/resources/ ethnicity-health/asian-american/suicide

Illich, P. (2004). *Suicide intervention training outcomes study: Summary report.* Research Consulting Services.

I Love Ancestry. (2014, July 2). A native teen's story. Native American Teen suicide epidemic [Video]. *YouTube.* www.youtube.com/watch?v=PfEwokj-eMA

Impey, M., & Heun, R. (2012). Completed suicide, ideation, and attempt in attention deficit hyperactivity disorder. *Acta Psychiatrica Scandinavica, 125*(2), 93–102. https://doi.org/10.1111/j.1600-0447.2011.01798.x

Indian Health Service (n.d.). *Indian Health Service.* www.ihs.gov/

Insalaco, S. (2019, October 18). TF-CBT LGBTQ implementation manual – trauma focus cognitive behavioral therapy certification program. *Trauma Focus Cognitive Behavioral Therapy Certification Program.*

Jimenez-Colon, G., & Duarte-Velez, Y. (2022). Raising children in different cultures: Working with Latinx youth with suicidal behaviors and their families. *Rhode Island Medical Journal, 105*(4), 31–35.

Joe, S. (2006). Implications of national suicide trends for social work practice with Black youth. *Child & Adolescent Social Work Journal, 23*(4), 458–471. https://doi.org/10.1007/s10560-006-0064-7

Joe, S. (2008). Chapter 14. Suicide patterns among Black males. (pp. 218–241). In Anderson, E. Against the wall. In University of Pennsylvania PresseBooks. https://doi.org/10.9783/9780812206951

Johns, M. M., Lowry, R., Haderxhanaj, L. T., Rasberry, C. N., Robin, L., Scales, L., Stone, D. L., & Suárez, N. M. (2020). Trends in violence victimization and suicide risk by sexual identity among high school students – youth risk behavior survey, United States, 2015–2019. *MMWR Supplements*, *69*(1), 19–27. https://doi.org/10.15585/mmwr.su6901a3

Joiner, T. E. (2005). *Why people die by suicide*. Harvard University Press.

Joiner, T. (2007). *Why people die by suicide*. Harvard University Press.

Katz-Wise, S. L., Rosario, M., & Tsappis, M. (2016). Lesbian, gay, bisexual, and transgender youth and family acceptance. *Pediatric Clinics of North America, 63*(6), 1011–1025. https://doi.org/10.1016/j.pcl.2016.07.005

Kidd, T. (2022). *Helping autistic teens to manage their anxiety: Strategies and worksheets using CBT, DBT, and ACT Skills*. Jessica Kingsley Publishers.

Kim, J. E., & Zane, N. (2016). Help-seeking intentions among Asian American and White American students in psychological distress: Application of the health belief model. *Cultural Diversity and Ethnic Minority Psychology, 22*(3), 311–321. https://doi.org/10.1037/cdp0000056

Kirby, A. V., Bakian, A. V., Zhang, Y., Bilder, D. A., Keeshin, B. R., & Coon, H. (2019). A 20-year study of suicide death in a statewide autism population. *Autism Research: Official Journal of the International Society for Autism Research, 12*(4), 658–666. https://doi.org/10.1002/aur.2076

Kirby, A. V., Bakian, A. V., Zhang, Y., Bilder, D. A., Keeshin, B. R., & Coon, H. (2019). A 20-year study of suicide death in a statewide autism population. *Autism Research, 12*(4), 658–666. https://doi.org/10.1002/aur.2076

Lang, W. A., Ramsay, R. F., Tanney, B. L., Kinzel, T., Turley, B., & Tierney, R. J. (2013). *ASIST trainer manual* (11th ed.). Living Works Education.

Lau, A. S., Jernewall, N. M., Zane, N., & Myers, H. F. (2002). Correlates of suicidal behaviors among Asian American outpatient youths. *Cultural Diversity and Ethnic Minority Psychology, 8*(3), 199–213. https://doi.org/10.1037/1099-9809.8.3.199

Lee, E. (2019). *America for Americans: A history of xenophobia in the United States*. Basic Books.

Lee, S., Juon, H., Martinez, G., Hsu, C. E., Robinson, E. S., Bawa, J., & Ma, G. X. (2009). Model minority at risk: Expressed needs of mental health by Asian American young adults. *Journal of Community Health, 34*(2), 144–152. https://doi.org/10.1007/s10900-008-9137-1

Leigh. (2017). Experiencing emotion: Children's perceptions, reflections, and self-regulation. *Body, Movement, and Dance in Psychotherapy, 12*(2), 128–144. https://doi.org/10.1080/17432979.2017.1303544

Lin, Y., & Bratton, S. (2015). A meta-analytic review of child-centered play therapy approaches. *Journal of Counseling and Development, 93*(1), 45–58. https://doi.org/10.1002/j.1556-6676.2015.00180.x

Lindsey, M. A., Sheftall, A. H., Xiao, Y., & Joe, S. (2019). Trends of suicidal behaviors among high school students in the United States: 1991–2017. *Pediatrics, 144*(5). https://doi.org/10.1542/peds.2019-1187

Llamas, J. D., & Alvarado, C. (2022). More than just a game: Using lotería in play therapy with Mexican/Mexican American clients. *International Journal of Play Therapy*. https://doi.org/10.1037/pla0000185

Madubata, I. J., Spivey, L. A., Alvarez, G., Neblett, E. W., & Prinstein, M. J. (2022). Forms of racial/ethnic discrimination and suicidal ideation: A prospective examination of African-American and Latinx Youth. *Journal of Clinical Child and Adolescent Psychology, 51*(1), 23–31. https://doi.org/10.1080/15374416.2019.1655756

Mahajan, S., Caraballo, C., Lu, Y., Valero-Elizondo, J., Lu, Y., Annapureddy, A., Roy, B., Roy, B., Murugiah, K., Onuma, O. K., Nunez-Smith, M., Forman, H. P., Nasir, K., Herrin, J., & Krumholz, H. M. (2021). Trends in differences in health status and health care access and affordability by race and ethnicity in the United States, 1999–2018. *JAMA, 326*(7), 637. https://doi.org/10.1001/jama.2021.9907

Marraccini, M. E., Ingram, K. H., Naser, S. C., Grapin, S. L., Toole, E. N., O'Neill, J. C., Chin, A., Martinez, R., & Griffin, D. (2022). The roles of school in supporting LGBTQ+ youth: A systematic review and ecological framework for understanding risk for suicide-related thoughts and behaviors. *Journal of School Psychology, 91*, 27–49. https://doi.org/10.1016/j.jsp.2021.11.006

Mayo, C. (2022). Gender diversities and sex education. *Journal of Philosophy of Education, 56*(5), 654–662. https://doi.org/10.1111/1467-9752.12686

McAuliffe, N., & Perry, L. (2007). Making it safer: A health center's strategy for suicide prevention. *Psychiatric Quarterly, 78*, 295–307. https://doi.org/10.1007/s11126-007-9047-x

McDonald, J. D., Gonzalez, J. M., & Sargent, E. M. (2019). Cognitive behavior therapy with American Indians. *American Psychological Association eBooks*, pp. 27–51. https://doi.org/10.1037/0000119-002

McGuire, T. G., & Miranda, J. (2008). New evidence regarding racial and ethnic disparities in mental health: Policy implications. *Health Affairs, 27*(2), 393–403. https://doi.org/10.1377/hlthaff.27.2.393

Mehl-Madrona, L., & Mainguy, B. (2020). Narrative approaches to North American indigenous people who attempt suicide. *The Permanente Journal, 24*(2). https://doi.org/10.7812/tpp/19.032

Merchant, C., Kramer, A., Joe, S., Venkataraman, S., & King, C. A. (2009). Predictors of multiple suicide attempts among suicidal Black adolescents. *Suicide & Life-Threatening Behavior, 39*(2), 115–124. https://doi.org/10.1521/suli.2009.39.2.115

Meyer, I. H. (1995). Minority stress and mental health in gay men. *Journal of Health and Social Behavior, 36*(1), 38. https://doi.org/10.2307/2137286

Mezzalira, S., Scandurra, C., Mezza, F., Miscioscia, M., Innamorati, M., & Bochicchio, V. (2022). Gender felt pressure, affective domains, and mental health outcomes among transgender and gender diverse (TGD) children and adolescents: A systematic review with developmental and clinical implications. *International Journal of Environmental Research and Public Health, 20*(1), 785. https://doi.org/10.3390/ijerph20010785

National Indian Child Welfare Association, & Sahota, P. (2019). Culture and emotional well-being in adolescents who are American Indian/Alaska Native: A review of current literature. *Child Welfare, 97*(3), 1–21. www.jstor.org/stable/48623655

O'Connor, K. (2001). Ecosystemic play therapy. *International Journal of Play Therapy, 10*(2), 33–44. https://doi.org/10.1037/h0089478

Oh, H., Waldman, K., Koyanagi, A., Anderson, R. E., & DeVylder, J. (2020). Major discriminatory events and suicidal thoughts and behaviors amongst Black Americans: Findings from the National Survey of American Life. *Journal of Affective Disorders, 263*, 47–53. https://doi.org/10.1016/j.jad.2019.11.128

O'Halloran, L., Coey, P., & Wilson, C. (2022). Suicidality in autistic youth: A systematic review and meta-analysis. *Clinical Psychology Review, 93*, 102144. https://doi.org/10.1016/j.cpr.2022.102144

O'Keefe, V. M., Waugh, E., Grubin, F., Cwik, M., Chambers, R., Ivanich, J., Weeks, R., & Barlow, A. (2022). Development of "CULTURE FORWARD: A strengths and culture-based tool to protect our native youth from suicide." *Cultural Diversity & Ethnic Minority Psychology, 28*(4), 587–597. https://doi.org/10.1037/cdp0000546

Olson, K. R., Durwood, L., DeMeules, M., & McLaughlin, K. A. (2016). Mental health of transgender children who are supported in their identities. *Pediatrics, 137*(3). https://doi.org/10.1542/peds.2015-3223

Opara, I., Assan, M. A., Pierre, K., Gunn, J. F., Metzger, I., Hamilton, J., & Arugu, E. (2020). Suicide among Black children: An integrated model of the interpersonal-psychological theory of suicide and intersectionality theory for researchers and clinicians. *Journal of Black Studies, 51*(6), 611–631. https://doi.org/10.1177/0021934720935641

Orbach, I., Seymour, F., Gabrielle, C., Hananyah, G., & Yigal, G. (1983). Attraction and repulsion by life and death in suicidal and in normal children. *Journal of Consulting and Clinical Psychology, 51*(5), 661–670. https://doi.org/10.1037/0022-006x.51.5.661

Parikh, S., Ceballos, P. L., & Post, P. (2013). Factors related to play therapists' social justice advocacy attitudes. *Journal of Multicultural Counseling and Development*. https://doi.org/10.1002/j.2161-1912.2013.00039.x

Perez, N. M., Jennings, W. G., Piquero, A. R., & Baglivio, M. T. (2016). Adverse childhood experiences and suicide attempts: The mediating influence of personality development and problem behaviors. *Journal of Youth and Adolescence, 45*, 1527–1545. https://doi.org/10.1007/s10964-016-0519-x

Perez-Rodriguez, M. M., Baca-Garcia, E., Oquendo, M. A., Wang, S., Wall, M. M., Liu, S. M., & Blanco, C. (2014). Relationship between acculturation, discrimination, and suicidal ideation and attempts among US Hispanics in the National Epidemiologic Survey of Alcohol and Related Conditions. *The Journal of Clinical Psychiatry*, *75*(4), 399–407. https://doi.org/10.4088/JCP.13m08548

Pew Research Center. (n.d.). *Hispanics/Latinos – research and data from Pew Research Center*. www.pewresearch.org/topic/race-ethnicity/racial-ethnic-groups/hispanics-latinos/

Play Therapy Best Practices Clinical, Professional & Ethical Issues. (2022). Association for Play Therapy. Retrieved September 13, 2023, from https://cdn.ymaws.com/www.a4pt.org/resource/resmgr/publications/best_practices.pdf

Polanco-Roman, L. (2020, January 5). Suicide-related risk among racial and ethnic minority youth: Important considerations. *Youth Suicide Research*. www.youthsuicideresearch.org/blog/suicide-related-risk-among-racial-and-ethnic-minority-youthnbspimportant-considerationsblog/youthresearchorg

Post, P. B., Phipps, C. B., Camp, A. C., & Grybush, A. L. (2019). Effectiveness of child-centered play therapy among marginalized children. *International Journal of Play Therapy*, *28*(2), 88–97. https://doi.org/10.1037/pla0000096

Price, J. H., & Khubchandani, J. (2022). Hispanic child suicides in the United States, 2010–2019. *Journal of Community Health*, *47*(1), 311–315. https://doi.org/10.1007/s10900-021-01054-4

Pronouns/Minus18. (n.d.). *Pronouns*. www.minus18.org.au/pronouns/

Ratts, M. J., Singh, A. A., Butler, S. K., Nassar-McMillan, S., & McCullough, J. R. (2016, January 27). Multicultural and social justice counseling competencies: Practical applications in counseling. *Counseling Today*. https://ct.counseling.org/2016/01/multicultural-and-social-justice-counseling-competencies-practical-applications-in-counseling/

Retrieved September 13, 2023, from https://cdn.ymaws.com/www.a4pt.org/resource/resmgr/publications/best_practices.pdf

Richa, S., Fahed, M., Khoury, E., & Mishara, B. (2014). Suicide in autism spectrum disorders. *Archives of Suicide Research: Official Journal of the International Academy for Suicide Research*, *18*(4), 327–339. https://doi.org/10.1080/13811118.2013.824834

Romanelli, M., Sheftall, A. H., Irsheid, S. B., Lindsey, M. A., & Grogan, T. M. (2022). Factors associated with distinct patterns of suicidal thoughts, suicide plans, and suicide attempts among US adolescents. *Prevention Science: The Official Journal of the Society for Prevention Research*, *23*(1), 73–84. https://doi.org/10.1007/s11121-021-01295-8

SAMHSA. (2022, March 28). Historical trauma: Understanding origins part 1 [Video]. *YouTube*. www.youtube.com/watch?v=5h5ZjhPOy30

Sarris, M. (2022). Autism and the troubling risk of suicide. *SPARK*. https://sparkforautism.org/discover_article/autism-suicide-risk/

Shannonhouse, L., Elston, N., Lin, Y., Mize, M. C., Rumsey, A., Rice, R., Wanna, R., & Porter, M. (2018). Suicide intervention training for counselor-trainees: Quasi-experimental study on skill retention. *Counselor Education and Supervision*, *57*(3), 194–210. https://doi.org/10.1002/ceas.12110

Shannonhouse, L., Lin, Y., Shaw, K., & Porter, M. J. (2017). Investigating the impact of ASIST training in K-12 Schools: A quasi-experimental research study. *Journal of Counseling and Development*, *95*, 3–13. https://doi.org/10.1002/jcad.12112

Sheftall, A. H., Asti, L., Horowitz, L. M., Felts, A., Fontanella, C. A., Campo, J. V., & Bridge, J. A. (2016). Suicide in elementary school-aged children and early adolescents. *Pediatrics*, *138*(4), e20160436. https://doi.org/10.1542/peds.2016-0436

Silverman, C. (2015). NeuroTribes: The legacy of autism and the future of neurodiversity by Steve Silberman. *Anthropological Quarterly*, *88*(4), 1111–1121. https://doi.org/10.1353/anq.2015.0057

Suicide Prevention Resource Center. (n.d.). www.sprc.org. Retrieved June 26, 2022, from www.sprc.org/

Suicide Prevention Resource Center. (2020). *Racial and ethnic disparities.* https://sprc.org/about-suicide/scope-of-the-problem/racial-and-ethnic-disparities/

Taylor, M. R., Boden, J. M., & Rucklidge, J. J. (2014). The relationship between ADHD symptomatology and self-harm, suicidal ideation, and suicidal behaviours in adults: A pilot study. *Attention Deficit and Hyperactivity Disorders, 6*(4), 303–312. https://doi.org/10.1007/s12402-014-0139-9

The Trevor Project. (2022). *2022 National survey on LGBTQ youth mental health.* www.thetrevorproject.org/survey-2022/

Thielemann, J., Kasparik, B., König, J., Unterhitzenberger, J., & Rosner, R. (2022). A systematic review and meta-analysis of trauma-focused cognitive behavioral therapy for children and adolescents. *Child Abuse & Neglect, 134,* 105899. https://doi.org/10.1016/j.chiabu.2022.105899

Thomason, T. (2011). Best practices in counseling Native Americans. *Journal of Indigenous Research, 1*(1), 3. https://doi.org/10.26077/ypcz-9x86

Toussaint, L., Nguyen, Q., Roettger, C., Dixon, K., Offenbächer, M., Kohls, N., Hirsch, J. K., & Sirois, F. M. (2021). Effectiveness of progressive muscle relaxation, deep breathing, and guided imagery in promoting psychological and physiological states of relaxation. *Evidence-Based Complementary and Alternative Medicine, 2021,* 1–8. https://doi.org/10.1155/2021/5924040

Troxell Klingenbjerg, P. M. (2017). Suicide in elementary school-aged children and early adolescents. *The Journal of Emergency Medicine, 52*(1), 125. https://doi.org/10.1016/j.jemermed.2016.11.037

van Manen, M. (2017). But is it phenomenology? *Qualitative Health Research, 27*(6), 775–779. https://doi.org/10.1177/1049732317699570

Walker, L. (2022). Autism paradigms and mental well-being among autistic adults: A quantitative exploration. *Antioch University ProQuest Dissertations Publishing.* https://www.proquest.com/openview/c747cf72ebd30e4805434746a3cfee29/1?pq-origsite=gscholar&cbl=18750&diss=y

Wamser-Nanney, R., & Steinzor, C. E. (2016). Characteristics of attrition among children receiving trauma-focused treatment. *Psychological Trauma, 8*(6), 745–754. https://doi.org/10.1037/tra0000143

Wei, C., & Liu, W. (2019). Coming out in Mainland China: A national survey of LGBTQ students. *Journal of Light Youth, 16*(2), 192–219. https://doi.org/10.1080/19361653.2019.1565795

Weniger, J., Young, S., & Hernandez, C. (2020). Risk and protective factors with Native American Indian and Alaska Native children who have a history of suicidal behavior. *Journal of Indigenous Research, 8,* 2. https://doi.org/10.26077/6qnp-z328

Whitten, C., & Thomas, C. (2023). Anti-queer policy & rural schools: A framework to analyze AntiQueer policy implementation in rural schools. *The Rural Educator, 44*(2), 7. https://doi.org/10.55533/2643-9662.1408

Williams, D., Hall, W. W., Dawes, H. C., Rizo, C. F., & Goldbach, J. T. (2022). An integrated conceptual model to understand suicidality among queer youth to inform suicide prevention. *Societies, 12*(6), 170. https://doi.org/10.3390/soc12060170

Wong, Y. J., Deng, K., & Li, Y. (2022). "Please forgive me:" Asian and Pacific Islander Americans' suicide notes. *Asian American Journal of Psychology, 13*(2), 158–167. https://doi.org/10.1037/aap0000234

Wong, Y. J., & Maffini, C. S. (2011). Predictors of Asian American adolescents' suicide attempts: A latent class regression analysis. *Journal of Youth and Adolescence, 40,* 1453–1464. https://doi.org/10.1007/s10964-011-9701-3

World Health Organization (WHO). (2024). *Mental health.* https://www.who.int/health-topics/mental-health#tab=tab_1

Xie, Y., & Goyette, K. (2003). Social mobility and the educational choices of Asian Americans. *Social Science Research, 32*(3), 467–498. https://doi.org/10.1016/S0049-089X(03)00018-8

Yip, T. (2015). The effects of ethnic/racial discrimination and sleep quality on depressive symptoms and self-esteem trajectories among diverse adolescents. *Journal of Youth and Adolescence, 44*(2), 419–430. https://doi.org/10.1007/s10964-014-0123-x

Yu, M., & Stiffman, A. R. (2007). Culture and environment as predictors of alcohol abuse/dependence symptoms in American Indian youths. *Addictive Behaviors, 32*(10), 2253–2259. https://doi.org/10.1016/j.addbeh.2007.01.008

Zayas, L. H., Gulbas, L. E., Fedoravicius, N., & Cabassa, L. J. (2010). Patterns of distress, precipitating events, and reflections on suicide attempts by young Latinas. *Social Science & Medicine, 70*(11), 1773–1779. https://doi.org/10.1016/j.socscimed.2010.02.013

CHAPTER 9

THE ROLE OF SCHOOLS IN SUICIDE

Response, Resourcing, and Prevention for Children

Nichole Vernon

BREAKING DOWN DENIAL AND MINIMIZATION

The crisis of suicide in children and adolescents is alarming and well noted by Gallo and Wachter (2022), who reported that death by suicide for individuals ages 10–24 increased by more than 40% for Hispanic females, 30% for Black females, 23% for Black males, and 20% for Hispanic males. School systems are working to identify the warning signs and risk factors for suicide, emphasizing prevention intervention that empowers school personnel to intervene. Suicide is a gamut of behaviors that include ideations, intent, and attempts. Not all children or adolescents advance through each stage, and the behaviors vary. Per Knipe et al. (2022), there has been a rise in concerns regarding the impact of the pandemic and the potential rise in suicide and self-harm. The occurrence of suicidal behaviors varies seasonally and increases rapidly at the onset age of puberty. Self-harm is self-directed behavior that deliberately results in injury or the potential to injure oneself. Self-injurious behavior occurs when there is evidence that the person has at least some intent to die. A suicide attempt may result in death, injuries, or no injuries. Suicidal behavior is developing a plan or strategy for suicide, gathering the means for a suicide plan, or any other overt action or thought indicating intent to end one's life. Suicidal ideation is planning or considering self-injurious behavior that may result in death.

In the school environment, students are exposed to traumatic events, which could lead to the reduction of resistance to suicide and increase the likelihood of attempts. Many students often elect not to tell anyone about their suicidal thoughts due to the stigma, not wanting to burden others with their situation, and believing these thoughts are fleeting as they are at low risk. Schools are often so focused on meeting district benchmarks that they neglect supporting social connections, mindfulness, and understanding the importance of addressing social-emotional behavior. The evolving period between childhood and adulthood is a period of critical changes in one's body, thoughts, and feelings.

Concealing and minimizing suicidal thoughts can lead mental health professionals to monitor and treat students experiencing a suicidal crisis improperly (Nagdimon et al., 2021). Within the school environment, determining what a crisis is often falls on the classroom teacher's responsibility to identify possible warning signs before connecting the student with the school-based mental health provider. A teacher with limited training may underestimate or poorly identify the warning signs. Their response may ignite shame or the stigma surrounding suicidal behavior. School counselors are hesitant to engage in suicide prevention efforts due to feelings of lack of recognition for their expertise (Whisenhunt et al., 2017). Many school systems are now implementing "gatekeeper training" to provide an individual with skills used in recognizing, responding to, and helping a suicidal person to get help (Becker, 2017).

DOI: 10.4324/9781003358565-19

Gatekeepers are people who know essential suicide prevention and intervention steps and strategies. Providing individuals with these skills is helpful and a step in the right direction. However, ongoing training occurs due to the high turnover rate of educators and the constant reinforcement of skill knowledge. Prevention tactics are often inadequately utilized due to students minimizing suicidal ideations and being prone to relay suicide intent to their peers. Most school systems classify suicide prevention and intervention as crisis management.

Crisis management is the application of strategies designed to help an organization manage unexpected, traumatic events. Crisis management applies before, during, and after a crisis. It affects each person differently and can potentially destroy their mental, physical, social, emotional, and spiritual well-being. Established training is vital for schools to focus on ongoing interventions and services.

Many districts have a district-wide crisis team. Crisis teams include mental health professionals, administrative leaders, school nurses, designated staff members, and resource officers. With these individuals identified, schools can develop crisis plans and execute them. Regarding developing consistent strategies, schools need to have clear guidelines and policies dictated in a designated response protocol.

With new and unfamiliar staff in the education environment, minimizing and denying symptoms is relatively common due to the lack of training and a limited understanding of crisis management (Sheftall et al., 2016). With this limited knowledge, newly minted educators may not fully understand the continuum of suicidal behaviors, what constitutes a crisis, social-emotional learning, and critical terminology. The emphasis on destigmatizing suicide in students is often not provided in the training. Training focuses on prevention and crisis management from a clinician's perspective. Teachers are required to focus on the curriculum, which now includes social-emotional learning. Crisis training is the responsibility of school-based mental health providers. These staff train and manage crises while being responsible for their designated duties.

Furthermore, training often does not provide enough information or consider anxiety from the adult's and student's perspectives. Encouraging dialogue on anxiety in students and adults as a way of sustaining rapport and detecting clues would also assist in breaking down the minimalization and denial of suicidal behaviors (Durlak et al., 2011). Schools that fully integrate a variety of learning supports that include social-emotional learning, instruction, and school management can foster a comprehensive, consistent tactic that enables multidisciplinary collaboration. Supporting this dialogue during training on social-emotional learning will help foster additional communication within the school environment.

Social-emotional learning is the process that assists individuals in developing a healthy sense of self, managing emotions, feeling empathy for others, maintaining supportive relationships with friends and loved ones, and making responsible decisions. Social-emotional learning incorporates goal setting and stress management, providing children and adults with tools to express themselves genuinely and appropriately. Moreover, social-emotional learning leads students to acquire techniques for processing and managing emotions and developing essential social skills that prevent suicidal ideation (Posamentier et al., 2022). It educates students on how to be more socially and emotionally aware. Social-emotional learning is essential for building healthy relationships, communicating efficiently, and living a fruitful and meaningful life.

PROVIDING A SAFE ENVIRONMENT FOR CHILDREN

Creating a safe and warm learning environment is critical to educating and preparing all students to achieve their highest potential and contribute to society. When we consider providing a safe environment for students, we should always consider skills often challenging to measure, such as critical thinking skills, emotional management, conflict resolution, emotional management, teamwork, and decision-making skills. Students need to learn a wide range of skills, attitudes, and behaviors that can impact students' success in school and life. To teach these skills, educators and school-based mental health providers should focus on curriculum components that can be incorporated into the curriculum to assist in creating a safe environment. Using age-approach language and strategies is imperative when designing a safe environment. In research from Marraccini et al., schools in high-poverty communities, those with greater racial diversity, and those in areas with poor infrastructure or high crime rates may face unique challenges in creating a safe environment (n.d.). Although there is a common goal of providing a safe environment and focusing on prevention, educators need to remember that elementary, middle, and high school students are all in different stages of life.

Components should focus on reflection, balance, coping strategies, physical well-being, identifying people who nurture healthy relationships, developing and connecting mentors, healthy activities, service, cultivating mindfulness, and strategically utilizing strengths. Developing an understanding of how we process information using our brains and bodies is a process that involves reflection and balance when responding to experiences. Students should learn to practice emotional regulation by utilizing their strengths and developing healthy coping strategies. Helping children to identify different methods of caring while increasing their physical well-being promotes understanding, emotional regulation, and self-care. When creating an environment, students should learn to identify the people who provide support, nurture, and care for them. When discussing positive relationships, educating students on identifying and promoting healthy friendships with people who uplift, encourage, and support them (Sheftall et al., 2016). Promoting healthy friendships teaches students how to navigate conflict, increase empathy, and understand perspective-taking.

Teachers are not licensed mental health professionals, but they can create a safe environment within their classroom for students. The challenge for most teachers is creating an emotionally safe environment without renouncing their role as teachers. Teachers should find the right balance of being emotionally open and authentic without sacrificing any boundaries. More school-based mental health clinicians are necessary to create and promote a safe environment for children. Developing and connecting with mentors in the school as well as in the community can assist with manifesting a safe environment and ensuring those components are transferred from school to home (Becker, 2017).

Additionally, drawing strength from various types of healthy activities that navigate life. Strategically utilizing strengths and coping skills to overcome expected and unexpected changes in life, whether big or small, to practice regulation and resilience. Students should be encouraged to examine what gives them a sense of purpose and connection to something larger than themselves, including engaging in kindness, practicing thankfulness, cultivating mindfulness, or participating in cultural traditions.

UNIQUE CHALLENGES AND VULNERABILITIES TO SCHOOL IDENTIFICATION

When we discuss warning signs and risk factors, we consider mental health disorders, substance use, family history, access to lethal means, exposure to the suicide of another person, and stress. Appropriate school-based mental health clinicians conduct risk assessments to gather data regarding the student's intent to die by suicide, previous history of suicide attempts, presence of a suicide plan, presence of support systems, level of vulnerability, mental status, and any additional relevant risk factors. Most often, several risk factors converge at the moment and may incorporate various factors depending on the student, his or her family, and the current environment. Clinicians should note that when factors are escalating, the likelihood of an attempt increases (Bridge et al., 2015). Furthermore, school-based mental health clinicians are imperative stakeholders in youth suicide prevention and postvention due to their propinquity to the at-risk population. Prevention are activities aimed at obstructing acts of suicide, and postvention is strategies implemented following an act of suicide to decrease the likelihood of contagion.

Although the goal is to become proactive and strive for a collaborative approach, some school districts operate on a reactive strategy (*A Model for School-based Crisis Preparedness and Response*, n.d.). Operating on such a strategy is counterproductive, highlights weaknesses, and further challenges systems currently in place. Schools lack support from staff, have limited resources, overextended staff, and staff burnout. Due to the latter, there has been a high turnover rate in the field of education, and newly hired educators often do not have the proper training or the necessary support to be successful within the field. This level of vulnerability impacts school-based mental health clinicians' and educators' ability to intervene and follow protocol. Additionally, some school-based mental health clinicians may perceive their confidence waver when intervening effectively due to a high caseload and many daily tasks. These deficits also impede the necessary training to effectively prevent, identify, and manage suicidal behavior in at-risk students.

Another challenge schools face is employing longer-term strategies that are effective, measurable, and flexible. Due to staffing shortages, resource access, funding, skills training, and education programs still need to be expanded. Longer educational sessions and ongoing skills training have demonstrated effective outcomes (Surgenor et al., 2016). Research has shown that amplified information is not a suitable learning outcome when the focus is prevention. Having clearly defined outcomes and observable measures will assist in determining the effectiveness of a suicide prevention program and resources. As issues arise, plans should be flexible and accommodating to address the needs of the target audience and the sensitivity of suicide-related topics. Tension and resistance are contributing factors that also place schools in challenging positions that daunt moral responsibility and critical engagement. Educators often need clarification about their roles, the referral process, and the additional available resources.

RESOURCES AND PREVENTION

Prevention is critical and requires support from all stakeholders, including students. Ogawa et al. (2022) researched community education programs utilized in preventing suicide with the expectation of reducing suicide risk ultimately. Schools offer consistent and direct contact with students in a greater capacity. Prevention starts with administrator and educator buy-in, empowerment, and training, as with all programs. Mental health concepts are introduced to destigmatize nurturing mental health and social-emotional behavior. Schools have become havens for students to feel cared for and safe. More schools are creating programs and systems that endorse resilience, healthy relationships, self-care, and mindfulness (Lottman et al., 2017) – in addition to staff training, designing classroom curricula on suicide prevention to educate students and incorporate with current educational programming. If designed and implemented correctly, schools would not fear the possibility of discussing suicidal behavior but rather seek support as well as engage in open conversations that suicide is a permanent solution to a temporary problem. Schools must recognize and utilize school-based mental health professionals to serve in critical leadership roles.

School-based mental health professionals possess training and expertise that links mental health, education, and environmental factors that support students. Additionally, each professional creates a school environment that promotes positive mental health and encourages safety and support favorable to learning (Posamentier, J. et al., 2022). School-based mental health professionals can provide counseling, social-emotional skill instruction, collaboration, complementary services, and consultation. With these known skills, school-based mental health professionals can assist with interventions and creating a curriculum that supports identifying emotions, relationship skills, social awareness, assertiveness training, self-management, psychoeducation, responsible decision-making, and coping skills.

A classroom curriculum on suicide prevention should be a collaborative effort between school-based mental health professionals, outside resources, and educators. Training should be held in small groups so that students can communicate their concerns. Building on essential knowledge and skills related to suicide prevention is vital when assessing learning objectives for the curriculum. Teaching problem-solving, coping skills, and conflict-resolution skills are essential elements that will help reduce the likelihood of suicide (Becker, 2017).

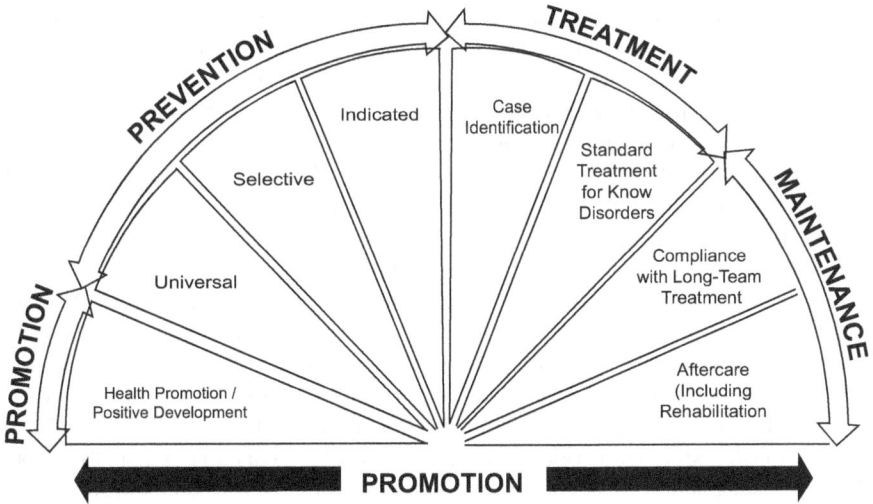

Figure 9.1 Mental Health Intervention Spectrum

Source: Mental health intervention spectrum. National Academies of Sciences, Engineering, and Medicine. 2016. Preventing Bullying Through Science, Policy, and Practice. https://doi.org/10.17226/23482. Reproduced with permission from the National Academy of Sciences, courtesy of the National Academies Press.

Cultivating a school-wide initiative and promoting tolerance within the curriculum and the gatekeeper training will aid in addressing the sensitive nature of the subject matter. Over time, schools can build this sense of belonging by incorporating student-led activities and clubs central to social-emotional learning. Activity networks create feelings of connectedness and desire to partake in an environment students enjoy. In addition, experts facilitate special intervention programs that focus on bullying prevention and peer victimization. These experts will confirm that disclosures and challenging questions about trauma triggers for suicidal thoughts and behaviors are addressed appropriately. Experts can also determine the need for support for identified students. Due to the involvement and collaboration of factors that may lead to suicidal ideation, prevention programs should focus on a broader range of factors to develop skills and awareness among students. Knowledge of risk factors is a vital component of the prevention program and building resilience in students to enable them to cope with the challenges they encounter during puberty. Schools that design and promote programs focusing on multi-components of prevention on various levels have proven more effective (Surgenor et al., 2016). Due to a plethora of limitations that may prevent ongoing and year-long training programs, there is a benefit in continuously revisiting and assessing the strategies, skills, and outcomes of designated programs.

CASE EXAMPLE BACKGROUND

Danielle is a 13-year-old female student with an educational diagnosis of Emotional Disturbance. Per the *Individuals With Disabilities Education Act (IDEA)* (2023), Emotional Disturbance is described as exhibiting one or more characteristics over a long period and to a marked degree that adversely affects a child's educational performance. These characteristics include an inability to learn that cannot be explained by intellectual, sensory, or health factors; an inability to build or maintain satisfactory interpersonal relationships with peers and teachers; inappropriate types of behavior or feelings under normal circumstances; a general pervasive mood of unhappiness or depression; a tendency to develop physical symptoms or fears associated with personal or school problems (Auer, 2014). In Danielle's case, she struggled with maintaining relationships with her peers and adults and exhibited severe emotional dysregulation during instructional and non-instructional activities. Due to her emotional instability, Danielle was not progressing academically, and her overall achievement was significantly below expectations. Often, Danielle avoided school, and her frequent emotional outbursts resulted in her removal from the classroom environment.

Danielle receives exceptional education support and attends general education courses with her non-disabled peers. Due to ongoing staff reports, Danielle was screened and found to be at risk for suicidal behavior. Danielle has had several emotional meltdowns within the past few months and has been removed from the instructional environment. Per a review of incident reports, Danielle's emotional breakdowns have occurred at various times and days of the week. Reportedly, triggers for Danielle's behaviors appear to be due to poor social skills, limited coping strategies, and a family history of mental illness. Per a review of teacher reports, Danielle exhibited at-risk behaviors last school year (i.e., crying spells, emotional outbursts, making statements about death, and attempting to wrap a belt around her neck while in the girls' bathroom). More recently, Danielle has often observed having fleeting suicidal thoughts ("I am going to kill myself," "I wish I were dead," "I hate my life, I am going to end it"). Per academic reports, Danielle has made some progress toward her educational goals. She can complete tasks, stay focused on select tasks within small settings, and transition from one task to another with verbal directions and encouragement.

When I worked with Danielle, she resided with her mother, stepfather, and adult brother in Washington, DC. Danielle's mother reported that Danielle had reached all of her developmental milestones within normal limits. Danielle had not received counseling or therapy before working with me. She has not taken any medication for sleep problems, mood, or behavior. Danielle's family history is significant for bipolar disorder, learning disabilities, substance abuse, and suicide. Danielle's biological father suffered from bipolar disorder and committed suicide when Danielle was 6 years old. Danielle's brother was diagnosed with anxiety and depression during his teenage years. He is currently taking 10mg of Lexapro per day. Danielle's biological mother has denied her son exhibiting suicidal behavior.

Danielle enjoys spending time with her family and tends to gravitate toward her biological mother when feeling uncomfortable. Danielle's mother and stepfather have denied observing similar behaviors at home that are reported at school. Reportedly, Danielle prefers to keep to herself when she is at home. Danielle's family noted that she does not have many friends and rarely attends social events outside of family outings. Danielle's family has expressed concerns regarding Danielle's emotional behavior at school and has worked with the school staff to support Danielle.

OBSERVED BEHAVIOR

During instructional activities, Danielle struggled to connect with her peers socially and manage her emotions. Danielle appeared to have a limited understanding of engaging with others and a sense of belonging. Danielle also struggled with consistently articulating her wants and needs in an age-appropriate manner. Teachers have noted that Danielle has attempted to engage positively with her peers during lunch, and her peers will reciprocate the greeting. When she can engage with others, Danielle has exhibited difficulty staying on topic, commented about wanting to hurt herself, and expressed that no one understands her. Danielle's professional school counselor has stated that Danielle has been working on positive self-talk strategies, social awareness, and peer engagement. Her progress has been inconsistent, according to the service progress notes. It appears Danielle has difficulty being consistent and adhering to appropriate therapeutic practices due to her disability.

Danielle could participate in the bell ringer activity during classroom observation and remain on task without prompting. Danielle's resource English/Language Arts class comprised twelve students and two adults. During the pair and share activity, Danielle struggled to remain on topic and display patience – she was redirected several times to wait her turn to speak. Danielle became visibly frustrated each time and said no one understood her. Danielle's teacher approached her twice and encouraged Danielle to take deep breaths and give herself some grace. As the class period progressed, Danielle attempted to engage with her peers by sharing her interests in television shows. When some of their peers did not reciprocate the conversation, Danielle became visibly upset and began writing in her notebook. Danielle expressed feeling lonely and isolated when asked to participate in a class discussion.

ANALYSIS

As a certified School Psychologist working on Danielle's case was referred to the office. Danielle was scheduled for a re-evaluation to determine her continued eligibility for specialized services as a student with an emotional disturbance. Per the collected data, I noticed a pattern of self-harm, suicidal ideations, and behavior patterns that classified Danielle as being at risk. Per a review of her service notes, Cognitive Behavior Therapy was implemented, but progress was inconsistent. Academic reports indicated that Danielle was making gains when assignments were modified to her current level of performance. Cognitively, Danielle was functioning in the low average range compared to same-age peers. Her developmental history was significant for mental illness, substance abuse, and learning disabilities, and there was a pattern of suicidal behavior. Per a comprehensive psychological report, Danielle was rated in the clinically significant range in functional communication, depression, anxiety, learning problems, adaptability, aggression, and somatization.

Based on the evaluation, I recommended teaching problem-solving strategies as directly and explicitly as you would any academic skill, providing instruction, ample guided and independent practice, and monitoring for misunderstandings and errors. Incorporate instruction and practice in when to apply the strategy. Due to Danielle's low cognitive abilities, I also recommended teaching various cognitive strategies so that she can actively monitor her comprehension. Danielle also appeared to be a suitable candidate for social skills group or individual play therapy sessions to teach problem-solving in social situations, including specific training in (a) identifying and defining the problem, (b) generating a variety of alternative solutions, (c) identifying the most likely outcomes of each alternative, and (d) selecting and implementing the appropriate solution. Danielle also needed clear rules and expectations within her learning environments. The skills group will assist her in managing her behavior and regulating her emotions and her responses to others during emotionally stressful periods. Students with inhibitory control difficulties often require additional structure in the environment at the outset to maintain more appropriately controlled behavior. Self-monitoring and response-delay techniques can be helpful for students who struggle with impulsivity and emotional deficits before responding verbally or physically. Stop-and-think methods help teach students to constrain their initial response, consider the potential consequences of their behaviors, and develop a plan of approach to a situation.

Given the staff's limited knowledge of suicide prevention and intervention techniques, a comprehensive approach was needed to address Danielle's suicidal behavior. It should be noted that the staff's attitudes about suicide influenced their approach and engagement with Danielle. With the appropriate training and education, the school staff is more likely to improve their attitudes, increase suicide intervention skills, and display a higher level of competence. When more school staff members are trained to provide suicide prevention and intervention, this allows for more comprehensive services within the school setting. The National Research Council and Institute of Medicine adopted a public health model focusing on the three prevention levels (Le Menestrel & Rivara, 2016). The levels of preventive interventions are universal, selective, and indicated. The main focus of this model is bullying prevention and mental health promotion. The universal prevention programs focus on community or school settings to minimize risks and improve students' skills. Selective prevention programs are designed for more intensive social-emotional skills and approaches for students who are at risk for engaging in bullying behavior or may be targeted. Indicated prevention programs focus on more intensive support and activities for individuals with a history of bullying. These supports thoroughly address behavioral health concerns with the support of community stakeholders, mental health professionals, and educators.

Danielle is not able to articulate herself or correctly identify her emotions. Providing her with the vocabulary to appropriately express herself will minimize her emotional outbursts, develop social connections, and teach Danielle how to engage in age-appropriate language skills. Based on the data collected, her developmental history, and her progress notes, play therapy appeared appropriate for Danielle to help her regulate her emotions,

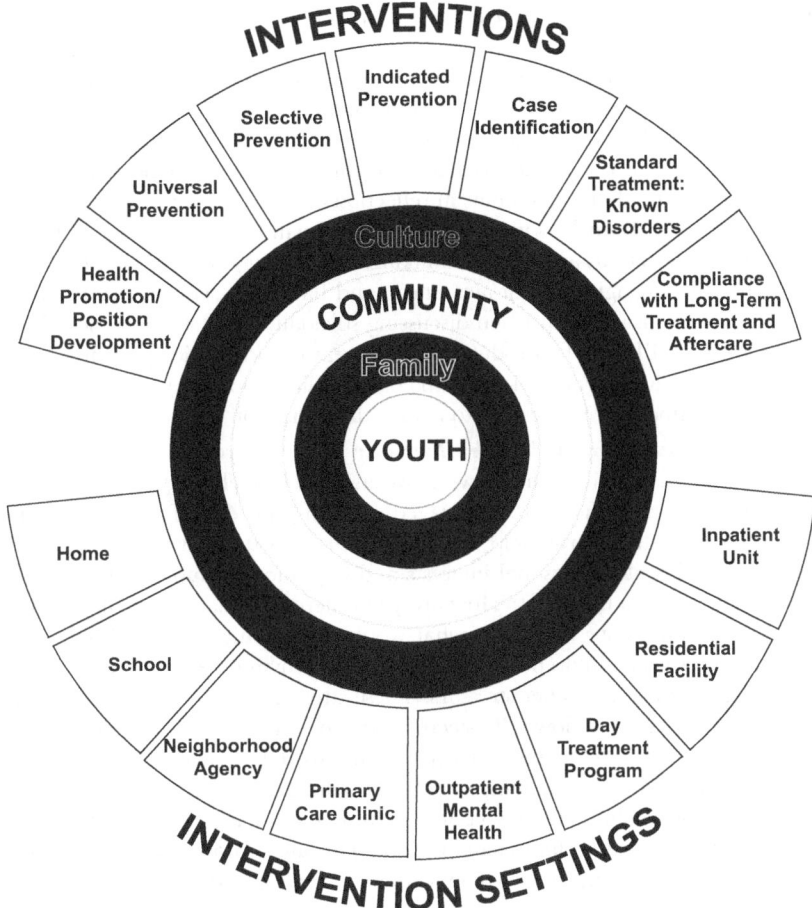

Figure 9.2 An Ecodevelopmental Model of Prevention

Source: An Eco Developmental Model of Prevention. National Academies of Sciences, Engineering, and Medicine. 2016. Preventing Bullying Through Science, Policy, and Practice. https://doi.org/10.17226/23482. Reproduced with permission from the National Academy of Sciences, courtesy of the National Academies Press.

problem-solve, improve social engagement, foster social connections, and develop the tools to express herself appropriately in her environment. With implementing interventions, there are benefits to layering various components to address the specific needs of the individual, the culture, the climate of the setting, and the growing level of support within the settings (Le Menestrel & Rivara, 2016).

APPLIED PLAY-BASED INTERVENTIONS

Danielle has difficulty managing emotions, social awareness, and social connections, improving her self-esteem, self-monitoring, problem-solving, and positive self-talk. During our sessions, Danielle was introduced to interventions that brought awareness to these areas.

- **Virtual Word Wall(s):** I provided Danielle with a visual word wall due to her academic and cognitive limitations. The visual word wall included the word and a picture of the word/action. I provided Danielle access to a virtual word wall with a visual, a picture of the word/action, and audio of the word's pronunciation (See it, Hear It, Say It). I asked her to review and describe select pictures on the virtual word wall(s). During this activity, Danielle selected specific pictures to describe again and used "I" statements in reflection of her description. The additional support assisted Danielle with developing and expanding her vocabulary to help foster social connections and flexible thinking. Developing the skills to utilize appropriate language, engaging in self-awareness, and having the vocabulary to process various situations will help when discussing suicidality with students. Social-emotional learning (SEL) can be productive in upstream youth suicide prevention (Posamentier et al., 2022). For students with cognitive limitations or who are visual learners, visual supports are necessary to help with application skills.

- **Self-empowerment/self-reflection:** Danielle created a self-portrait of her views in this activity. In a follow-up, we engaged in a self-reflection discussion (About Me). The dialogue was encouraged with the use of self-exploration cue cards. Self-exploration cards help students understand themselves, discover self-awareness, and explore personal interests and hopes for the future. Example questions: Where are you the safest? How are you different? What do you like to do for fun? If you could have one wish, what would it be? Suicidal thoughts and behaviors are often from children coping with a home environment, parental conflicts, bullying, trauma, and other stressors. These stressors can result in youth feeling overwhelmed, suffering low self-esteem, and experiencing coping difficulties. Research suggests that self-esteem-related interventions reduce suicidal ideation (Dat et al., 2022). Students experiencing suicidal thoughts and behaviors believe suicide is their only option. This activity will help them regain their perspective and promote an understanding that things can improve. This intervention empowers individuals to consider deepening positive connections within support groups.

- **Sandtray Therapy:** This activity allows individuals to construct their community or world using miniature toys and colored sand. The scene created acts as a reflection of the individual's own life and allows them to resolve conflicts, remove obstacles, and gain acceptance of self (Homeyer & Sweeney, 2022). Danielle used a variety of miniatures to create her world (i.e., animals, elves, mythical creatures, skeletons, elements, and trees) to help with difficulties with socializing. Sandtray is also helpful for Danielle as she has difficulty verbalizing her thoughts and experiences. It may be a challenge to talk about suicidal thoughts and feelings, and others may not understand how the youth's thoughts and feelings are connected to suicidal behaviors. Utilizing Sandtray Therapy, a projective method, can allow youth to share their thoughts and feelings. Additionally, with this type of therapy, youths can select objects representing a range of feelings like fear, confusion, distrust, thoughts of death, safety, security, community support, and connection to others. Before using Sandtray Therapy, specific training is required to use and understand what the youth creates appropriately.

- **Emotions Charade:** Danielle and the school-based therapist introduced emotions and identified characteristics of those emotions (facial expressions, body language, and statements) through emotion cards. Emotions Charade requires students to act out emotions in front of group members, who then guess the emotions and describe the clues that help to identify the emotions correctly. Studies suggest that a strong level of emotional intelligence (EI) is crucial in safeguarding individuals against suicidal behavior (Domínguez-García & Fernández-Berrocal, 2018). This intervention can be supplemented by a conversation on emotional triggers, coping skills, building strengths, the development of self-efficacy, and connectedness, which can aid in prevention.

OTHER SUGGESTED INTERVENTIONS

- *My Own Superhero*: Create your superhero comic book based on positive behavior and characteristics that reflect the child or adolescent. Materials needed: blank comic book strips, blank drawing paper, superhero coloring sheets or pictures of various superheroes (some students may want to draw their own), and sentence starters. This activity focuses on developing/enhancing positive language, our views, and social competence. For youth who experience STB and social isolation, developing and understanding the skills needed for social adaptation and self-perception improves social connectedness, which can help reduce STBs. Utilizing explicit socio-emotional techniques is vital to character development in middle childhood (Thomas et al., 2022).
- *Discovering Gratitude*: This intervention focuses on thinking about the positive things in our lives and being grateful. Individuals work towards expressing thankfulness and understanding. Gratitude can change our outlook on life and shift toward more positive thinking. This intervention will also assist in fostering dialogue on how we understand ourselves and relate to others. A recent review of gratitude interventions found that gratitude interventions consistently show that psychological well-being is improved; however, there are minor positive effects on depression and anxiety (Boggiss et al., 2020). Practicing gratitude can promote positive emotions, increase optimism, and may lower the risk of depressive symptoms associated with STBs.

    - Sample questions/prompts:
        a. Something you treasure.
        b. Your favorite smell.
        c. Someone who brings you joy.
        d. Something that brings you joy.
        e. A memory that makes you feel warmth or pride.

CONCLUSION

This chapter focused on discussing a trend of denial and minimization of suicide in students within the school setting. Prevention and intervention strategies focus on providing a safe environment for children and fully integrating a variety of learning supports (e.g., behavioral, mental health, and social services), instruction, and school management can foster a comprehensive, consistent tactic that enables a multidisciplinary collaboration. Improving a school-wide initiative and promoting tolerance within the curriculum and educator training will support various strategies. Crisis influences each person differently and has the potential to destructively impact a youth's overall wellness and the complex interactions that contribute to one's quality of life. Many schools have a crisis team, and many districts have a district-wide crisis team. Schools are uniquely positioned as a supportive structure to identify and assist a child or adolescent until help is accessed and the suicidal ideation is sufficiently managed.

REFERENCES

A Model for School-based Crisis Preparedness and Response. (n.d.). https://ovc.ojp.gov/sites/g/files/xyckuh226/files/publications/bulletins/schoolcrisis/pg3.html

Auer, S. L. (2014). *Teachers expectations for students with externalizing and internalizing behaviors*. https://core.ac.uk/download/215261315.pdf

Becker, M. (2017, June 8). Why schools need to step up suicide prevention efforts. *Brookings*. Retrieved May 28, 2023, from www.brookings.edu/articles/why-schools-need-to-step-up-suicide-prevention-efforts/

Boggiss, A., Consedine, N. S., Brenton-Peters, J., Hofman, P. L., & Serlachius, A. (2020). A systematic review of gratitude interventions: Effects on physical health and health behaviors. *Journal of Psychosomatic Research, 135*, 110165. https://doi.org/10.1016/j.jpsychores.2020.110165

Bridge, J. A., Asti, L., Horowitz, L. M., Greenhouse, J. B., Fontanella, C. A., Sheftall, A. H., Kelleher, K. J., & Campo, J. V. (2015). Suicide trends among elementary school–aged children in the United States from 1993 to 2012. *JAMA Pediatrics, 169*(7), 673. https://doi.org/10.1001/jamapediatrics.2015.0465

Dat, N. T., Mitsui, N., Asakura, S., Takanobu, K., Fujii, Y., Toyoshima, K., Kako, Y., & Kusumi, I. (2022). The effectiveness of self-esteem-related interventions in reducing suicidal behaviors: A systematic review and meta-analysis. *Frontiers in Psychiatry, 13*, 925423. https://doi.org/10.3389/fpsyt.2022.925423

Domínguez-García, E., & Fernández-Berrocal, P. (2018). The association between emotional intelligence and suicidal behavior: A systematic review. *Frontiers in Psychology, 9*. https://doi.org/10.3389/fpsyg.2018.02380

Durlak, J. A., Weissberg, R. P., Dymnicki, A. B., Taylor, R. D., & Schellinger, K. B. (2011). The impact of enhancing students' social and emotional learning: A meta-analysis of school-based universal interventions. *Child Development, 82*(1), 405–432. https://doi.org/10.1111/j.1467-8624.2010.01564.x

Gallo, L., & Wachter Morris, C. A. (2022). Suicide intervention in schools: If not school counselors, then who? *Teaching and Supervision in Counseling, 4*(2), Article 6. https://doi.org/10.7290/tsc043z3v

Homeyer, L. E., & Sweeney, D. S. (2022). *Sandtray therapy* (4th ed.). Routledge.

IDEA Individuals with Disabilities Education Act. (2022, December 20). *U.S. Department of Education's individuals with disabilities education act*. Retrieved May 25, 2023, from https://sites.ed.gov/idea/

Knipe, D., John, A., Padmanathan, P., Eyles, E., Dekel, D., Higgins, J. P. T., Bantjes, J., Dandona, R., Macleod-Hall, C., McGuinness, L. A., Schmidt, L., Webb, R. T., & Gunnell, D. (2022). Suicide and self-harm in low– and middle-income countries during the COVID-19 pandemic: A systematic review. *pLoS Global Public Health, 2*(6), e0000282. https://doi.org/10.1371/journal.pgph.0000282

Le Menestrel, S., & Rivara, F. (Eds.). (2016). *Preventing bullying through science, policy, and practice*. National Academies Press (US). www.ncbi.nlm.nih.gov/books/NBK390407/

Lottman, T. J., Zawaly, S., & Niemiec, R. (2017). Well-being and well-doing: Bringing mindfulness and character strengths to the early childhood classroom and home. *Positive Psychology Interventions in Practice*, 83–105. https://doi.org/10.1007/978-3-319-51787-2_6

Marraccini, M. (n.d.). *Practice experiences for school reintegration: An immersive virtual reality program to enhance skill development of adolescents hospitalized for suicidal thoughts and behaviors* (By University Of North

Carolina, Chapel Hill). reporter.nih.gov. Retrieved September 29, 2023, from https://reporter. nih.gov/search/4PfSukBEhEKqJdktOODeAQ/project-details/10456729#description

Nagdimon, J., McGovern, C., & Craw, M. (2021). Addressing concealed suicidality: A flexible and contextual approach to suicide risk assessment in adults. *Journal of Contemporary Psychotherapy*, *51*(3), 241–250. https://doi.org/10.1007/s10879-021-09493-9

National Academies of Sciences, Engineering, and Medicine. (2016). *Preventing bullying through science, policy, and practice*. National Academies Press.

Ogawa, S., Suzuki, H., Takahashi, T., Fujita, K., Murayama, Y., Sato, K., Matsunaga, H., Motohashi, Y., & Fujiwara, Y. (2022). Suicide prevention program with cooperation from senior volunteers, governments, and schools: A study of the intervention effects of "educational lessons regarding SOS output" focusing on junior high school students. *Children*, *9*(4), 541. https://doi.org/10.3390/children9040541

Posamentier, J., Seibel, K., & DyTang, N. (2022). Preventing youth suicide: A review of school-based practices and how social–emotional learning fits into comprehensive efforts. *Trauma, Violence, & Abuse*. https://doi.org/10.1177/15248380211039475

Sheftall, A. H., Asti, L., Horowitz, L. M., Felts, A., Fontanella, C. A., Campo, J. V., & Bridge, J. (2016). Suicide in elementary school-aged children and early adolescents. *Pediatrics*, *138*(4). https://doi.org/10.1542/peds.2016-0436

Surgenor, P. W. G., Quinn, P., & Hughes, C. (2016). Ten recommendations for effective school-based, adolescent, suicide prevention programs. *School Mental Health*, *8*(4), 413–424. https://doi.org/10.1007/s12310-016-9189-9

Thomas, K. J., Da Cunha, J. M., & Santo, J. B. (2022). Classroom relationships drive changes in character virtues: A longitudinal study of elementary school children. *School Mental Health*, *14*(2), 266–277. https://doi.org/10.1007/s12310-022-09511-8

Whisenhunt, J. L., DuFresne, R. M., Stargell, N. A., Rovnak, A., Zoldan, C. A., & Kress, V. E. (2017). Supporting counselors after a client suicide: Creative supervision techniques. *Journal of Creativity in Mental Health*, *12*(4), 451–467. https://doi.org/10.1080/15401383.2017.1281184

CHAPTER 10

TECHNOLOGY'S EMERGING ROLE FROM ASSESSMENT TO PREVENTION IN CHILDREN AND ADOLESCENTS

Jessica Stone

INTRODUCTION

Suicide evokes emotional and behavioral responses from all who are touched by it. Children and adolescents comprise a vulnerable group who are particularly impacted by suicidal ideations, communications, threats, attempts, plans, and completion for oneself or others. Understanding a young person's worldview and perspective is critical in supporting them through these tumultuous times. Currently, these worldviews are often expressed, communicated, and exhibited through their digital play. We must recognize and implement mental health services that acknowledge, include, and incorporate the digital culture of so many of our clients' lives, especially when working with clients who are impacted by suicidality. This chapter introduces Digital Play Therapy™ (DPT) as an emerging and viable tool within this important work's assessment, intervention, and prevention phases.

DIFFERENCES IN THE 21ST CENTURY

Ending one's own life or dying by suicide is an event that has happened throughout the history of human beings. Over the generations, a variety of professionals have striven toward further understanding of and assistance for those who have contemplated suicide on any level. The topic of suicide is complicated by many things, including history, experiences, emotions, environment, perceptions, development, mental health, physical health, support, connectedness, and more. The responsibility, complexities, and loss levels create difficult experiences for anyone involved, including clinicians – the proverbial question of "why" is at the foundation of these contemplations.

Suicide at any age elicits many emotions and reactions; however, suicidality in children and adolescents creates exponentially fearful situations. It is common for much care and effort to be expended to avoid both the pain and experience of suicidality and the finality of completed suicide. Professional assistance from a mental health clinician can be critical for the client, family, and caregivers during these times. Beyond the primary goal of the safety of the client and addressing any acute situations, the clinician is faced with three primary tasks: assessment, treatment, and prevention. The clinician must enter a client's carefully guarded world to accomplish these tasks. Understanding the client's genuine worldview, perceptions, understandings, emotions, and experiences, as much as possible, assists tremendously in the clinical treatment of suicidality. Who are they? What is important to them? What are they experiencing? How can assistance be presented in a way that can be accepted?

DOI: 10.4324/9781003358565-20

DIGITAL AGE

The digital age of the 21st century includes not only a plethora of tools and possibilities but also a new culture and way of life. Termed "Gen Z" and "Gen Alpha (α)," children born after 1997 have little to no recollection of life before devices that bring information and experiences to their fingertips (Eldridge, 2022; McCrindle & Fell, 2020). Much debate has occurred about the pros and cons of these advancements, but the reality is that digital tools are here to stay. In therapeutic settings, an important query arises: How can we enter our clients' digital worlds and understand their perceptions, understandings, emotions, and experiences to assist them in therapeutic, customized, unique ways tailored to their needs? Specifically for suicidality, how can we understand our clients in culturally appropriate ways that allow us to intervene and prevent a young person from ending their life? Trust and safety arise from feeling seen, heard, understood, and accepted; how do we provide this environment for our clients, particularly when the struggle is so precariously important?

SUICIDALITY

Suicidality is defined as "the risk of suicide, usually indicated by suicidal ideation or intent, especially as evident in the presence of a well-elaborated suicidal plan" (American Psychological Association, 2022a). Miller breaks down suicidality into different levels of suicidal behavior: suicidal ideations, suicide-related communications (suicide threats), suicide attempts, repeated suicide attempts, and suicide (2021). Historically believed to be a negative aspect of a person's fortitude, as shown by physician Dr. Pierre Janet in 1901, "Death seems so easy a means for lazy people to solve all life's problems" (Janet, 1901, p. 220), more modern science yearns to understand the underlying components which can lead a person to any or all aspects of suicidality. Once believed to derive from a severe level of depression, suicidality is now thought to have elements of any of the following: severe psychological distress, pain, emotional suffering, severe dysfunction, genetics, environment, and pathology of the family system (Miller, 2021); genetic, neurobiological, cultural, and social influences (U.S. Department of Health and Human Services & Centers for Disease Control and Prevention, 2022); legal difficulties, interpersonal relationship issues, stressful life events, social isolation, absence of school and/or work, hopelessness (Brown et al., 2000) and unsupported gender identification (Shain & AAP, 2016). "[E]ach suicidal death is a multifaceted event – that biological, biochemical, cultural, sociological, interpersonal, intrapsychic, logical, philosophical, conscious, and unconscious elements are always present" (Shneidman, 1996, p. 5).

The "why" underneath suicidality is not simplistic; however, understanding it is critical for treatment. In the digital play, as in all others, it is important to understand the underlying components to train the therapeutic eyes and ears toward recognition of themes, patterns, and communications. The client will allow the clinician to enter their world, see through their eyes, show their response patterns, and express their worldview in environments and interactions that are safe and meaningful to them – it is the clinician's job to be open, receptive, accepting, and observant. Shneidman, the founder of the American Association of Suicidology (AAS), "posited that individuals engage in suicidal behavior because of severe and intolerable psychological pain" (Miller, 2021, p. 21). He named this psychological pain *psychache* – the psychological pain that causes suicide (Shneidman & Farberow, 1956).

He states that "this psychache stems from thwarted or distorted psychological needs" (p. 4). This anguish, combined with lethality, can result in suicidality. Per Schneidman, "Suicide happens when the psychache is deemed unbearable and death is actively sought to stop the unceasing flow of painful consciousness" (p. 13). He continues, "What my research has taught me is that only a small minority of cases of excessive psychological pain result in suicide, but every case of suicide stems from excessive psychache" (p. 13). Youth suicide is believed to be a desire to escape psychache and not a desire to die. Per Miller, "most suicidal youths don't want to die as much as they want their suffering to end" (Miller, 2021, p. 211).

DIGITAL TECHNOLOGY AND DIGITAL PLAY THERAPY™

Digital Technology

At this point in history, digital technology is ubiquitous. Not only is it a set of tools used in one's day-to-day life, but digital technology also comprises a culture; "the shared patterns of behaviors and interactions, cognitive constructs, and affective understanding that are learned through a process of socialization. These shared patterns identify the members of a culture group while also distinguishing those of another group" (CARLA, 2022, para. 1). The culture of those who use digital technology as an integrated way of life is different from those of previous generations who did not.

Gen Z (born 1997–2012) and Gen Alpha (born 2012–2027) are inherently digital natives (Prensky, 2001; Eldridge, 2022; McCrindle & Fell, 2020). Digital natives have learned to communicate, seek, acquire, and share information, work, play, relax, and learn through digital tools. Clients who are minors at the time of this publication were born within these generations and are, therefore, by default, part of the digital generation. Clinicians must strive toward cultural inclusion and humility regarding a minor client's way of life. This is important in general and particularly in delicate situations where a lack of understanding of a client's needs could be life-altering.

Prensky introduced the concept of digital natives in 2001 to highlight a discrepancy between how teachers learned to teach the material and the evolution of the child into one who needs to be instructed differently. This digital divide is impacting the interactions between different generations in many ways. From communication and connection styles, coping skills, and approaches toward problem-solving, digital natives often exhibit different ways of conceptualizing scenarios and addressing any needs. As an example, digital natives often exhibit a different approach to novel situations by trying out the unknown. In DPT, digital natives often start clicking on items to see what they do, what they might hold, what their purpose is, etc. Digital immigrants, those who are not native but have adopted such tools into their lives, most often avoid such explorations for fear of doing something "wrong." As a fundamental concept, these are very different approaches to novel situations and will impact every facet of moving forward. Teachers and mental health clinicians alike will benefit from recognizing the different ways digital natives process stimuli and adjust approaches accordingly (Prensky, 2016; Stone, 2022).

Digital Play Therapy™

In recognition of the shift toward the incorporation of digital tools into numerous facets of day-to-day life, Digital Play Therapy™ was created to provide a culturally sensitive structure through which a clinician can connect with a client, enter their world, and identify clinically relevant themes and patterns within the digital play (Stone, 2019a, 2022, 2023b).

> Digital play therapy is a modality that utilizes highly motivating, immersive activities to incorporate areas of client culture and interest into the play therapy process to deepen relationships, gather information, implement interventions, and advance the treatment plan forward.
>
> (Stone, 2022, p. 16)

Forward-thinking clinicians such as Russoniello et al. (2009), Ceranoglu (2010), and Granic et al. (2014) recognized the therapeutic power embedded in video game play, and Stone culminates these concepts into a structured modality for use in therapy (2019a, 2022, 2023b). The modality incorporates fundamentals of prescriptive therapy (Beutler, 1979; Beutler & Harwood, 2000), the Therapeutic Powers of Play (Schaefer & Drewes, 2014), and the DPT 5 Cs: competency, culture, comfort, congruence, and capability (Stone, 2019a, 2022). With three levels of incorporation, DPT provides multiple ways for a clinician to invite the digital play aspects of a client's life into the session. For more detailed information, please refer to the text *Digital Play Therapy™* by Stone (2022). Per Stone, "The digital tool is merely a medium for the expression, creation, communication, relationship, understanding, assessment, and intervention within the therapy" (Stone, 2019b, pp. 107–108).

USING DIGITAL PLAY THERAPY™ WITH CLIENTS EXPERIENCING SUICIDALITY

A clinician who has achieved DPT competency through education, research, training, supervision, consultation, and experience will have the skills to identify and incorporate the themes and expressions communicated through digital play. By utilizing a variety of hardware, such as mobile devices (phones, tablets), consoles (Xbox, Nintendo Switch, Steam Deck, etc.), virtual reality headsets (Quest, Vive, etc.), and computers (laptop, desktop) along with software (games, apps, programs, etc.), a clinician can expand the assessment, intervention, and prevention aspects of the therapeutic process while incorporating the digital native client's culture and interests.

As described previously, it is believed that clients who are experiencing suicidality are experiencing a high level of psychological pain. This pain can lead to suffering, which can be experienced as "unendurable" (Miller, 2021, p. 29). To further explore the components a clinician would seek to understand and identify within the digital play, we can look to possible risk factors and warning signs of suicidality (please refer to Tables 10.1 and 10.2).

Clinicians can apply the knowledge regarding the personal, interpersonal, and environmental factors contributing to suicidality, along with the warning signs, to address and triage acute care needs. Beyond the acute, these components can assist the clinician in moving forward toward clinical assessment, treatment, and prevention during DPT.

Table 10.1 Risk Factors Chart

Risk Factors	Family history of suicide, suicidal behavior, or psychiatric diagnosis
	A history of physical or sexual abuse
	A history of exposure to violence or bullying
	Substance use disorder
	Suicide of a family member or friend
	Loss of close friends or family members
	Conflict with close friends or family members
	Physical or medical concerns
	Previous suicide attempts

Table 10.2 Warning Signs

Warning Signs	Making plans for suicide
	Isolation
	Mood swings
	Increased use of drugs or alcohol
	Feeling hopeless and or helpless
	Sleeping, too litle or too much
	Looking for ways to access lethal means
	Talking about being a burden
	Increased anxiety or agitation

ASSESSMENT

The assessment of suicidality is initially focused on the acute needs of the client. Care should be taken to ensure any imminent dangers are addressed appropriately. If there are no acute considerations, the focus of the assessment is to understand the history of the child, particularly from a systems perspective (home, school, etc.), the current environment(s) and relationships, and the internal, emotional, and salient experiences of the child. Caregivers and young people alike can vary in their ability and/or willingness to provide information. Additionally, as stated earlier in the chapter, numerous considerations for the etiology of suicidality can complicate the history-taking process. The components can be arduous, multi-dimensional, and layered. Ultimately, the clinician performs due diligence to collate the information provided and works to incorporate what is understood through direct session experiences with what is discovered through formal and informal assessments.

SELF-HELP

Digital tools such as mobile apps can provide self-assessments for levels of depression, anxiety, and even Adverse Childhood Experiences (ACES). Numerous questionnaires can be found through internet searches. Some programs will even map reported levels over time and provide a summary. When used in conjunction with mental health therapy at the request of the clinician, these tools can provide invaluable information about the functioning of the client outside of the treatment space. For children, self-report measures can prove difficult in dissecting the true experience of the child from the involvement of the parent in completing the reported information. However, results from self-help apps and programs can be shared with the clinician, and areas of strength and difficulty can be processed in the session.

PROFESSIONAL ASSESSMENT

Professional assessment of suicidality includes formal, informal, and clinical components. For this chapter, we will focus on the clinical components of the professional assessment. Within DPT, the clinician can engage with the client in any of the three levels of DPT engagement (see Table 10.3) to assess suicidality risk factors listed earlier in this chapter.

Professional clinical assessment in DPT focuses on two primary components: 1) creating, communicating, and providing a safe, supportive, and nurturing environment and 2) attending to the verbal and non-verbal communications of the client while understanding these communications in the context of the client's history, culture, identity and representation, experiences, and worldview. The context within which the client has experienced and understood their world allows the clinician to incorporate the client's perspective, thereby understanding the client at a fundamental level necessary for the deep and vulnerable work of suicidality. The assessment process is traditionally believed to be in the initial stages of the therapeutic process, but realistically, the foundation is built in the beginning. This foundation is added to and altered over time and should be conceptualized, at least in part, as a fluid, living document.

INTERVENTION

The intervention components of DPT in suicidality treatment incorporate the themes, metaphors, creations, projections, and processes of traditional play therapy – through a digital medium. As the clinician is attending to the play interactions and styles, the Mayo Clinic (2023) risk factor and warning sign components are presenting themselves where applicable. This play can be general, client-driven and non-directive, therapist-driven and directive, or a combination of both. Once the client's worldview is better known to the clinician, the interventions can be tailored to the client's needs, interests, etc. Additionally, as the client interacts within the digital world, the client's worldview becomes more well-known to the clinician; a continuation of the fluid, living assessment occurs.

Opportunities to incorporate interventions can arise in a game, app, or program chosen by the client or the clinician. Understanding what that gameplay means to the client is an important first step in the process. After that, experiencing how the client presents their character, interacts within the gameplay, approaches tasks, organizes, strategizes, and moves through the environment provides a further understanding of the client and opportunities for intervention. The interventions here mirror many of those within traditional play therapy; these include anything from introducing a helping character or dynamic to intentionally creating a dynamic for the client to respond to/interact within, etc. The beauty of using digital tools is the customizability of many programs and the plethora of different games available. Intervention goals can include topics such as identifying emotions, identifying

Table 10.3 Levels of Engagement in Digital Play

DPT Level	Description
Level 1	Any inclusion of the client's interests in digital tools directly in the session. The clinician is open to the client discussing, drawing: and or recreating any components of their digital tool interest and or use. The client is provided with a safe and accepting environment in which they can share their digital interests and experiences.
Level 2	In addition to the safe and accepting environment in Level 1, Level 2 includes and incorporates digital tools in the sharing and discussing of digital interests. This can include sharing videos, webpages, song lyrics, and more.
Level 3	Level 3 incorporates all components of the previous levels and includes the clinician and client joining in active digital co-play utilizing both digital hardware and software.

Source: Levels of Engagement of Digital Play. Adapted from: Stone, J. (2022). Digital play therapy: A clinician's guide to comfort and competence, 2nd ed. Routledge, p. 18.

stressors, increasing self-esteem, increasing problem-solving skills, improving interpersonal communication, increasing self-control, setting goals, improving decision-making, and/or eliminating self-destructive behaviors (Miller, 2021), as well as the well-known Therapeutic Powers of Play 20 agents of change (Schaefer & Drewes, 2014).

PREVENTION

A significant shift in the conceptualization of suicidality has been from a focus on pathology to psychological resilience (Sánchez-Teruel et al., 2021; Masten, 2019). Protective factors, such as resilience, assist in preventing suicidality (Miller, 2021). Understanding resilience and incorporating components within the treatment strategy for suicidality can help to prevent future occurrences. If suicidality is anchored in psychache and hopelessness, as is believed, then resiliency and hope should be key components in the treatment and prevention of suicidality.

The medical community has defined resilience as having a "high energy barrier between the health and the disease state" (Kalisch et al., 2019, p. 8). Applying this to psychology, we certainly strive to have a strong barrier between the client and suicidality. Psychological resilience has been defined by many throughout the decades. Generally, the definition includes components of recognizing, utilizing, and adapting internal and external resources to recover after stressful events. The APA defines resilience as "the process and outcome of successfully adapting to difficult or challenging life experiences, especially through mental, emotional, and behavioral flexibility and adjustment to external and internal demands" (American Psychological Association, 2022b, para. 1). APA attributes one's adaptability to adversities to "how individuals view and engage with the world, the availability and quality of social resources, and specific coping strategies" (American Psychological Association, 2022b, para. 2). For our purposes, young people who can experience connection, support, mutual respect, participation in decision-making, share positive norms, employ problem-solving and coping skills, and positive relationships can build resilience and therefore combat and prevent suicidality. Utilizing digital tools in therapy presents ample opportunities for building resilience (Zaera, 2022b).

SUICIDE ASSESSMENT APPS

Current professional and self-help trends include using applications, or apps, for assessing, monitoring, communicating, and understanding symptoms and experiences. While it is acknowledged that the digital development world is fast-moving, the following apps are offered as examples of what might be used when assessing suicidality digitally.

For Clinicians

Suicide Safe Mobile App by SAMHSA (Substance Abuse and Mental Health Services Administration, n.d.)

- No cost/free
- Ages 12+
- English language
- Copyright 2015

This app was released as a learning tool for primary and behavioral health care providers who are working with people at risk of suicide. This app is based on the SAMHSA Suicide Assessment

Five-Step Evaluation and Triage, or "Safe-T," protocol:

1. Identify and modify risk factors.
2. Identify and enhance protective factors.
3. Conduct suicide inquiry (ideation, plan, etc.).
4. Determine risk level/choose appropriate intervention(s).
5. Document assessment, treatment rationale, intervention(s), and follow-up.

(Substance Abuse and Mental Health Services Administration, 2009)

Offering tips for providers to communicate effectively with clients/patients and their families, assisting with treatment plans, and making referrals to community resources, this app serves as a suicide prevention learning tool.

Features include:

- Learn the five steps of the SAFE-T approach
- Easily download resources for use offline
- Study interactive sample case studies
- Browse conversation starters that provide sample language and tips
- Explore clinical and educational resources
- Share crisis line phone numbers and other patient-focused materials
- Use SAMHSA's Behavioral Health Treatment Services Locator

(App Store Preview, 2023a)

For Clients

Suicide Safety Plan App by Inquiry Health, LLC (App Store Preview, 2022a). This app is intended to support anyone who is experiencing suicidal thoughts and help to prevent suicide. Features of the app aim to help the user recognize that suicidal thoughts and feelings will pass with time.

- No cost/free
- Age rating 12+
- English language
- Copyright 2020

Once the user fills in the requested information, this app serves as a guide in the moment of struggle and/or crisis. This action plan and resource guide provide information when the client is unable to formulate well due to distress. The requested information can be completed on one's own or with the guidance of a clinician.

Features include:

- Designing a safety plan
- Customize warning signs
- Develop coping strategies
- Develop own resource list/contacts
- Making the environment safe
- List important reasons for living
- Easy-to-access list of emergency resources
- Guide to dealing with suicidal thoughts

The **Suicide Safety Plan App** is open source and looking for contributors (more information here: https://github.com/suicidesafetyplan/safetyplan-ios/).

Columbia Protocol App by PSS Chute Software (App Store Preview, 2022b):

- No cost/free
- Age rating 12+
- English language
- Copyright 2020

The *Columbia Protocol App* is based on the traditional Columbia-Suicide Severity Rating Scale (C-SSRS), which includes a series of six simple questions intended to screen a person's risk of suicide (Columbia-Suicide Severity Rating Scale, n.d.). The publicly available screening questions are as follows:

1. Have you wished you were dead or wished you could go to sleep and not wake up?
2. Have you had any thoughts about killing yourself?
   a. If yes to 2, ask questions 3, 4, 5, and 6.
   b. If no to 2, skip to question 6.
3. Have you been thinking about how you might do this?

4. Have you had these thoughts and had some intention of acting on them?
5. Have you started to work out or worked out the details of how to kill yourself? Did you intend to carry out this plan?

Always ask question 6

6. Have you done anything, started to do anything, or prepared to do anything to end your life?

(Columbia-Suicide Severity Rating Scale (C-SSRS), n.d., para. 1)

Claimed to be the most evidence-supported tool of its kind, the C-SSRS has been included in numerous studies. Please refer to the Columbia Lighthouse Project for more information (Columbia Lighthouse Project, 2016).

The ***Stanley-Brown Safety Plan*** app by Two Penguins Studios, LLC assists with creating a suicide safety plan by a user alone or in conjunction with a clinician. The suicide plan is a brief emergency plan in the user's own words, intended to provide a list of supports and strategies for suicide crises or extreme distress. It is:

- No cost/free
- Age rating 4+
- English language
- Copyright 2013

The developers suggest the user 1) assess the likelihood that the plan will be used, 2) problem-solve to identify any barriers or obstacles, 3) determine how to eliminate barriers, and 4) review the plan periodically for any necessary revisions.

Features include:

- Design a safety plan
- Identify warning signs
- Recognize internal coping strategies
- Identify social supports and social settings
- Identify contacts, family, and/or friends for help in a crisis
- List professionals and agencies
- Make the environment safe
- Steps to take after the plan is created

(App Store Preview, 2023b)

Applications for use in suicide assessment, intervention, and prevention will certainly continue to develop. The clinician must incorporate the needs, style, and interests of the client into the selection and use of any digital software, particularly in delicate situations, along with relevant clinical information and treatment needs.

CASE EXAMPLE

Allison is a 13-year-old, tenth-grade student. She is intellectually gifted and transgendered, having transitioned over ten months before presenting to this therapist for services. It was reported that a connection was initially established with her previous therapist of approximately 12 months, but it declined as she transitioned from identifying as male to female. Allison is successful academically in her advanced grade but struggles socially, as she is more intellectually advanced and two to three years younger than her same-grade peers. Her parents, who were divorced and had difficulty communicating, reported that Allison began withdrawing, dressing differently, refusing to go to her ballet class (which she previously loved), and had been treating her younger sister poorly over the last two months of work with the previous therapist.

Allison presented for services during the COVID-19 pandemic and was met virtually. She would log on per her parent's request but placed tape over the camera to blur her image. The shadowy figure on the screen was dressed in dark colors and slumped. Her verbal responses were mumbled and sounded like irritated whispers. It was nearly impossible to engage with her.

The therapist noted that the name she used for her Zoom identification was "Peely." Knowing this was a character within Fortnite, the therapist hoped to have a connection point. "Peely! No way!" the therapist exclaimed. The slumped, shadowy blob of a figure moved. The therapist began a bit of a monologue about a new skin and emote she had gotten recently in the game and how bad she is at playing Fortnite, but she enjoyed going around and collecting resources. The shadowy figure typed in the chat box, "Wait – you're telling me you play Fortnite? You're a therapist and you play Fortnite? WTH? (What the hell)," "Oh, yes!" the therapist responded verbally, "I play all sorts of games with my clients. I can learn a lot about someone by the way they play, what games they play, what skins they use, etc. Plus, it is a lot of fun." Allison responded, "Weird." "I guess so – want to play anyway?" the therapist asked. After some time and thought, the word "sure" appeared in the chat box.

Allison and the therapist met up in Fortnite for level 3 DPT play. Her character's skin (the character's outward appearance: gender, hair, skin color, clothing, etc.) depicted a strong, powerful woman. The emote (action/dance, etc.) she kept playing over and over is called the *Azarath Metrion Zinthos*. It depicted her character as having magical abilities to suspend particles, group them, and use them to attack. The therapist stayed with a silly emote of her character, knitting a Christmas sweater. She could imagine Allison rolling her eyes at the therapist's lameness. The therapist explained that she was not good at several things in the game but enjoyed collecting resources. She offered to work to find items for Allison if desired. Allison did not respond.

Fortnite includes several different ways to play and interact. Allison chose to play a duo in Battle Royale. This game includes 100 people playing to be the last one standing. A duo means two people are playing as a team and hope to be the last team standing. Over time, a storm circle encloses and forces remaining players to a smaller circumference of the play area (map). During this play, Allison repeatedly allowed her character to perish in the storm. She would play until the storm approached and then activate her emote as her character's body emitted smoke from the storm damage. The therapist encouraged her to "Run, get out of the storm!" but Allison remained, and her character died. Once the character dies, the duo partner can shadow the remaining character and watch the gameplay from a ghost-like perspective. The therapist would be attacked shortly after, and the gameplay would end. The therapist had observed that one of Allison's approaches was to be involved if it was little effort – little expenditure of her resources – but once an external force presented itself, she surrendered and no longer would fight. The therapist wondered how this might play out in Allison's day-to-day life.

Many themes and approaches like this appeared throughout the gameplay. The therapist took notes and worked to bridge what Allison's parents and teachers reported with what was experienced during the play. At one point, Allison typed into the Zoom chat: "She just wants to die." The therapist attended to this statement and began to weave questions from the C-SSRS about suicide, ideation, and plan(s) into the conversation to both ascertain the level of seriousness and risk and to let Allison know this was a very important topic. Per Miller (2013), questions should be direct and specific to ascertain risk and establish clear communication. Allison's life included several risk factors: gender identity, acrimoniously divorced parents, anhedonia, and difficulty connecting with peers. After some initial questions, to which Allison responded in the Zoom chat, the therapist requested that Allison remove the tape from the camera. She refused.

It did not appear that the risk was imminent. Allison expressed her character's suicidal ideation surrounding a desire to escape. She did not like the life she was living. She wanted to be accepted and fit in, at least with a best friend. The therapist offered parallel-play, monologue-type narration regarding the importance of her Fortnite character as a partner, a friend in this duo who was important. Each time the therapist's character would perish, the therapist would lament that it is so very hard to do this alone, that support from a partner would make such a difference in this loneliness inside the circle. The therapist was working to verbally acknowledge what Allison's character was feeling, to identify the impact on the gameplay, and to highlight some components of resilience (social connection, support, engagement, skills ⟶ increased self-efficacy).

Over a few additional sessions, Allison began to place herself closer to the therapist's character and ran away from the storm in tandem. This was a huge statement by Allison – her character was worth self-preservation and she felt connected to the therapist's character in some way and wanted to pair up. She began responding verbally over time and ultimately took the tape off the camera. There was a lot of work to be continued and still continues as of the time of this writing.

The connection created through the mutual medium of a digital video game allowed Allison to depict her character in a way that was meaningful to her. She changed her emotes and her skins to express herself – the way she was feeling, the way she saw herself, and the way she wished she could be seen. She could change these very quickly in response to her internal state or the situation at hand. Video games allow for these rapid depiction options. Her coping skills, styles, expressions, actions, inactions, and approaches to the gameplay communicated with the therapist about her internal state, her worldview, and her understanding of herself in it. The ability to be relatively invisible and engage on her terms via telemental health proved invaluable in allowing her to progress as her comfort level improved. The inclusion of her interest, as depicted by her chosen Zoom name identifier, increased her level of initial comfort and ultimately led to safety and belonging within the therapist-client dyad. Creating this space and safety within the digital environment allowed for the expression and exploration of suicidal ideation and the underlying emotions and experiences within Allison's preferred language and culture.

INTERVENTIONS

Table 10.4 101 Digital Play Therapy™ Games

Animal Crossing	Tetris	Jenga	SwapTales Leon!
Legend of Zelda	Trivia Royale	Yahtzee with Buddies	Cramble
Minecraft	Tsuro	Roll the Pigs	Big Brain Academy
Fortnite	Twenty	Finger Twister	Mario Party Superstars
Skribbl.io	Forbidden Desert	Battle Slimes	WarioWare: Get it Together
Unofreak	Space Team	6 Takes!	Super Mario 3D World + Bowsers Fury
Virtual Sandtray	Battleship	Who Can't Draw?	Clubhouse Games
FIFA 22	Fingle	Keep Talking and Nobody Explodes	
Thisissand	Magic: Manastrike	Jackbox Games	ManoCart 8 Deluxe
Boardgamearena	Heads up	The Game of Life	Super Mario Party
Roblox	Words With Friends	June's Journey	Overcooked 2
Bitmojl	Mad Libs	Plants v Zombies	Super Smash Bros
FlipAnim	Bounden	Drop the Number	Super Mario Maker
Silk	Scrabble	Slime Simulator	Luigi's Mansion 3
Quick Draw	Reverse Charades Jr	Paint by Number	Pikmin 3 Deluxe
Jamboard	Ticket to Ride	Joy Doodle, and all of the Doodle family of apps	Yoshi's Crafted World
Music Lab	Teledoodle	Procreate	Fast RMX
Real Dnve 3D	Psych!	Halloween - Where Is My Hat?	Mano Tennis Aces
Crossword Jam	Catan	Marble Mixer	Marvel ultimate Alliance 3
Words with Friends	Shakepop	RelationShapes	Snipperclips
wordle	Space Team	Silly Street Learn & Play	Puyo Puyo Tetris
Diamondcoloring	Uno & Friends	Duel 1st, 2nd, 3,d, 4th Grade Math Games for Kids	Google Blob Opera
Snake.lo	Battleships - Fleet Battle	Montesson Nature	Cool Math Games
Slither.io	Carcassonne	The Game of Life	
Paper.io	King of Opera	Connect Four	
Google Play a Kandinsky			
Ⓒ www.jessicastonephd.com			

Source: 101 Digital Play Therapy™ Games. Stone, J. (2023a) 101 Digital Play Therapy™ Games [Graphic] [Unpublished].

CONCLUSION

Clinicians who work with young people who struggle with suicidality are tasked with simultaneously assessing levels of safety, understanding the client's worldview, intervening where appropriate, and building resiliency skills to prevent future suicidality. Incorporating the client's interests and culture in digital technology can increase acceptance and safety within the therapeutic dynamic. The ability to enter a client's world through digital tools and experience their approaches to many environments, scenarios, interactions, and tasks allows the clinician to gain a more holistic view of the client and their needs. Assessment, intervention, and prevention methods incorporating digital tools activate the many components within the treatment of suicidality identified through decades of research.

REFERENCES

American Psychological Association. (2022a). APA dictionary of psychology: Suicidality. *American Psychological Association*. https://dictionary.apa.org/suicidality

American Psychological Association. (2022b). APA dictionary of psychology: Resilience. *American Psychological Association*. www.apa.org/topics/resilience/

App Store Preview. (2022a). Suicide safety plan. *Apple*. https://apps.apple.com/us/app/suicide-safety-plan/id1003891579

App Store Preview. (2022b). Columbia protocol. *Apple*. https://apps.apple.com/us/app/columbia-protocol/id1450966911?platform=ipad

App Store Preview. (2023a). Suicide safe by SAMHSA. *Apple*. https://apps.apple.com/us/app/suicide-safe-by-samhsa/id968468139

App Store Preview. (2023b). Stanley-Brown safety plan. *Apple*. https://apps.apple.com/us/app/stanley-brown-safety-plan/id695122998

Beutler, L. E. (1979). Toward specific psychological therapies for specific conditions. *Journal of Consulting and Clinical Psychology*, *47*(5), 882–897. https://doi.org/10.1037/0022-006x.47.5.882

Beutler, L. E., & Harwood, T. M. (2000). *Prescriptive psychotherapy: A practical guide to systematic treatment selection*. Oxford University Press.

Brown, G. M., Beck, A. T., Steer, R. A., & Grisham, J. R. (2000). Risk factors for suicide in psychiatric outpatients: A 20-year prospective study. *Journal of Consulting and Clinical Psychology*, *68*(3), 371–377. https://doi.org/10.1037/0022-006x.68.3.371

Center for Advanced Research on Language Acquisition (CARLA). (2022). *What is culture?* University of Minnesota. https://carla.umn.edu/culture/definitions.html

Ceranoglu, T. A. (2010). Video games in psychotherapy. *Review of General Psychology*, *14*(2), 141–146. https://doi.org/10.1037/a0019439

Columbia-Suicide Severity Rating Scale (C-SSRS) (n.d.). C-SSRS. *Columbia.edu*. https://cssrs.columbia.edu/wp-content/uploads/Columbia_Protocol.pdf

Eldridge, A. (2022). Generation Z: Demographic group. *Britannica*. www.britannica.com/topic/Generation-Z

Granic, I., Lobel, A., & Engels, R. C. M. E. (2014). The benefits of playing video games. *American Psychologist*, *69*(1), 66–78. https://doi.org/10.1037/a0034857

Janet, P. (1901). *The mental state of hystericals: A study of mental stigmata and mental accidents*. G.P. Putnam's Sons.

Kalisch, R., Cramer, A. O. J., Binder, H., Fritz, J., Leertouwer, I., Lunansky, G., Meyer, B., Timmer, J., Veer, I. M., & Van Harmelen, A. (2019). Deconstructing and reconstructing resilience: A dynamic network approach. *Perspectives on Psychological Science*, *14*(5), 765–777. https://doi.org/10.1177/1745691619855637

Masten, A. S. (2019). Resilience from a developmental systems perspective. *World Psychiatry*, *18*(1), 101–102. https://doi.org/10.1002/wps.20591

Mayo Clinic. (2023). *Teen suicide: What parents need to know*. www.mayoclinic.org/healthy-lifestyle/tween-and-teen-health/in-depth/teen-suicide/art-20044308

McCrindle, M., & Fell, A. (2020). *Understanding generation alpha*. https://mccrindle.com.au/app/uploads/reports/Understanding-Generation-Alpha-Report-2020.pdf

Miller, D. N. (2013). Assessing risk for suicide. In S. H. McConaughy (Ed.), *Clinical interviews for children and adolescents: Assessment to intervention* (2nd ed., pp. 208–227). Guilford.

Miller, D. N. (2021). *Child and adolescent suicidal behavior: School-based prevention, assessment, and intervention* (2nd ed.). Guildford.

Prensky, M. (2001). *Digital natives, digital immigrants*. www.marcprensky.com/writing/Prensky%20-%20Digital%20Natives,%20Digital%20Immigrants%20-%20Part1.pdf

Prensky, M. (2016). *Education to better their world: Unleashing the power of 21st-century kids*. Teachers College Press.

Russoniello, C. V., O'Brien, K., & Parks, J. M. (2009). EEG, HRV, and psychological correlates while playing Bejewelled II: A randomized control study. *Student Health Technology Information*, *144*, 189–192. https://pubmed.ncbi.nlm.nih.gov/19592761/

Sánchez-Teruel, D., Robles-Bello, M. A., Muela-Martínez, J. A., & García-León, A. (2021). Resilience assessment scale for the prediction of suicide reattempt in a clinical population. *Frontiers*. www.frontiersin.org/articles/10.3389/fpsyg.2021.673088/full#B33

Schaefer, C. E., & Drewes, A. A. (2014). *The therapeutic powers of play: 20 core agents of change* (2nd ed.). Wiley.

Shain, B., & AAP Committee on Adolescence. (2016). Suicide and suicide attempts in adolescence. *Pediatrics*, *138*(1), e20161420, e1–e11. www.cpaawa.org/wp-content/uploads/2017/09/02_AU_AdolescentSuicide_AmerAcadPediatrics2016.pdf

Shneidman, E. S. (1996). *The suicidal mind*. Oxford University Press.

Shneidman, E. S., & Farberow, N. L. (1956). Clues to suicide. *Public Health Reports*, *71*(2), 109. https://doi.org/10.2307/4589373

Stone, J. (2019a). *Digital play therapy: A clinician's guide to comfort and competence* (1st ed.). Routledge.

Stone, J. (2019b). Digital games. In J. Stone & C. E. Schaefer (Eds.), *Game play: Therapeutic use of games with children and adolescents* (3rd ed., pp. 99–120). Routledge.

Stone, J. (2022). *Digital play therapy: A clinician's guide to comfort and competence* (2nd ed., p. 18). Routledge.

Stone, J. (2023a). 101 Digital Play Therapy™ games [Graphic] [Unpublished].

Stone, J. (2023b). *Technology in mental health: Foundations of clinical use*. Routledge.

Substance Abuse and Mental Health Services Administration (n.d.). *Publications and digital products: Suicide Safe Mobile App*. https://store.samhsa.gov/product/suicide-safe

Substance Abuse and Mental Health Services Administration. (2009). *SAFE-T*. https://store.samhsa.gov/sites/default/files/sma09-4432.pdf

The Columbia Lighthouse Project. (2016). The Columbia Suicide Severity Rating Scale (C-SSRS): Psychometric evidence. *Columbia.edu*. https://cssrs.columbia.edu/the-columbia-scalecssrs/evidence/#:~:text=Numerous%20studies%20support%20the%20psychometric%20properties%20of%20the,inter-rater%20reliability%2C%20cross-cultural%20and%20multi-lingual%20application%2C%20and%20more

U.S. Department of Health and Human Services & Centers for Disease Control and Prevention. (2022). Adolescent behaviors and experiences survey — United States, January–June 2021. *Morbidity and Mortality Weekly Report*, *71*(3), 1–40. https://www.cdc.gov/mmwr/volumes/71/su/pdfs/su7103a1-a5-H.pdf

Zaera, A. (2022a). Did you know these surprising benefits of playing video games? *Ugami*. https://ugami.com/gaming-lifestyle/did-you-know-these-surprising-benefits-of-playing-video-games/

Zaera, A. (2022b). How to build resilience with video games. *Forbes EQ*. www.forbes.com/sites/forbeseq/2022/09/30/how-to-build-resilience-with-video-games/?sh=1580aef76a29

EPILOGUE

Mary Ruth Cross and Leslie W. Baker

As we come to a close in assisting play therapists in conceptualizing how to assess and treat children with obvious or hidden signs of suicidal thinking, we want to highlight a few points.

Breaking down the denial and stigma that youth suicide exists and is impacted by awareness so assessment, treatment, and prevention can occur is vital. We cannot apply adult perspectives of suicide to youth as they are developmentally different and process the world from distinct perspectives. Change happens through compassion and connection. Children and adolescents suffer from emotional pain so deeply that sometimes, they feel numb. Self-harm may be a response to numbness, an effort to feel something other than emotional pain. Parents and caregivers deserve compassionate support as they manage the needs of their suicidal youth and cope with their own needs.

Play therapists and mental health professionals need to create the safety of the relationship, a place in times of pain built on trust, empathy, and respect. Clinicians must develop an awareness of the intricacies of working with youth suffering from suicidal thoughts and behaviors and learn to manage their countertransference effectively. Sometimes, words fail with youth; when this happens, let play take over. Through the Therapeutic Powers of Play and applying the 20 core agents of change, play therapists and other mental health providers can create a treatment strategy that is mindful of the many cultures and dynamics within today's society. Taking a comprehensive look at selected theoretical perspectives enables the clinician to understand and utilize inclusive therapies for diverse populations. Successful prevention efforts require a multifaceted approach. The solution calls for everyone to work together in the Zero-Suicide system and honor diversity on multiple levels: leading, training, identifying, engaging, transitioning, and improving. Parents, caregivers, and all allied professionals have the potential to impact prevention by increasing their knowledge about suicide. Indeed, more research is needed as we grow in our understanding of suicidal children and adolescents. Through diligent collaboration, we can achieve the goal of Zero Suicide.

Thank you for sharing this journey with us. Please take care of yourselves because you are essential and needed. You are the light that guides children through the darkest days, and even momentarily, you shine hope over despair.

~ Mary Ruth Cross and Leslie W. Baker

APPENDIX

Leslie W. Baker and Mary Ruth Cross

There is no accepted nomenclature for suicide terms; however, the article by Crosby et al. (2011) developed a glossary of accepted terms regarding uniform definitions created in partnership with the Department of Veterans Affairs. A cohesive language may assist play therapists, school counselors, parents, and caregivers in communicating more clearly and remove the stigma and blame that has existed in the terminology for decades. Explicit language is a positive step toward reducing the guilt and shame of suicide and other mental health issues; for example, "died by suicide" or "died of suicide" denotes that a person has died by suicide versus "committed suicide." This previous term is no longer used due to stigmatization and the implication that suicide is a crime (as involuntarily incarcerated in a mental health facility) or a sin, as the word "commit" is commonly used in connection with religious offenses (Beaton et al., 2013). We included definitions of terms to assist in understanding the LGBTQIA+ community; however, this list is not exhaustive. Lastly, we included terms to understand bullying victimization better.

UNDERSTANDING CONCEPTS THROUGH DEFINITIONS

Agender refers to individuals who do not identify with any gender group or feel such identification is irrelevant to their sense of self (Antonsen et al., 2020).

An *aromantic* person does not experience romantic attraction to others or experiences little to no desire for romantic relationships. Aromatic does not necessarily preclude sexual interest in one or more gender groups.

Asexuality refers to a complete or partial lack of sexual attraction or lack of interest in sexual activity with others. The level of disinterest can vary among individuals (Antonsen et al., 2020).

Bereaved by suicide refers to the relatives, acquaintances, and others impacted by a loved one's suicide (often termed as those who have survived after a suicide loss) (Crosby et al., 2011).

A *Bisexual* is a person of any gender who is attracted to more than one sex, gender, or gender identity, though not necessarily simultaneously, in the same way, or to the same degree (Hrc.org. n.d.).

Bullying is unwanted aggressive actions from one young individual or a group, excluding siblings or those in a romantic relationship, that show a noticeable power disparity and either occur repeatedly or have a high likelihood of reoccurrence. "Bullying may inflict harm or distress on the targeted youth, including physical, psychological, social, or educational harm" (Gladden et al., 2014, p. 7).

Comprehensive suicide prevention plans that use a multifaceted approach to addressing the problem include interventions targeting biopsychosocial, social, and environmental factors (Crosby et al., 2011).

Cyberbullicide describes suicides directly or indirectly influenced by online aggression or cyberbullying (Hinduja & Patchin, 2010; Hinduja & Patchin, 2018).

Cyberbullying is bullying that occurs online or through technology (Schonfeld et al., 2023).

Fatal or non-fatal attempts: Non-fatal suicidal behaviors are suicidal thought, specific suicidal plan, and suicide attempt. Prospective studies have emphasized the high subsequent suicide rates in clinically presenting suicide attempters (Jena & Sidhartha, 2004).

A fatal attempt is when a person dies by suicide. Applying the general principle of speaking about suicide using illness-based language, fatal and non-fatal, is in line with a terminal or non-fatal heart attack or other illness (Centers for Disease Control and Prevention & National Center for Injury Prevention and Control, 2023).

A ***gay*** man is a male who is emotionally, romantically, or sexually attracted to men (hrc. org. n.d.).

Gender refers to the socially constructed characteristics of women, men, girls, and boys. Gender includes norms, behaviors, and roles associated with being a woman, man, girl, or boy, as well as relationships with each other. As a social construct, gender varies from society to society and can change over time (World Health Organization, 2023).

Gender expression is the external appearance of one's gender identity, usually expressed through behavior, clothing, body characteristics, or voice, and which may or may not conform to socially defined behaviors and characteristics typically associated with being either masculine or feminine (Hrc.org. n.d.).

A ***gender-fluid*** person does not identify with a single fixed gender or has a fluid or unfixed gender identity (Hrc.org. n.d.).

Gender identity is one's innermost concept of self as male, female, or a blend of both or neither – how individuals perceive themselves and what they call themselves. One's gender identity can be the same or different from the sex assigned at birth (Hrc.org., n.d.).

Intersex is a term used to describe a person born with physical sex characteristics that do not conform exclusively to the male or female. Approximately one in 2,000 individuals are estimated to be born with a combination of male and female sex characteristics, such as ambiguous genitalia, reproductive organs that are not fully formed, or an ambiguous set of chromosomes (*How Common Is Intersex: Intersex Society of North America*, 2008).

A ***lesbian*** is a woman who is emotionally, romantically, or sexually attracted to other women (Hrc.org., n.d.).

"Lived experience" of suicide with suicidal thoughts, a suicidal crisis, or a suicide attempt is a term that refers to someone's experience (Lived Experience Programs, 2022).

Means for suicide refers to the tools or items utilized to execute a self-harming action (for instance, chemicals, prescription drugs, illegal substances, or a weapon) (Crosby et al., 2011).

The term ***non-binary*** is used by people who experience gender identity and gender expression as falling outside the binary gender categories of "man" and "woman" (Hrc.org., n.d.).

***Nonsuicidal* self-injury** (NSSI) is self-harm behavior linked with no intention to cause death. The act is solely performed for other motives, either to alleviate distress (commonly known as "self-mutilation," examples include shallow cuts or scratches, hitting/banging, or burns) or to induce changes in others or the surrounding environment (Posner et al., 2007).

Pornography depicts erotic behavior intended to cause sexual excitement (The Editors of Encyclopedia Britannica, 2003, May 14).

Protective factors pertain to interactive elements that mitigate the adverse effect of a risk factor on an undesirable outcome, also referred to as resilience (Luthar & Cicchetti, 2000).

Queer is a term people often use to express a spectrum of identities and orientations counter to the mainstream, especially among youth who do not identify with narrower categories. Queer is often used as a catch-all to include people who are not exclusively straight and folks with non-binary or gender-expansive identities (Hrc. org., n.d.).

Questioning is a term used to describe people exploring their sexual orientation or gender identity (Hrc.org., n.d.).

Roasting (also known as "flaming") relates to posts that contain offensive, hostile, intimidating, insulting, satirical, or unfriendly content. Typical behaviors include posting provocative or abusive posts to social media platforms, with information often being characterized by extensive use of punctuation marks and capital letters (Zhang et al., 2022).

A ***safety plan*** is a documented listing of a person's warning signs, coping strategies, and assistance sources that someone can use to prevent or handle a suicidal situation (Crosby et al., 2011).

Safety planning is a collaborative approach in which a therapist and a patient construct a plan of action for implementation should the patient experience suicidal ideation, ordered from least to most intense responses (Moscardini et al., 2020).

Sex assigned at birth is the sex, male, female, or intersex, that a doctor or midwife uses to describe a child at birth based on their external anatomy (Hrc.org., n.d.).

Sexting is a term to describe the combination of "sex" and "texting" – it refers to the sending and/or receiving via digital media of sexually explicit messages and partial or fully nude photos and/or videos with sexual connotations (Ragona et al., 2023).

Sex trafficking is the recruitment, harboring, transportation, provision, obtaining, patronizing, or soliciting of a person for a commercial sex act in which the commercial sex act is induced by force, fraud, or coercion or in which the person induced to perform such an act has not attained 18 years of age (22 U.S.C. § 7102(11)(A) ("*Human Trafficking*," 2023).

Sexual orientation is an inherent or immutable enduring emotional, romantic, or sexual attraction to others. Note: An individual's sexual orientation is independent of gender identity (Hrc.org., n.d.).

Suicidal behavior refers to actions and preparations leading to a suicide attempt, instances of attempted suicide, and instances of death by suicide (Crosby et al., 2011).

> ***Other suicidal behavior, including preparatory acts,*** refers to acts or preparation towards making a suicide attempt, but before the potential for harm has begun. A suicide behavior can include anything beyond a verbalization or

thought, such as assembling a method (e.g., buying a gun, collecting pills) or preparing for one's death by suicide (e.g., writing a suicide note or giving things away) (Posner et al., 2007).

Suicidal ideation refers to thinking about or planning suicide. The thoughts lie on a continuum of severity from a wish to die with no method, plan, intent, or behavior to active suicidal ideation with a specific plan and intent (Posner et al., 2011).

> ***Active suicidal ideation (thoughts)*** is when a person thinks about *specific ways* to end their life (Posner et al., 2011).

> ***Passive suicidal ideation*** is when someone thinks about or wishes for death without planning to end their life (Posner et al., 2007).

Suicidality is often used to refer simultaneously to suicidal thoughts and suicidal behaviors. These phenomena are vastly different in occurrence, associated factors, consequences, and interventions, so they should be addressed separately – *alternate terms*: suicidal thoughts and suicidal behavior (Crosby et al., 2011).

Suicide is a death caused by self-directed injurious behavior with any intent to die due to the behavior (Posner et al., 2007).

Suicide attempt (SA) is a behavior that could cause self-harm, linked with at least a minimal intention to die due to the action. Proof that the individual intended to end their own life, at least to a certain extent, can be explicitly stated or implied from the behavior or situation. A suicide attempt may lead to actual harm, but this is not always the case (Posner et al., 2007).

A ***suicide cluster*** is a group of suicides, suicide attempts, or self-harm events occurring closer together in time and space than expected in a given community (Niedzwiedz et al., 2014).

Suicide contagion is a phenomenon whereby susceptible persons are influenced toward suicidal behavior through knowledge of another person's suicidal acts (Crosby et al., 2011).

Suicide intent refers to evidence, either explicit or implied, suggests that when the injury occurred, the person had the intent to end their own life or had the desire to die, and they comprehended the likely outcomes of their actions (Crosby et al., 2011).

Suicide intervention is a direct effort to stop an individual from attempting suicide. A suicide intervention is a method designed to avert a specific result or modify the progression of a current situation (like administering lithium for bipolar conditions, training professionals on preventing suicide, or limiting the availability of lethal means for those at risk of suicide) (Crosby et al., 2011).

A ***suicide note*** is a note or letter explaining why one died by suicide (Merriam-Webster, n.d.-a).

A ***suicide pact*** is an agreement between two or more people to kill themselves simultaneously (Merriam-Webster, n.d.-b).

Suicide postvention is support and care given to people impacted following a suicide attempt or the death of someone due to suicide (Crosby et al., 2011).

Suicide prevention is to reduce factors that increase risk and increase factors that promote resilience (Crosby et al., 2011).

Transgender is an umbrella term for people whose gender identity or expression differs from cultural expectations based on the sex they were assigned at birth.

It is important to note that being transgender does not imply any specific orientation. Therefore, transgender people may identify as straight, gay, lesbian, etc. (Hrc.org., n.d.).

Trolling is an umbrella term for online multidimensional, antagonistic, antisocial, or deviant online behaviors and motivations (Ortiz, 2020).

REFERENCES

Antonsen, A. N., Zdaniuk, B., Yule, M. A., & Brotto, L. A. (2020). Ace and aro: Understanding differences in romantic attractions among persons identifying as asexual. *Archives of Sexual Behavior, 49*(5), 1615–1630. https://doi.org/10.1007/s10508-019-01600-1

Beaton, S., Forster, P., & Maple, M. (2013). *Suicide and language: Why we shouldn't use the "C" word*. Australian Psychological Society. https://eprints.worc.ac.uk/2237/

Centers for Disease Control and Prevention & National Center for Injury Prevention and Control. (2023, March 8). Suicide prevention: Facts about suicide. *CDC.gov*. Retrieved March 31, 2024, from https://www.cdc.gov/suicide/facts/index.html#:~:text=Suicide%20is%20death%20caused%20by,a%20result%20of%20their%20actions

Crosby, A. E., Ortega, L., & Melanson, C. (2011). *Self-directed violence surveillance: Uniform definitions and recommended data elements, Version 1.0*. Centers for Disease Control and Prevention, National Center for Injury Prevention and Control. www.cdc.gov/violenceprevention/pdf/self-directed-violence-a.pdf

Editors of Encyclopedia Britannica. (2003, May 14). Pornography summary. *Encyclopedia Britannica*. www.britannica.com/summary/pornography

Gladden, R. M., Vivolo-Kantor, A. M., Hamburger, M. E., & Lumpkin, C.D. (2014). *Bullying surveillance among youths: Uniform definitions for public health and recommended data elements* (Version 1.0, pp. 1–116). National Center for Injury Prevention and Control, Centers for Disease Control and Prevention and the United States Department of Education. www.cdc.gov/violenceprevention/pdf/Bullying-Definitions-FINAL-a.pdf

Hinduja, S., & Patchin, J. W. (2010). Bullying, cyberbullying, and suicide. *Archives of Suicide Research, 14*(3), 206–221. https://doi.org/10.1080/13811118.2010.494133

Hinduja, S., & Patchin, J. W. (2018). Connecting adolescent suicide to the severity of bullying and cyberbullying. *Journal of School Violence, 18*(3), 333–346. https://doi.org/10.1080/15388220.2018.1492417

How common is intersex? | Intersex Society of North America. (2008). InterACT Advocates for Intersex Youth. Retrieved April 8, 2023, from https://isna.org/faq/frequency/

HRC.org. (n.d.). Glossary of terms. *Human Rights Campaign*. Retrieved April 8, 2023, from www.hrc.org/resources/glossary-of-terms

Human trafficking. (2023, May 13). United States Department of Justice. www.justice.gov/humantrafficking#:~:text=Human%20Trafficking%20Defined

Jena, S., & Sidhartha, T. (2004). Non-fatal suicidal behaviors in adolescents. *Indian Journal of Psychiatry, 46*(4), 310–318.

Lived experience programs. (2022, March 30). American Foundation for Suicide Prevention. https://afsp.org/lived-experience-programs/

Luthar, S. S., & Cicchetti, D. (2000). The construct of resilience: Implications for interventions and social policies. *Development and Psychopathology, 12*(4), 857–885. https://doi.org/10.1017/s0954579400004156

Merriam-Webster. (n.d.-a). Suicide note. *The Merriam-Webster.com*. Retrieved July 18, 2023, from www.merriam-webster.com/dictionary/suicide%20note

Merriam-Webster. (n.d.-b). Suicide pact. *The Merriam-Webster.com*. Retrieved July 18, 2023, from www.merriam-webster.com/dictionary/suicide%20pact

Moscardini, E. H., Hill, R. M., Dodd, C. G., Do, C., Kaplow, J. B., & Tucker, R. P. (2020). Suicide safety planning: Clinician training, comfort, and safety plan utilization. *International Journal of Environmental Research and Public Health, 17*(18), 6444. https://doi.org/10.3390/ijerph17186444

Niedzwiedz, C. L., Haw, C., Hawton, K., & Platt, S. (2014). The definition and epidemiology of clusters of suicidal behavior: A systematic review. *Suicide and Life Threatening Behavior, 44*(5), 569–581. https://doi.org/10.1111/sltb.12091

Ortiz, S. M. (2020). Trolling as a collective form of harassment: An inductive study of how online users understand trolling. *Social Media and Society, 6*(2). https://doi.org/10.1177/2056305120928512

Posner, K., Brown, G. M., Stanley, B., Brent, D. A., Yershova, K., Oquendo, M. A., Currier, G. W., Melvin, G. A., Greenhill, L. L., Shen, S., & Mann, J. J. (2011). The Columbia–Suicide Severity Rating Scale: Initial validity and internal consistency findings from three multisite studies with adolescents and adults. *American Journal of Psychiatry, 168*(12), 1266–1277. https://doi.org/10.1176/appi.ajp.2011.10111704

Posner, K., Oquendo, M. A., Gould, M., Stanley, B., & Davies, M. (2007). Columbia Classification Algorithm of Suicide Assessment (C-CASA): Classification of suicidal events in the FDA's pediatric suicidal risk analysis of antidepressants. *The American Journal of Psychiatry, 164*(7), 1035. https://doi.org/10.1176/appi.ajp.164.7.1035

Ragona, A., Mesce, M., Cimino, S., & Cerniglia, L. (2023). Motivations, behaviors, and expectancies of sexting: The role of defensive strategies and social media addiction in a sample of adolescents. *International Journal of Environmental Research and Public Health, 20*(3), 1805. https://doi.org/10.3390/ijerph20031805

Schonfeld, A., McNiel, D. E., Toyoshima, T., & Binder, R. L. (2023). Cyberbullying and adolescent suicide. *PubMed, 51*(1), 112–119. https://doi.org/10.29158/jaapl.220078-22

World Health Organization. (2023). *Gender and health.* Author. www.who.int/health-topics/gender#tab=tab_1

Zhang, W., Huang, S., Lam, L., Evans, R., & Zhu, C. (2022). Cyberbullying definitions and measurements in children and adolescents: Summarizing 20 years of global efforts. *Frontiers in Public Health, 10.* https://doi.org/10.3389/fpubh.2022.1000504

INDEX

6PSM 74

AACAP 4, 37
AAPI 148
ableism 160, 164
abuse 17, 19–24, 33, 64, 67, 70–71, 88–90,
    94, 100–101, 133, 143, 145–146, 161,
    181–182, 192, 195
academic stress 23, 151
academic support 147
acculturation 131, 148–153
acquired 22
activity therapy 141
ADHD 16–17, 61, 99, 160–163, 165
adolescents 3–8, 14–19, 21–26, 33, 39–41,
    48, 62–63, 66–70, 76, 78–79, 84, 90–96,
    99–107, 112, 118–119, 122–124, 129,
    133, 138, 145, 148, 154, 159, 165, 175
adolescent suicide 20, 116, 148
adverse outcomes 112
affirmation 82, 84–87, 93–94, 106–107,
    109–111, 160, 165
affirmation interventions 86
aftercare 6, 69, 179, 183
Alaskan native 8, 129, 143
alcohol 33, 62, 71, 139, 145, 154–155, 192
alexithymia 160–161, 163–164
alliance 7, 14, 40–41, 44, 49, 52, 64, 70, 80,
    82, 101, 104, 116, 156, 200
American Academy of Child & Adolescent
    Psychiatry (AACAP) 4, 37
anxiety 5, 18, 26, 32–34, 41–42, 70–73, 99,
    101–102, 112, 119, 133, 136, 139, 141,
    146–147, 155, 161–164, 176, 181–182,
    185, 192
applied suicide intervention skills training
    (ASIST) 150
art therapy 78, 90, 109, 146, 152–153
Asian American 7, 146, 148
Asian Americans and Pacific Islanders (AAPI)
    148
ask suicide-screening questions (ASQ) 62–63
ASQ 62–63
assessing for medication 33
assessments 7, 12, 59, 62, 69–70, 94,
    131–133, 138–140, 150–151
assessment tools 62, 82
attention deficit 61, 133, 160, 163, 178, 192
autism 159, 161–163
autistic individuals 161

AutPlay® therapy 162, 164
Axline, Virginia 78, 80

bag of marbles 111
barriers to prevention services 120
Beck, Aaron 84
behavioral interventions 84
behavioral therapy 6, 69, 93, 106, 107, 142,
    145, 155
beneficence and maleficence 12
bereavement 26, 45, 48, 119
biodiversity 159
BIPOC 8
Black Indigenous People of Color (BIPOC) 8
boundaries 44, 48, 81, 83, 101, 132, 144, 177
brain development 7, 102
bullying 20–23, 27, 85, 100, 113, 133, 146,
    150, 154–158, 163, 179, 182–184, 192,
    204
bullying prevention 156, 180, 182
burnout 39, 44, 55, 178

caregivers 3–8, 18, 20–21, 25–26, 32,
    44–46, 48, 52, 60–62, 66–70, 79, 84,
    93, 99, 104, 107, 109, 111–112, 115,
    117–119, 120–124, 139, 150, 154, 190,
    192
CBPT 6, 22, 72, 84, 106, 112
CBT 6, 69, 93, 97, 106–107, 142, 145, 155
CCPT 6, 78–81, 92, 96, 101, 132, 140–142
Centers for Disease Control and Prevention
    (CDC) 4, 16–19, 30, 148, 150, 167, 189,
    202, 205
chain analysis 89, 93, 107
Child-Centered Play Therapy (CCPT) 6,
    78–81, 92, 96, 101, 132, 140–142
child development 104, 166
child exploitation 22
child suicide 3, 19
Child Therapists 78, 99
church 44, 145, 157
clinical components 193
cognitive behavioral play therapy (CBPT) 6,
    22, 72, 84, 106, 112
cognitive behavioral therapy (CBT) 6, 69, 93,
    97, 106–107, 142, 145, 155
cognitive interventions 84
Cognitive Play Therapy 96
cognitive restructuring 135
cognitive therapy 84

collaboration 8, 36–37, 74, 116–117, 124, 145, 176, 179–180, 185
collage affirmation cards 85–86
Columbia Protocol 63, 67–68, 94, 196
Columbia Protocol app 94, 196
Columbia-Suicide Severity Rating Scale (C-SSRS) 68, 196–197
community support 44, 184
compassion fatigue 39, 42, 44
comprehensive treatment 35, 78, 124, 158
confidentiality 12, 14, 45, 83, 94, 140
continuing bond 50
coping mechanisms 65, 87, 119
coping skills 6, 41, 70, 76, 93–94, 107, 146, 155, 164, 177, 179, 185, 190, 194, 199
coping strategies 4, 52, 62, 64–65, 72, 83, 94, 119, 147, 152, 176, 180, 194–197
counseling 6, 12, 17, 45, 62, 64, 68, 80, 85, 94, 106, 121, 130, 141, 152–153, 155–156, 179, 181
countertransference 5, 39–44, 52, 144
creative arts 6
creative expression 90–91
crisis 5–7, 11, 15, 18, 25, 39, 42–45, 59, 65–69, 88, 94, 106, 117, 119, 124, 147, 150, 154, 175–176, 185–186, 195–197
crisis care 45
crisis intervention 88, 154
crisis management 43–44, 106, 176
crisis team 7, 65–68, 176, 186
C-SSRS 68, 196–197
cultural awareness 146
cultural competence 130, 137
cultural considerations 138
cultural factors 5, 23
cultural heritage 147, 148
cultural identity 61, 130, 134, 139
cultural inclusion 190
culturally appropriate treatment 145
cultural model of suicide 23
cultural perceptions 131
cultural research 17, 27
cultural sensitivity 130, 143, 150, 166
curriculum 6, 176–177, 179–180, 185
cyberbullying 20–21, 27, 113, 205
cyber victimization 20, 27

DBT 6, 68–70, 87–90, 93, 95–96, 106–124
DBT-A 6
deaths by suicide 17, 84
decriminalization of suicide 12
denial 3, 7, 118, 175–176, 185
depression 3, 15–17, 20, 26, 33, 36–37, 42, 46, 61, 70, 112, 119, 133, 143, 146–147, 157, 161–164, 180, 182–185, 189, 192

developmental history 5, 59, 60, 93, 182
developmental stage 7, 15–16, 75, 131
developmental trauma 102–103
diagnosis 12, 16, 32–36, 92, 159, 161, 180, 192
diagnostic overshadowing 160
Dialectical Behavior Therapy (DBT) 6, 68–70, 87–90, 93, 95–96, 106–124
digital age 189
digital culture 188
digital gaming 112
Digital Play Therapy™ 8, 165, 188, 190–191, 194, 200
digital technology 190, 201
digital tools 8, 189–195, 201
directive play therapy 6, 78–79, 136
discrimination 13, 130–131, 138–139, 150, 155, 160, 164
distress tolerance 87
diverse cultural groups 130
diversity 8, 18, 90, 129, 132, 157, 159–160, 163, 165, 177
double empathy problem 160–161
dual-process model 47

ecosocial theory 134
educational advocacy 147
educational therapy 84
elder mentors 147
electronic record systems 59
emotional disturbance
emotional expression
emotional intelligence
emotional pain 4, 7, 27, 47, 76, 102, 116, 203
emotional regulation 180–181
emotion regulation 48, 87
empathy 40, 42, 82–83, 100–101, 109, 117, 141, 156, 160–161, 176–177
equity 18, 90, 149
ethical challenges 12–13, 27
ethical responsibilities 12–13
ethics 12–13, 27, 45, 67
ethnicity 18–19, 24, 159
evaluation 7, 32–36, 43, 61–62, 67–69, 75, 81, 93, 117, 133, 147, 164, 181–182, 195
evidence-based practices 6–7, 14, 15–16, 25, 63, 89, 93, 96, 108, 117, 124, 145, 155
expressive art therapy 146, 152–153
expressive play 5–8, 22, 48, 60, 68–70, 76, 79–80, 90–93, 96, 105, 107–108, 112, 114, 120, 122, 145–146
expressive play-based interventions 7, 22, 70, 76, 80, 114, 120
expressive play-based theory 6, 69, 79, 90–91, 108

expressive play therapy 6, 8, 47, 76, 79, 107, 146
expressive therapy 41

fairy tale test 139
family acceptance 155, 157–158
Family Acceptance Project (FAP™) 155
family aquarium project 114
family cohesiveness 111
family dynamics 36–37, 47, 60, 114, 118
family history 17, 33, 36, 59–62, 93–94, 178, 180–181, 192
family intervention 112
family involvement 70, 124
family play genogram 60
Family Play Therapy 37, 107–109, 111, 114
family relationships 109, 148–149
family systems 109, 141
Family Systems theory 109
filial play therapy 79
Fortnite 198–200
Freud, Anna 78
Freud, Sigmund 12, 39, 78–79

gaming addiction 21, 111–112
gaming disorder 112
gatekeeper 7, 175–176, 180
gen alpha 189–190
gender and sexuality alliances 156
gender identity 139, 154–158, 199, 204–207
genogram 60
Gen Z 189–190
gratitude interventions 185
grief and loss 4, 42, 46, 52–53, 119
grief sculpture mobile 119
Guerney, Bernard and Louise 79

help-seeking stigma 149
Hispanic 8, 138, 175
historical trauma 131, 143
history of play therapy 78
human trafficking 21

ICD-11 16, 112
IEP 70
immersive activities 191
immigration status 139
impacts of suicide 25
improved diagnostics 158
inclusiveness 8, 90
indigenous practices 145
indirect teaching 100, 121
Individualized Education Program (IEP) 70
individuation 15
informed consent 14

insurance 32, 70
integrative expressive play-based therapy 105, 108
internal coping strategies 65, 197
internalized ableism 164
International Classification of Diseases (ICD-11) 16, 112
intersectionality 156, 1341
intervention programs 180
interventions 5–7, 13, 21, 32, 37, 39, 45, 48, 60, 68, 70–76, 82–89, 92–96, 99–109, 114, 117, 120, 122–124, 131, 134, 137, 141, 145, 154, 157, 164, 176–179, 182–186, 193, 200
intervention strategies 185
intervention techniques 182
involuntary hospitalization (5585 hold) 68, 144

Kalff, Dora M. 78

lack of control 112
Lakota Nation 111
Landreth, Garry 79
Latine 138–141
law 6, 12–13, 19, 22, 27, 40, 43, 66–69, 76, 100
legal responsibilities 14
Lego 101, 136–137
Levy, David 78
LGBTQ community 155, 157
LGBTQIA 8, 130, 154, 156, 204
LGBTQ youth 154–155, 157–158
long-term support 152–153
Lowenfeld, Margaret 78–79, 102, 127

marginalized children 130
masking (neurodivergence) 160–161, 164
meaning reconstruction 47, 54
media 11, 20–21, 23, 79–80, 108, 112, 146, 206
medications 18, 32–35, 45, 67, 70
mental health and suicide 17, 150
mental health issues 12, 138, 204
mental health professionals 3–8, 27, 70, 79, 112, 131, 153, 175–177, 179
mental health promotion 182
mental health services 90, 94, 119–122, 131–132, 138–139, 149, 152, 188, 195
mental health stigma 135
mental health support 44
mental health training 163
mental status examination 33
mindfulness 26, 42–44, 87–90, 93, 95–96, 104, 106–107, 115, 175, 177, 179

minority stress 23, 154–156
mnemonics 15
mood changes 34
Moustakas, Clark 79
multicultural competence 130
multi-faceted 5–6, 8, 87, 90

neurobiology 101, 104
neurocognitive functioning 159–160
neurodivergence 159–161, 163–165
neurodivergent 159–165
neurodivergent identity 164–165
neurodiversity 159–160, 163, 165
neurosequential model 7, 102–104
Neurosequential Model of Therapeutics
    (NMT) 7, 104, 126
Neurosequential Therapeutics 124
neurotypical 159–162, 164–165
non-suicidal self-injury (NSSI) 138, 142

Pacific Islanders 148
PAL Model (pathway for assisting life)
    148–153
pandemic 5, 18–19, 27, 175, 198
Papageno effect 23
parental support 118, 121
parenting programs 145, 153
peer relationships 131, 149
peer support 21
peer victimization 180
phase-based treatment 120
phenomenological 81, 90
play activities 80
play-based interventions 7, 22, 70, 76, 80,
    114, 120, 183
play therapists 3–8, 16, 21, 32, 35, 40–49,
    52–53, 59–69, 73, 78, 80, 92, 99, 104,
    112–118, 124, 130–132, 141–142, 165
play therapy continuum 89, 105
play therapy interventions 48, 76
PMR 44, 157, 173
pornography 20–21, 206
positive transformation 51
post-traumatic 155
posttraumatic growth 51
postvention 45–46, 117, 152, 178, 207
PPT 6, 92–96, 107
Prescriptive Play Therapy (PPT) 6, 92–96,
    107
pre-treatment 87
prevention strategies 23, 72, 116, 118, 145
problem-solving skills 61–62, 194
Progressive Muscle Relaxation (PMR) 44,
    157, 173
projection 40, 52, 75, 193

protective factors 6, 8, 14, 33, 60–65, 85, 90,
    93, 105, 109, 130–133, 144–145, 155,
    161–162, 194–195, 206
PSS Chute software 196
psychache 190, 194
psychiatric clinical interview 33
psychiatric evaluation 32, 35–36, 69
psychoanalysis 39
psychoeducation 117, 121, 135–136, 152,
    157, 179
psychological pain 151, 190–191
psychotherapeutic interventions 161

quality of life 35, 46, 87, 156, 186
Queer Prysm 155–156

race 17–19, 24, 131, 133
racial disparity 17
racism and discrimination 150
recommendations 24, 26, 89, 139, 142
referral to psychiatry 32
relational epistemic humility 165
release therapy 78
religious participation 134
resilience 19, 52, 62, 76, 118, 133, 156, 177,
    179–180, 194–195, 199
resilience factors 118
risk assessment 12, 41, 59, 62–66, 73, 178
risk factors 4, 14, 17, 21, 23, 33, 60–66, 85,
    90, 105, 109, 118, 130–133, 139, 142,
    144–145, 148, 161, 163, 175, 178, 180,
    191–196, 199
risk factors for suicidal youth 33
risk management 14, 82
Rogers, Carl 78, 80

sad persons scale 15
safe environment 71, 81, 177, 185
safe space 49, 101, 156
safety plan 7, 14, 64–67, 73–74, 88, 94,
    96, 116, 142, 152, 163–164, 196–197,
    206
safety planning 14, 64, 94, 96, 116, 206
SAMHSA suicide safe mobile app 90, 94,
    195
Sandplay 78–79, 102
Sandtray 79–83, 99, 102, 145, 152–153,
    184, 200
Sandtray therapy 145, 184–185
school-based counselors 32, 124
school-based interventions 141
school counseling 85
school counselors 7, 16–17, 45, 48, 52,
    59–60, 66–67, 76, 99–100, 114,
    117–118, 124, 166, 175, 205

School Psychologist 119, 146, 181
school safety 158
school settings 150, 152, 182
screening tools 6, 59, 63, 67
self-acceptance 48
self-awareness 42, 101, 112, 121, 130, 184
self-care 5, 41–44, 52, 73, 123, 177, 179
self-esteem 21, 26, 80, 87, 95, 99, 110, 141,
    183–184, 194
self-expression 6, 40, 79, 83, 100, 102, 121,
    132
self-harm 3, 8, 11–13, 16, 20, 23–24, 35–37,
    42–45, 62–67, 82–83, 87, 93, 116, 118,
    154, 155, 175, 182, 203
self-help 192–195
self-poisoning 18
severity 23, 32, 59–63, 68, 94, 140, 196–197,
    206
sexting 20–21, 107, 111, 113, 206
sexual abuse 8–9, 21, 33 21, 27, 100, 161,
    192
sexual exploitation 21–22, 27
SI see suicidal ideation
Six Part Story Making (6PSM) 74
sleep 34, 36, 42–45, 62, 67–68, 71, 100, 112,
    121, 123, 145, 154, 181, 192, 196
social connections 158, 163, 176, 182–184
social-emotional learning 176, 180, 184
social influence 40, 189
social injustice 130
social isolation 4, 154, 185, 189
social media 20–21, 27, 112, 146, 206
social skills group 182
social supports 197
SOGICE (Sexual Orientation & Gender
    Identity Change Efforts) 154
stability and homeostasis 119
standard of care 14, 25
Stanley-Brown safety plan app 197
STB see suicidal thinking and behaviors
stigma 12, 16, 23, 26, 46, 48, 50–51, 66, 120,
    131, 135, 138, 141, 143, 149, 156, 175
stigma and shame 48
Stone, Jessica 8, 188, 200
Stop & Calm Intervention 106–107
storytelling 74, 108, 132, 135–137, 139, 145
strategies
stress 5, 7, 15, 20, 23, 39, 44, 47, 52, 62,
    86, 100, 102–107, 111, 135–137, 139,
    149–152, 155–156, 164, 176, 178
stress management 100, 176
structured play therapy 79
structuring 83, 93
substance abuse 64, 70–71, 90, 94, 143, 145,
    181–182, 195

suicidal behavior 8, 14, 20, 22–23, 36, 45,
    63, 82, 86, 89, 94, 96, 116, 119, 131–133,
    142, 155, 160, 175–176, 179–185, 189,
    192, 206
Suicidal Behaviors Questionnaire-Revised
    (SBQ-R) 63
suicidal ideation (SI) 3–8, 12, 20–23, 33, 40,
    45, 59–63, 66, 68, 70–72, 81–84, 87, 96,
    99–103, 108–109, 120–121, 130–133,
    144, 146–147, 148–156, 160–161, 165,
    188–189, 180, 199, 207
Suicidal Thinking and Behaviors (STB) 3–4,
    19–21, 27, 34, 37, 39–40, 76, 84, 90–97,
    99, 106, 118–120, 124, 130, 138, 141,
    158, 185
suicidal thoughts in young individuals 121,
    151
suicide assessment 3, 8, 23, 42–43, 60,
    63–64, 84, 94, 122–123, 130, 140, 143,
    150–151, 195, 197
suicide assessment apps 195
suicide crisis 25, 39, 66
suicide hotline 11
suicide prevention efforts (US) 16, 96, 175
suicide prevention strategies 23, 145
suicide rates 4, 16–19, 23–24, 148, 205
suicide risk assessment 64, 66, 187
suicide risk factors 17, 118, 148
suicide safety plan app 196–197
suicide screening 118
suicide warning signs 150–151
suicidology 14–15, 45, 99, 150, 189
superhero 101, 185
symptom assessment 34

task theory 46
techno home activity board 112–113
telemental health 199
TF-CBT (Trauma-Focused Cognitive
    Behavioral Therapy) 155–158
therapeutic alliance 7, 14, 41, 49, 70, 80, 82,
    104, 116
therapeutic interventions 22, 161
therapeutic modalities 79
therapeutic play 120
therapeutic powers 6, 8, 100, 132, 191, 194
therapeutic powers of play 6, 8, 100, 132,
    191, 194
therapeutic process 44, 52, 75, 79, 136, 191,
    193
therapeutic rapport 136
therapeutic relationship 12, 39, 52–53,
    75, 78–83, 99, 104, 121, 130, 144,
    164, 166
therapist protocol 45

therapy approaches 7, 92, 132, 145
threat 36, 45, 48, 67, 69, 71, 86–88, 109,
    112, 118, 188–189
transference 39–40, 52
transphobic legislation 154
trauma 4, 17, 24, 26, 39, 45–48,
    50–55, 69, 74, 78, 88–89, 93,
    99, 101–105, 120–121, 131,
    143–146, 155, 157, 158, 166, 176,
    180, 184
trauma recovery 157
traumatic loss 39, 45–46, 48–53
treatment interventions 93, 106–107, 134,
    137
Trevor Project 154–155
tribal environment 44
tribal-specific teachings 145

trigger 39–40, 62, 89, 116–117, 120, 180,
    185
Two Penguins Studios 64, 197

validation 51, 87
values affirmation 110–111
victimization 21, 23, 27, 133, 154, 180, 204
video gaming 112
vulnerability factors 89

warning signs 5, 14, 15, 33, 46, 60–66,
    72, 76, 85, 90–93, 105, 118, 130–131,
    143–144, 150–151, 154, 162, 175, 178,
    191–192, 196–197
Werther Effect 23, 28, 30
world health organization 16, 26, 133
worldview 19, 188–189